Series Title: Immune Response to Parasitic Infections

Immunity to Helminths and Novel Therapeutic Approaches
(Volume 2)

Edited By

Emilio Jirillo
Department of Basic Medical Sciences
Neuroscience and Sensory Organs
University of Bari
Bari (Italy)

Thea Magrone
Department of Basic Medical Sciences
Neuroscience and Sensory Organs
University of Bari
Bari (Italy)

&

Giuseppe Miragliotta
Department of Interdisciplinary Medicine
University of Bari
Bari (Italy)

Bentham Science Publishers Ltd.
Executive Suite Y - 2
PO Box 7917, Saif Zone
Sharjah, U.A.E.
subscriptions@benthamscienc.org

All rights reserved-© 2014 Bentham Science Publishers Ltd.

Please read this license agreement carefully before using this eBook. Your use of this eBook/chapter constitutes your agreement to the terms and conditions set forth in this License Agreement. This work is protected under copyright by Bentham Science Publishers Ltd. to grant the user of this eBook/chapter, a non-exclusive, nontransferable license to download and use this eBook/chapter under the following terms and conditions:

1. This eBook/chapter may be downloaded and used by one user on one computer. The user may make one back-up copy of this publication to avoid losing it. The user may not give copies of this publication to others, or make it available for others to copy or download. For a multi-user license contact permission@benthamscience.org

2. All rights reserved: All content in this publication is copyrighted and Bentham Science Publishers Ltd. own the copyright. You may not copy, reproduce, modify, remove, delete, augment, add to, publish, transmit, sell, resell, create derivative works from, or in any way exploit any of this publication's content, in any form by any means, in whole or in part, without the prior written permission from Bentham Science Publishers Ltd..

3. The user may print one or more copies/pages of this eBook/chapter for their personal use. The user may not print pages from this eBook/chapter or the entire printed eBook/chapter for general distribution, for promotion, for creating new works, or for resale. Specific permission must be obtained from the publisher for such requirements. Requests must be sent to the permissions department at E-mail: permission@benthamscience.org

4. The unauthorized use or distribution of copyrighted or other proprietary content is illegal and could subject the purchaser to substantial money damages. The purchaser will be liable for any damage resulting from misuse of this publication or any violation of this License Agreement, including any infringement of copyrights or proprietary rights.

5. The following DRM (Digital Rights Management) policy is applicable on this eBook for the non-library / personal / single-user. Library / institutional / multi-users will get a DRM free copy and they may implement their own institutional DRM policy.

• **25 'Copy' commands can be executed every 7 days.** The text selected for copying cannot extend to more than one single page.

• **25 pages can be printed every 7 days.**

• **eBook files are not transferable to multiple computer/devices.** If you wish to use the eBook on another device, you must send a request to support@benthamscience.org along with the original order number that you received when the order was placed.

Warranty Disclaimer: The publisher does not guarantee that the information in this publication is error-free, or warrants that it will meet the users' requirements or that the operation of the publication will be uninterrupted or error-free. This publication is provided "as is" without warranty of any kind, either express or implied or statutory, including, without limitation, implied warranties of merchantability and fitness for a particular purpose. The entire risk as to the results and performance of this publication is assumed by the user. In no event will the publisher be liable for any damages, including, without limitation, incidental or consequential damages and damages for lost data or profits arising out of the use or inability to use the publication. The entire liability of the publisher shall be limited to the amount actually paid by the user for the eBook or eBook license agreement.

Limitation of Liability: Under no circumstances shall Bentham Science Publishers Ltd., its staff, editors and authors, be liable for any special or consequential damages that result from the use of, or the inability to use, the materials in this site.

eBook Product Disclaimer: No responsibility is assumed by Bentham Science Publishers Ltd., its staff or members of the editorial board for any injury and/or damage to persons or property as a matter of products liability, negligence or otherwise, or from any use or operation of any methods, products instruction, advertisements or ideas contained in the publication purchased or read by the user(s). Any dispute will be governed exclusively by the laws of the U.A.E. and will be settled exclusively by the competent Court at the city of Dubai, U.A.E.

You (the user) acknowledge that you have read this Agreement, and agree to be bound by its terms and conditions.

Permission for Use of Material and Reproduction

Permission Information for Users Outside the USA: Bentham Science Publishers Ltd. grants authorization for individuals to photocopy copyright material for private research use, on the sole basis that requests for such use are referred directly to the requestor's local Reproduction Rights Organization (RRO). The copyright fee is US $25.00 per copy per article exclusive of any charge or fee levied. In order to contact your local RRO, please contact the International Federation of Reproduction Rights Organisations (IFRRO), Rue Joseph II, 9-13 1000 Brussels, Belgium; Tel: +32 2 234 62 60; Fax: +32 2 234 62 69; E-mail: secretariat@ifrro.org; url: www.ifrro.org This authorization does not extend to any other kind of copying by any means, in any form, and for any purpose other than private research use.

Permission Information for Users in the USA: Authorization to photocopy items for internal or personal use, or the internal or personal use of specific clients, is granted by Bentham Science Publishers Ltd. for libraries and other users registered with the Copyright Clearance Center (CCC) Transactional Reporting Services, provided that the appropriate fee of US $25.00 per copy per chapter is paid directly to Copyright Clearance Center, 222 Rosewood Drive, Danvers MA 01923, USA. Refer also to www.copyright.com

CONTENTS

Foreword — i

Preface — iv

List of Contributors — vii

CHAPTERS

1. **Neuroendocrine Control of the Immune Response During Helminth Infections** — 3
   Karen Nava-Castro, Julieta Ivone Castro, Elizabeth Langley and Jorge Morales-Montor

2. **The Immune Response During Toxocariosis by *Toxocara Canis*** — 27
   Fernando Alba-Hurtado, Lorena Chávez-Guitrón, Victor Hugo del Río-Araiza, Karen Nava-Castro and Jorge Morales-Montor

3. **Mechanisms of Immune Modulation by *Fasciola Hepatica*: The Impact of Innate Immune Cells on the Developing Adaptive Immune Response** — 51
   Sandra M. O'Neill and Sheila Donnelly

4. **Parasite-Mediated Immune Modulation During the Development of Human Cystic Echinococcosis** — 69
   Elisabetta Profumo, Alessandra Ludovisi, Brigitta Buttari, Maria Angeles Gomez Morales and Rachele Riganò

5. **The Immunobiology of Urogenital Schistosomiasis** — 93
   Luke F. Pennington and Michael H. Hsieh

6. **The Translational Immunology of Trichinellosis: From Rodents to Humans** — 125
   Fabrizio Bruschi and Maria Angeles Gómez-Morales

7. ***Anisakis Simplex* Infestation and Immune-Mediated Responses** — 163
   Ventura M. Teresa, Buquicchio Rosalba, F. Gatti, F.L. Traetta and G. Iadarola

8. **Immunomodulation by Parasitic Helminths and its Therapeutic Exploitation**   175
Miguel Angel Pineda and William Harnett

9. **Parasites-Based Immunotherapy to Treat Allergies and Autoimmune Diseases**   213
Camila Alexandrina Figueiredo, Valdirene Leão Carneiro, Ryan Santos Costa, Leonardo Nascimento Santos, Raimon Rios and Neuza M Alcantara Neves

10. **The Impact of Helminths on the Human Microbiota: Therapeutic Correction of Disturbed Gut Microbial Immunity**   235
Thea Magrone, Emilio Jirillo and Giuseppe Miragliotta

Subject Index   255

FOREWORD

This eBook, edited by Jirillo E, Magrone T and Miragliotta G, is the second volume of a series on immune response to parasitic infections. The book consisting of 10 chapters provides an overview of the recent advances on immunity to helminthic parasites, which are among the most prevalent infectious agents in the world. The widespread prevalence of helminths worldwide is due to their ability to manipulate host immunity by secreting molecules with immunomodulatory activity. The ability of helminths to escape host immune response leads to establishment of long term chronic infections both in human and animal hosts. The interactions between host and helminths are more complex than previously thought. As discussed in Chapter 1 by Nava-Castro and Morales-Montor, helminthic parasites not only evade immune response, but are also able to activate a complex neuroendocrine network, that produces strong behavioural changes in the infected host favouring the establishment, growth and reproduction of parasites. In Chapter 2 (by Alba-Hurtado *et al.*) and Chapter 3 (by O'Neill and Donnelly) the innate and adaptive immune responses towards *Toxocara canis* and *Fasciola hepatica*, two important zoonotic helminths in both humans and animals, are discussed. *F. hepatica* is an excellent model to elucidate mechanisms involved in Th1-immune suppression and the induction of Th2/Treg immune responses, while the importance for Th1 and Th2 immune responses is well highlighted in all models of Toxocara parasitic disease. Chapter 4 (by Profumo *et al.*) illustrates the current findings about the complex host-parasite interaction during hydatidosis, a helminth disease caused by *Echinococcus granulosus* with a worldwide prevalence of approximately 3 million cases. In particular, great emphasis has been given to a number of molecules of *E. granulosus* that are able to modulate the host immune response and to favour its survival. The analysis of parasite-mediated immune modulation during the development of human cystic echinococcosis is crucial to improve research on vaccines and control of this infection. In Chapter 5 Pennington and Hsieh provide an excellent coverage on the immunobiologic events that occur during *S. haematobium* infection from human and rodent studies.

The knowledge of the host immune response to the different species of Trichinella both in humans and rodents is reviewed in Chapter 6 by Bruschi and *Gómez-Morales*. The authors described the different effector mechanisms involved in the control and elimination of this intracellular nematode. Particular attention has been paid not only to mechanisms of evasion and immunomodulation, but also to the evaluation of the humoral immune response with the aim to improve the development of diagnostic tests for trichinellosis.

Anisakis simplex is the main causative agent of Anisakiasis, an underestimated infestation that is acquired through the consumption of raw parasitized fish. Chapter 7 by Ventura *et al.* focuses on the immunopathogenesis of the disease, taking into account the role of gastrointestinal inflammatory response that involves the massive recruitment of eosinophils at the site of infection. The concept of manipulation of host immunity by helminths is widely discussed in Chapter 8 by Pineda and Harnett. The identification of helminth-derived molecules involved in immunoregulation is of great importance to understand immunopathogenesis of helminth infections. Paradoxically, these secreted products could represent the basis for the development of innovative strategies for the treatment of allergic and autoimmune diseases. The same topic is further discussed in Chapter 9 by Figueiredo *et al.* which reviewed epidemiological and experimental evidences whereby helminth infections are able to protect their hosts from immune mediated diseases. Studies that assess the development of parasites-based immunotherapy to treat immune-mediated disorders should be strongly encouraged. Finally, the editors of this e-book (Chapter 10) provide new insights in the interaction between helminths and human microbiota. In particular, they suggest that therapeutic correction of altered gut microbial immunity may interfere with helminth development. The authors reported their recent findings on the effect of polyphenols to downregulate the immunopathology in helminth infection. On these grounds, daily intake of polyphenols may be beneficial in chronic helminth infections by directly inducing parasite death and shaping the gut microbiota.

In conclusions, the present e-book provides key advances in our knowledge of the immunlogic mechanisms involved in the helminth infections. Importantly, this eBook integrates both basic and clinical immunology with relevant implications for the development of protective and therapeutic strategies for helminthiasis.

Claudio M. Mastroianni
Department of Public Health and Infectious Diseases
Sapienza University
Rome
Italy

PREFACE

Helminths can survive in the host for years in view of their ability to elude immune responses through various strategies. Therefore, a better knowledge of the immune mechanisms elicited by the host against invading helminths is fundamental for understanding pathogenesis of parasitoses as well as elaborating therapeutic measures to control or eradicate worm infections. At the same time, helminth-mediated immune response can be exploited to treat other human chronic diseases.

All these concepts will be illustrated in the present ebook, entitled "Immunity to Helminths and Therapeutic Novel Approaches".

Karen Nava-Castro and Jorge Morales-Montor in their chapter entitled "Neuroendocrine control of the immune response during helminth infections" will elucidate how the host neuroendocrine system may favor the establishment of parasitic infections, thus emphasizing interesting perspectives into the host parasite relationship field.

Fernando Alba-Hurtado, Lorena Chávez-Guitrón, Victor Hugo del Río-Araiza, Karen Nava-Castro and Jorge Morales-Montor in their chapter entitled "The immune response during toxocariosis by *Toxocara canis*" will review the major immunological responses that participate in the infection development with the aim to design more accurate immunodiagnostic methods and develop new vaccines.

Sandra M. O'Neill and Sheila Donnelly in their chapter entitled "Mechanisms of immune modulation by *Fasciola hepatica*: the impact of innate immune cells on the developing adaptive immune response" will examine the crosstalk between *F. hepatica* and dendritic cells, macrophages and mast cells with special reference to the development of Th1/Th17 immune responses.

Elisabetta Profumo, Alessandra Ludovisi, Brigitta Buttari, Maria Angeles Gomez Morales and Rachele Riganò in their chapter entitled "Parasite-mediated immune modulation during the development of human cystic echinococcosis" will discuss current findings about the human immune response during the development of cystic echinococcosis and the ability of *Echinococcus granulosus* to regulate as well as to exploit the host's immune system.

Luke F. Pennington and Michael H. Hsieh in their chapter entitled "The Immunobiology of Urogenital Schistosomiasis" will illustrate the immunological mechanism during *S. haematobium* infection and novel *S. haematobium* infection models for a better understanding of disease pathogenesis.

Fabrizio Bruschi and Maria Angeles Gómez-Morales in their chapter "The Translational Immunology of Trichinellosis: from Rodents to Humans" describe different aspects of the host innate and adaptive immune response to the different species of *Trichinella* in humans, as well as in rodents which are one of the most studied experimental models.

Ventura MT, Buquicchio R, Gatti F, Traetta FL and Iadarola G, in their chapter entitled *"Anisakis simplex* Infestation and Immune-Mediated Responses" report that *Anisakis (A.)* can trigger different kinds of hypersensitivities and, in particular, the I, III and IV type. The involvement of eosinophils in tissue lesions will also be discussed.

Miguel Angel Pineda and William Harnett in their chapter entitled "Immunomodulation by Parasitic Helminths and its Therapeutic Exploitation" summarize the current molecular mechanisms of worm infections and their potential clinical application for treatment of allergy and autoimmune diseases, like asthma, rheumatoid arthritis, inflammatory bowel disease and multiple sclerosis.

Camila Alexandrina Figueiredo, Ryan Santos Costa, Leonardo Nascimento Santos and Neuza M Alcantara Neves in their chapter entitled "Parasites-Based Immunotherapy to Treat Immune Mediated Diseases" will review the mechanisms which allow helminths to protect the host from immune-mediated diseases and the development of biological products for treatment and prophylaxis of various immunopathologies.

Thea Magrone, Emilio Jirillo and Giuseppe Miragliotta in their chapter entitled "The impact of helminths on the human microbiota: therapeutic correction of disturbed gut microbial immunity" will focus on the therapeutic potential of polyphenols that have been shown to modulate gut microbiota, also interfering with helminth development. In this context, polyphenols possess anti-inflammatory activities, even including expansion and activation of Treg cells which may attenuate immunopathology in the later phase of helminth infections.

Emilio Jirillo
Department of Basic Medical Sciences
Neuroscience and Sensory Organs
University of Bari
Bari (Italy)

Thea Magrone
Department of Basic Medical Sciences
Neuroscience and Sensory Organs
University of Bari
Bari (Italy)

&

Giuseppe Miragliotta
Department of Interdisciplinary Medicine
University of Bari
Bari (Italy)

List of Contributors

Alba-Hurtado Fernando
Departamento de Parasitología, Facultad de Estudios Superiores Cuautitlán, Universidad Nacional Autónoma de México, Mexico

Alcantara Neves Neuza M.
Instituto de Ciências da Saúde, Universidade Federal da Bahia, Salvador-Bahia, Brazil

Bruschi Fabrizio
Department of Translational Research, N.T.M.S., Università di Pisa, Scuola Medica, Pisa, Italy

Buquicchio Rosalba
Unit of Dermatology, University of Bari Medical School, Policlinico, Bari, Italy

Buttari Brigitta
Dipartimento di Malattie Infettive, Parassitarie ed Immunomediate, Istituto Superiore di Sanità, Rome, Italy

Chávez-Guitrón Lorena
Departamento de Parasitología, Facultad de Estudios Superiores Cuautitlán, Universidad Nacional Autónoma de México, Mexico

del Río-Araiza Victor Hugo
Departamento de Inmunología, Instituto de Investigaciones Biomédicas, Universidad Nacional Autónoma de México, México

Donnelly Sheila
School of Biotechnology, Faculty of Science and Health, Dublin, Ireland, and the i3 Institute, University of Technology Sydney, Ultimo, New South Wales, Australia

Figueiredo Camila Alexandrina
Instituto de Ciências da Saúde, Universidade Federal da Bahia, Salvador-Bahia, Brazil

Gatti F

Unit of Gastroenterology and Digestive Endoscopy, S. Camillo De Lellis Hospital, Manfredonia, Foggia, Italy

Gomez Morales Maria Angeles

Department of Infectious, Parasitic and Immunomediated Diseases, Istituto Superiore di Sanità, Rome, Italy

Harnett William

Strathclyde Institute of Pharmacy and Biomedical Sciences, University of Strathclyde, Glasgow, G4 0RE, UK

Hsieh Michael H.

Department of Urology, Stanford Immunology, Stanford University, Stanford, California, USA

Iadarola G

Department of Internal Medicine, Clinical Immunology and Allergology of Foggia General Hospital, University Medical School, Foggia, Italy

Jirillo Emilio

Department of Basic Medical Sciences, Neuroscience and Sensory Organs, University of Bari, Bari, Italy

Ludovisi Alessandra

Dipartimento di Malattie Infettive, Parassitarie ed Immunomediate, Istituto Superiore di Sanità, Rome, Italy

Magrone Thea

Department of Basic Medical Sciences, Neuroscience and Sensory Organs, University of Bari, Bari, Italy

Miragliotta Giuseppe

Department of Interdisciplinary Medicine, University of Bari, Bari, Italy

Morales-Montor Jorge
Departamento de Inmunología, Instituto de Investigaciones Biomédicas, Universidad Nacional Autónoma de México, México

Nascimento Santos Leonardo
Instituto de Ciências da Saúde, Universidade Federal da Bahia, Salvador-Bahia, Brazil

Nava-Castro Karen
Facultad de Química, Departamento de Biología, Universidad Nacional Autónoma de México, México DF 04510, México

O'Neill Sandra
Departamento de Inmunología, Instituto de Investigaciones Biomédicas, Universidad Nacional Autónoma de México, México

Pennington Luke
Stanford Immunology, Stanford University, Stanford, California, USA

Pineda Miguel Angel
Division of Immunology, Infection and Inflammation, University of Glasgow, Glasgow, G12 8TA, UK

Profumo Elisabetta
Dipartimento di Malattie Infettive, Parassitarie ed Immunomediate, Istituto Superiore di Sanità, Rome, Italy

Riganò Rachele
Dipartimento di Malattie Infettive, Parassitarie ed Immunomediate, Istituto Superiore di Sanità, Rome, Italy

Santos Costa
Instituto de Ciências da Saúde, Universidade Federal da Bahia, Salvador-Bahia, Brazil

Traetta PL

Unit of Clinical Immunology and Allergology, "Miulli" Hospital, Acquaviva delle Fonti, Bari, Italy

Ventura Maria Teresa

Interdisciplinary Department of Medicine, University of Bari Medical School, Policlinico, Bari, Italy

CHAPTER 1

Neuroendocrine Control of the Immune Response During Helminth Infections

Karen Nava-Castro[1], Julieta Ivone Castro[1], Elizabeth Langley[2] and Jorge Morales-Montor[3,*]

[1]*Center of Investigation for Infectious Disease, National Institute of Public Health, Morelos, Mexico;* [2]*National Institute of Cancerology, Morelos, Mexico and* [3]*Department of Immunology, Institute of Biomedical Investigations, Autonomous National University of Mexico, AP 70228, Mexico DF, Mexico*

Abstract: The physiological interactions during the course of the immune response to helminths are complex. As our understanding of the neuroendocrine system grows, it has become increasingly clear that this complex network of neurotransmitters, hormones, and cytokines plays an important role in mediating immunity. Helminths present an especially complex relationship between parasites and their physiological systems, with neuro and hormone dependent host factors such as sex, age, and physiological status that correlate with parasite success. On top of the effect that this particular type of parasite may have on the invaded host, recent experimental evidence suggests that helminth parasites not only actively evade immune response, but are also able to exploit the hormonal microenvironment within their host to favor their establishment, growth and reproduction. Additionally, the close interaction of the worm with the host's homeostatic systems, the molecules produced by them, and the activation of immune mediated mechanisms to eliminate it, activate a complex neuroendocrine network, that produces strong behavioral changes in the infected host. Understanding how the host neuroendocrine system can, under certain circumstances, favor the establishment of a parasitic infection, opens interesting perspectives into the host parasite relationship. This chapter focuses on the host-parasite neuroendocrine network activated by parasitic worm infections.

Keywords: Helminthes, immunoendocrine, neuroimmune, neuroimmunoendocrine, network, parasite infections, neurotransmitters, cytokines, sex steroids, behaviors, parasites, immune response, hormones, modulation, Th1, Th2, Th17, immunoregulation.

THE HOST-PARASITE NEUROIMMUNOENDOCRINE NETWORK

The relationship between parasites (P), particularly helminths, and their hosts (H)

---

*Corresponding author Jorge Morales-Montor: Department of Immunology, Institute of Biomedical Research, U.N.A.M., AP 70228, México D.F. 04510; Tel: (525)622-3854; Fax: (525)622-3369; E-mails: jmontor66@biomedicas.unam.mx or jmontor66@hotmail.com

Emilio Jirillo, Thea Magrone and Giuseppe Miragliotta (Eds)
All rights reserved-© 2014 Bentham Science Publishers

implies biochemical coevolution and communication between their complex physiological and metabolic systems and with the environment, at all levels of biological organization [1]. Hormones regulate a variety of cellular and physiological functions such as growth, reproduction and differentiation. Hormones and immune actors are prominent in H-P relationships. The comparatively sophisticated immune systems of vertebrates add complexity to the H-P interactions. Mammals sense and react with their innate and acquired immunological systems to the presence of a parasite and the parasite is also sensitive and reactive to the host's immune system effectors. Host hormones are also involved in the modulation of the immune system's protective or pathogenic functions as well as on the parasite's metabolism and reproduction [2, 3]. Host adrenal hormones are well known immune modulators [3], while sex steroids (estradiol, progesterone and testosterone) are progressively being recognized as players that significantly affect the immune system's functions [4]. More recently, the ability of hormones to affect the immunological response directed against pathogenic agents has gained attention [5]. This is clearly evident during various parasitic diseases including malaria, schistosomiasis, toxoplasmosis, cysticercosis, trypanosomiasis, and leishmaniasis [5-13], where strong hormonal regulation of the immune response has been described [14]. However, other factors besides the immunoendocrine response affect the course of a parasitic infection (Fig. **1**).

A striking example of exploitation of host molecules is the ability of a number of parasites to use host-synthesized cytokines as indirect growth factors [8]. Mammals sense and react with their innate and acquired immunological systems to the presence of a parasite and the parasite is also sensitive and reactive to the host's immune system's effectors. Host's hormones are also involved in the modulation of the immune system's protective or pathogenic functions as well as in the parasite's metabolism and reproduction. Host's adrenal hormones are well known immune modulators, while sex steroids (estradiol, progesterone and testosterone) are progressively being recognized for their role in significantly affecting the immune system's functions.

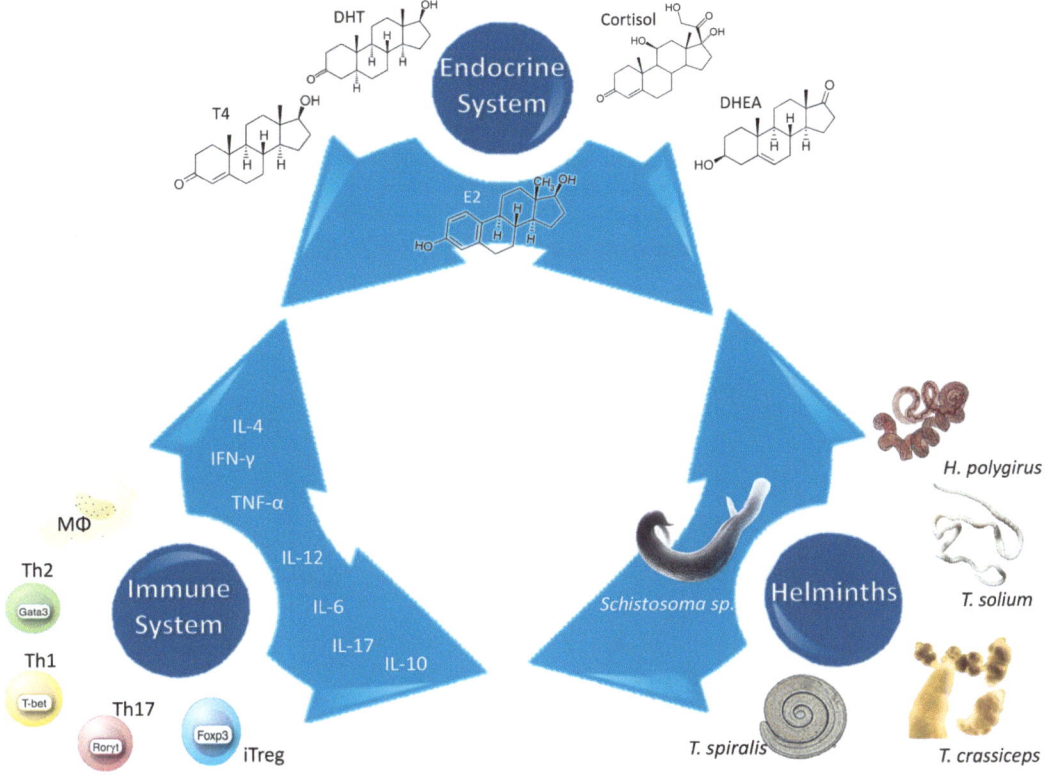

Figure 1: Immunoendocrine interactions in helminthic infections.

THE CASE OF HELMINTHS

Helminths are estimated to include 18000 to 24000 species, and are divided into two subclasses. Nearly all trematodes are parasites of molluscs and vertebrates. The smaller Aspidogastrea, comprising about 100 species, are obligate parasites of molluscs and may also infect turtles and fishes, including cartilaginous fishes. The Digenea, which constitute the majority of trematode diversity, are obligate parasites of both molluscs and vertebrates, but rarely occur in cartilaginous fishes. One-quarter of a billion people are infected with parasitic trematode worms worldwide. Disease-associated symptoms occur in 120 million people, and 20 million people suffer from severe morbidity. The three most important human schistosomes are *Schistosoma haematobium*, *Schistosoma japonicum*, and *Schistosoma mansoni* [15, 16].

Cestoda is the class of parasitic flatworms, commonly called tapeworms that live in the digestive tract of vertebrates as adults and often in the bodies of various animals as juveniles. There are two subclasses in class Cestoda, the Cestodaria and the Eucestoda. By far the most common and widespread are the Eucestoda, with only a few species of unusual worms in subclass Cestodaria. The cyclophyllideans are the most important to humans because they infect people and livestock. Two important tapeworms are the pork tapeworm, *Taenia solium*, and the beef tapeworms, *T. saginata* [17, 18].

Taennids, particularly *Taenia solium* (causal agent of porcine cysticercosis and human neurocysticercosis) and *Taenia crassiceps* (causal agent of murine cysticercosis) are highly evolved parasites that have developed diverse mechanisms of survival within the host that facilitate their establishment. These mechanisms can be roughly grouped into two types. The first is evasion of the immune response by molecular mimicry or by inactivating effector immune processes (*i.e.*, complement inhibition) [5, 19]. In the second mechanism, the parasite exploits the host system to its benefit in its establishment, growth or reproduction [20]. This exploitation mechanism provides parasites with a dual benefit: first, obtaining amino acids for metabolism and second, preventing the surface-bound antibody from interfering with the interaction of cytotoxic cells with the parasite [19].

EFFECT OF HORMONES DURING HELMINTH INFECTIONS

In last years, research has proved the influence of hormones in immune system regulation [21], and the idea of a neuroimmunoendocrine network was put forth. Since then, research has been focused on the role of these hormones and their possible mechanisms to intervene in the host susceptibility or resistance [22]. It is well known that males of vertebrate species tend to exhibit higher rates of parasite infections than females and that sex-associated hormones may influence immunocompetence and are hypothesized to lead to this bias [23]. Considering this point, females have also been shown to have higher resistance to many parasitic infections, a finding particularly striking in helminth infections such as *Schistosoma mansoni* and *Trichinella spiralis* [24]. Thus, research carried out recently proves and explains some of these phenomena associated with hormones, specifically, steroid hormones and their effect on some helminth infections (Table 1).

Table 1: Effect of hormones in both parasite biology and the immune response

Parasite	Hormone	Effect on immune system	Effect on the parasite
Schistosoma mansoni	DHEA-S	↑ Th2-driven antibody isotypes ↓ Proinflammatory cytokines	Kills larval and adult parasites in culture at physiologic concentrations
	DHEA	↑ TNF-α	Inhibits parasite oviposition
Brugia malayi	Prolactin	↑ TNF-α / IL-6	
	T4	↓ IFN-γ / IL-6	
Stronguloides ratti	T4	Inhibits macrophage function	
Taenia crassiceps	E2	• Decreases numbers of $CD3^+$, $CD4^+$ and $CD8^+$ in the thymus • Promotes Th2 type response • ↓ IL-2/ IFN-γ • ↑ IL-6, IL-10 and IL-4 • ↑ Parasite-specific IgG	Increases parasite loads
	T4 DHT	Increases spleenocyte proliferation ↑ IL-2 / IFN-γ	Decreases parasite loads
Taenia solium	E2		Increases parasite growth
	P4	↑ IL-4 / IL-6 /TNF-α	Increases parasite growth Promotes scolex evagination
Trichuris muris	E2	↑ Th2 response *in vitro*	
	DHT	Inhibits T-stimulatory capacity of DC's ↓ IL-18 mRNA	
Trichinella spiralis	Pituitary hormones	↓ Th1 cytokines in the duodenum ↑ IL-5 / IL-13	

There is enough evidence about corticoids and their influence on regulation of the immune response involved in parasitic infections [25]. However, there is recent data about their influence on the growth of the parasite, without an immune explanation. This is the case of *Echinococcus multiloclaris,* in which the effects of cortisone treatment on the number and size of primary *E. multilocularis*cysts developing in a moderately resistant strain of mice, was studied. The cortisone-treated mice became infected with hydatid cysts. Cortisone treatment significantly increased the average number of cysts, the average area of each cyst, and the total surface area occupied by cysts when compared with the untreated mice. Treatment of an *E. multilocularis* resistant mouse strain with cortisone drastically increased both the number of cysts and the average size of each cyst if the treatment occurred early in the infection. Consequently, this treatment increases the susceptibility of mice to primary infections with *E. multilocularis*. Based on these results, it could not be determined whether the increased susceptibility results from physiological or immunological effects caused by the cortisone treatments [26].

These results agree with other findings using the trichostrongyloid nematode *Heligmosomoides polygyrus*. In this study, peripheral immune responsiveness in male mice was reduced by infection with the parasite. Responsiveness was also lower among high-rankers or aggressive males regardless of infection status. Reduced responsiveness in infected animals and high rankers was associated with elevated serum corticosterone concentrations and was compounded among high-ranking males. Although glucocorticoids have a stimulatory effect on the initial cell proliferation phase of T lymphocytes, and thus some elevation might have been expected on this account, the change in corticosterone concentration during the infection phase was the best hormonal predictor of eventual worm burden. The negative relationship between these two parameters is more related with the later impact of glucocorticoids on the secretion of Th2 cytokines and thus depression of the Th2 arm of the immune response. This is consistent with the effects of glucocorticoid drugs in prolonging intestinal nematode infections, increasing the susceptibility of rodent hosts to *H. polygyrus* and depressing the expression of acquired resistance to *H. polygyrus*. There was no testosterone-dependent increase in parasite burden among high rankers in the experiment, perhaps because resistance to the parasite relies on the different emphasis on the Th1 and Th2 arms of the acquired immune response [27]. Schistosomiasis is another example in which steroids play an important role in host susceptibility. According to Kurtis *et al.*, the disproportionately high intensity and prevalence of schistosome infection in children, compared with adults, has been documented for decades, so understanding the mechanisms of this naturally occurring protection may guide efforts to develop a vaccine for schistosomiasis [28]. Thus, the importance of the hormonal changes during pubertal development, including increases in the levels of the adrenal hormones, dehydroepiandrosterona-sulfate (DHEA-S) and dehydroepiandrosterona (DHEA), which can be metabolized in peripheral tissues to androstenedione (A), testosterone (T4), dihydrotestosterone (DHT), and estrogens since they circulate at low levels in prepubescent children and the concentration of these steroids increases during puberty, plateaus during early adulthood, and decreases during senescence, so DHEA and DHEA-S may be partly responsible for the dramatic reduction in susceptibility to schistosome infection (Fig. **2**).

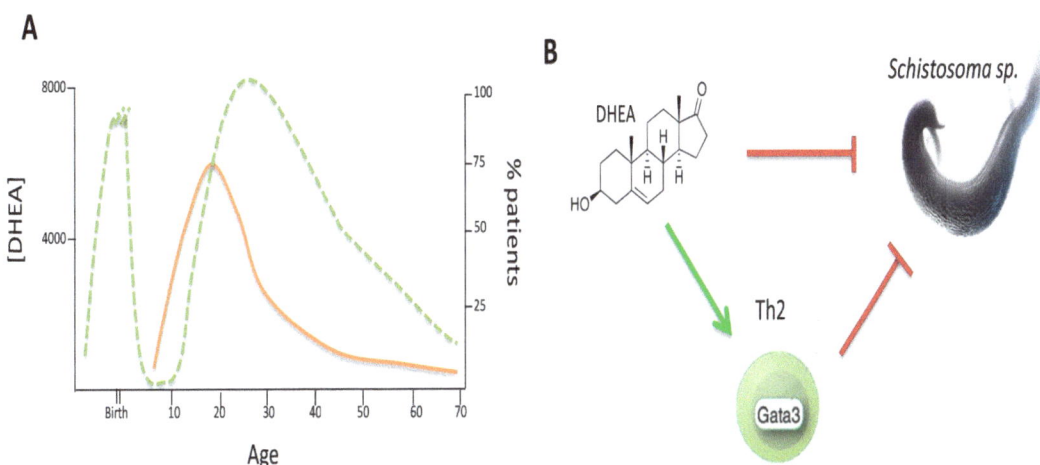

Figure 2: Schistosomiasis and DHEA/DHEA-S. (A) Comparison of serum DHEA levels (dotted line) and incidence of schistosomiasis (continued line) according to age. (B) DHEA-S induces the activation of a Th2 immune response that promotes the elimination of Schistosoma, but also has a suppressive effect on parasite proliferation *in vitro*.

Other evidence points to the relationship between increasing pubertal development, DHEA-S levels, and resistance to schistosome infection: (1) in mice, exogenous administration of DHEA-S leads to decreased schistosome worm burdens after challenge infection. Dehydroepiandrosterone sulfate treatment of mice modulates infection with *Schistosoma mansoni;* (2) DHEA-S kills larval and adult parasites in culture at physiologic concentrations; (3) in another two cross-sectional studies, increased DHEA-S levels are associated with decreased intensity of infection in humans; and (4) increased DHEA-S levels are associated with decreased intensity of reinfection after treatment with Praziquante l (PZQ) [28].

DHEA-S is known to have potent immunomodulatory activities, including up-regulation of Th2-driven antibody isotypes and down-regulation of proinflammatory cytokines. Finally if DHEA-S mediates resistance through a direct antiparasitic effect or *via* innate immune mechanisms, such as host skin thickness or fat deposition, then capitalizing on these mechanisms for vaccine development will be difficult. However, if DHEA-S mediates resistance *via* enhancement of acquired protective immune responses, then vaccine strategies designed to induce and augment these protective acquired immune responses, including hormonal adjuvants, may be promising [28].

Finally, the prediction of male biased parasitism was tested in free ranging chamois, which are intensely infested by gastrointestinal and lung helminthes, by investigating sex differences in faecal androgen (testosterone and epiandrosterone), cortisol and estrogen metabolites using enzyme immunoassays to evaluate the impact of these hormones on sex dependent parasite susceptibility. Male chamois had a higher output of gastrointestinal eggs and lungworm larvae when compared to females. Male biased parasitism originating in sex related hormone levels was confirmed for the elevated output of lungworm larvae, but not for the gastrointestinal nematodes. The faecal output of lungworm larvae was significantly correlated with androgen and cortisol metabolite levels. The immunosuppressant effects of these hormones may explain the greater susceptibility of males to infection by parasites and developing disease. The stress of the rutting season with elevated glucocorticoid levels is hypothesized to reduce humoral antibodies and to enhance larval output of nematodes in males but it should be considered that the subset samples were collected predominantly around the period when androgen levels between sexes differ most significantly. In contrast to the output of lungworm larvae, the male bias in quantitative gastrointestinal nematode output was not significantly correlated with sex differences in steroid levels [23]. Cytokines, peptide hormones and their shared receptors/ligands are used as a common biological language for communication within and between the immune and neuroendocrine systems. Such communication suggests an immunoregulatory role for the brain and a sensory function for the immune system. Then, it is evident that the immune system is widely related with the endocrine system and hormones. To prove this, researchers used a radioimmunoassay to measure the concentrations of steroid hormones (cortisol, testosterone, estradiol) in peripheral blood plasma from Gabonese women with chronic filarial infections and determined the concentrations of proinflammatory cytokines TNF-α, IFN-γ, IL-1 and IL-6 in the same plasma samples; concentrations were higher in microfilaremic women. A strong negative correlation was found between steroid hormones and pro-inflammatory cytokines. Cortisol was similar in the two groups. Plasma samples from amicrofilaremic men contained less testosterone and estradiol than those from microfilaremic women. A strong negative correlation was found between some steroid hormones from microfilaremic women, mainly human chorionic gonadotropin (HCG), testosterone and estradiol, and pro-inflammatory cytokines. Testosterone was also negatively correlated with IL-6, as was estradiol with IFN-γ. Furthermore, a positive correlation was found between prolactin and TNF-α and between prolactin and IL-6. The fact that cortisol concentrations were not elevated in women with filariasis may be related to the chronic nature of the disease. Hormone levels can be altered by long periods of disease [20]. In this case, the effect and changes between steroid hormones levels as related to some cytokines involved in the immune response activated against an infection by parasite in women is proven.

Another study that focused on the immune-endocrine system relationship in a helminth infection challenge was designed in rodents infected with *Stronguloides ratti*, in which a sex-related difference in host susceptibility was previously known. Here, male mice were more susceptible to *S. ratti* infection and the difference was seen comparing migrating larvae under the regulation of testosterone. To examine the effect of testosterone on macrophages, female mice were treated with testosterone and/or carbon to block the function of macrophages. Mice were then infected with third-stage larvae *of S. ratti*. Testosterone had a negative effect after macrophages were blocked. It has been shown that natural immunity against migrating larvae of *Strongyloides ratti* is chiefly regulated by macrophages. In the small intestine, host mast cells were related to adult worm expulsion. In the *S. ratti*-mouse model, male mice are more susceptible to *S. ratti* than are female mice [29]. According with this study, the sex-related difference is clearly mediated by testosterone during the migration of larvae, suggesting that testosterone renders mice susceptible to migrating larvae by modulating their natural defense mechanisms.

Investigators have shown that testosterone affects various cell functions. This finding means that testosterone can affect natural defense mechanisms after macrophage blockade. Testosterone may affect either other cells contributing to natural immunity against migrating larvae or L3 of *S. ratti* directly, by affecting the migrating ability of *S. ratti* L3. Testosterone treatment in mice has an additive effect on the numbers of *S. ratti* migrating larvae and testosterone can alter the susceptibility of female mice to *S. ratti* infection after macrophages have been blocked. Therefore, the effect of testosterone on worm recovery is partially independent of macrophage function [29].

Adrenal steroid hormones have been implicated, as some of the most important host factors controlling the onset, establishment, and pathogenesis of schistosomiasis, thus, adrenalectomy would greatly affect the course of the murine schistosomiasis infection. Adrenalectomized mice infected with *S. mansoni* were compared with intact infected and sham-infected controls and observed for their mortality rate, numbers of male and female worms, number of eggs, and liver pathology. There is evidence that lack of adrenal steroids mediates an increase in the adult worm burden and promotes worm fecundity *in vivo* [30].

Steroid hormones produced by the adrenal cortex, such as (DHEA-S) and cortisol, influence the intensity of the immune response during *S. mansoni* infections and have been implicated as being among the most important host factors controlling the onset, establishment, and pathogenesis of schistosomiasis. These hormones inhibit oviposition by *S. mansoni* both *in vitro* and *in vivo*. The adrenal steroid hormone DHEA is implicated in age-related changes in the immune system and in susceptibility to schistosomiasis [31, 32]. For instance, a relationship has been shown between DHEA-S, intensity of *S. mansoni* infection, and humoral immune response in human infections. A significant increase in DHEA-S serum levels in teenagers (15-19 years) was accompanied by a progressive decline in the intensity of infection [30].

The increased numbers of worms, larger number of eggs and more vigorous hepatic granulomas can be related to the lack of circulating glucocorticoids, whose presence in some way ameliorates the inflammatory immune response in the liver. The effect of adrenalectomy produced high levels of infection and more severe pathology, a fact that can be related to the well-known glucocorticoid anti-inflammatory effect. Low levels of cortisol could promote vigorous granuloma formation and the production of cytokines necessary for schistosome reproduction, such as TNF-α. The immunosuppressive effects of hydrocortisone and dexamethasone are counteracted by DHEA, suggesting a tightly controlled balance in the secretion of these hormones to regulate the inflammatory response. An intriguing question is how the lack of adrenal hormones affects the infection in the parasitized host. Host derived candidates that could possibly be affected by adrenalectomy are the interleukins (ILs), which are known to be altered during schistosomiasis. Potential endocrine-immune mediators of this process are IL-1, IL-6, TNF-α and macrophage migratory inhibitory factor (MIF), all known regulated by adrenal steroids. The changes produced in the infected adrenalectomized host herein could thus be cytokine mediated. Further work could elucidate the mechanism by which adrenalectomy induces changes in the immune function during disease progression and could establish causal links, if indeed they exist [30].

SEX STEROIDS IN MURINE AND PORCINE CYSTICERCOSIS

Taenia Crassiceps and the Murine Model

In *T. crassiceps* cysticercosis, females of all strains of mice studied sustain greater intensities of infection than males, but during chronic infection (more than 4 weeks) this difference disappears and the BALB/c males show a feminization process, characterized by high serum estrogens levels (200 times the normal values) while testosterone levels are 90% decreased. The target organs for testosterone action, testes and seminal vesicles, have a 50% weight reduction [33]. At the same time, the cellular immune response (Th_1) is markedly diminished in both sexes and the humoral response is enhanced (Th$_2$) [34]. Estradiol is involved in the immunoendocrine regulation of murine *T. crassiceps* cysticercosis as a major protagonist in promoting cysticercus growth and interfering with the thymus dependent cellular immune mechanisms that obstruct parasite growth [35]. Gonadectomy alters this resistance pattern and makes intensities equal in both sexes by increasing that of males and diminishing it in females [12], while serum sex steroid levels are not detectable in these animals. However, the absence of estrogens does not prevent parasite growth in both genders, demonstrating that although estradiol favors *Taenia crassiceps* development, it is not indispensable for rapid parasite growth [33].

A new round of *in vitro* and *in vivo* experiments was designed and performed in an effort to explore the mechanisms by which sex steroids act upon *T. crassiceps* cysticercus asexual reproduction: A) through the host's immune system mediation and/or B) directly through the parasite's own physiological systems.

The changes in steroid production of infected male mice were found to be associated with tissue damage in their reproductive system [36], together with a specific change in mRNA levels of the enzymes involved in normal male steroid metabolism: a decrease of the expression of 5α-reductase type II (the enzyme in charge of conversion from testosterone to DHT) and an increase in the expression of P450-aromatase (responsible for the conversion of testosterone to estradiol) [37]. Moreover, when the expression pattern of *c-fos* and *c-jun*, two estradiol-regulated genes, as well as that of *p53* and *bcl2* genes in the testes, spleen, and thymus of male mice infected with *T. crassiceps* cysticerci was studied, it was found that in infected animals the *c-fos* mRNA content was significantly increased in all tissues studied, whereas the *c-jun* mRNA content was increased only in the thymus. The p53 mRNA content was markedly reduced in all tissues of the parasitized animals analyzed, whereas bcl-2 gene expression was abolished only in the thymus [38].

Conversely, thymic cell analysis performed by flow cytometry showed a reduction in the content of $CD3^+$, $CD4^+$, and $CD8^+$ subpopulations in the infected mice. This suggests that the increase in estradiol levels of the host may change the expression pattern of several genes that participate in regulation of apoptosis in the thymus of male mice during chronic infection with *T. crassiceps* cysticerci, and that estrogens could inhibit the specific cellular immune response to the parasite [38]. Previous immunological experiments had led to suspect that estradiol positively regulates parasite reproduction in hosts of both sexes, presumably by interfering with the thymus-dependent cellular immune mechanisms that obstruct parasite growth (Th1) and favoring those that facilitate it (Th2) [35, 39]. A specific shift from a Th1 to a Th2 immune response in the course of infection was found, which coincided with an initial low rate of reproduction that accelerates at later times of infection. The shift is characterized by a marked decrease of IL-2 and IFN-γ in both sexes, while the secretion of cytokines involved in the specific humoral response (IL-6, IL-10 and IL-4) is enhanced [34, 40]. Thus, striking differences in susceptibility to cysticercosis between male and female mice may involve the joint action of the immune system and the gonads, both driven by the parasite, which is able to change the parasite's restrictive male normal hormonal milieu during chronic infection to a more female environment permissive for the parasite (Fig. 3).

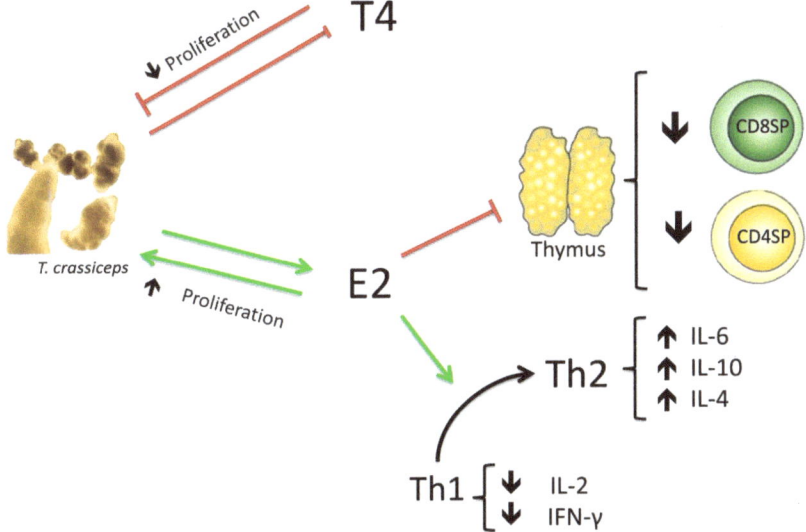

Figure 3: Bidirectional interaction between *T. crassiceps* and sex hormones and its effect on the immune response. Sex hormones play a dual role during *T. crassiceps* infection. Estradiol (E2) induces parasite-reproduction, which is accompanied by the polarization of a permissive Th2-immune response and the suppression in thymic development. In contrast, T4 and DHT inhibit parasite reproduction.

To strengthen the above notions and in an effort to identify the sex steroids involved, we studied the effects of testosterone, dihydrotestosterone, and 17β-estradiol in castrated mice of both sexes infected with *Taenia crassiceps* cysticerci [41]. In this study, we found that castration and treatment with either testosterone or dihydrotestosterone before infection markedly decreased parasite loads in both genders of mice, while the treatment with 17β-estradiol increased it in both genders [1]. The specific splenocyte cell proliferation, IL-2 and IFN-γ production were depressed in infected-castrated mice of both genders, while treatment with testosterone or dihydrotestosterone produced a significant recovery of cell proliferation and enhanced production of IL-2 and IFN-γ[41]. An opposite effect of the same sex steroids was found on the humoral response: it was unaffected with testosterone or dihydrotestosterone restitution, while treatment with estradiol in both genders augmented the levels of anti-cysticerci IgG, as well as IL-6 and IL-10 production. These results suggest that androgens mediate immune functions which protect mice from cysticercosis, possibly through the stimulation of the specific cellular immunity of the host [41].

Immunoendocrine interactions during cysticercosis are the cornerstone of the feminization of male mice. When the infected male mice have an intact immune system, there is an increase in serum estradiol levels and a decrease in levels of testosterone and DHT. However, when the immune system is knocked down by total irradiation or neonatal thymectomy, there is no change in the levels of serum steroids in chronically infected male mice, and the levels remain steady between infected and uninfected male mice [42]. IL-6 was demonstrated to be a key factor in this puzzle: IL-6$^{-/-}$ (KO) infected mice do not develop the feminization process, while restitution with IL-6 again allows the feminization. The expression of the IL-6 gene in the testes of parasitized mice was enhanced, a fact that can explain the primordial role of the testes in the feminization process produced by cysticercosis [41, 42]. Thus, IL-6 activates aromatase expression in the testes of the cysticercotic mice and produces active aromatization from androgens to estrogens. The increased serum levels of follicle stimulating hormone (FSH), the natural activator of aromatase expression, found in the chronically infected mice, supports the notion that FSH could be also a factor involved in the feminization process of the male mouse [42]. To further study the role of interleukin-6 (IL-6) and macrophage-migration inhibitory factor (MIF), known to be involved in immunoendocrinological processes during sex-associated susceptibility in cysticercosis, IL-6 and MIF gene knockout (KO) mice were infected, and the number of parasites and serum sex-steroid levels were measured. It was found that IL-6 and MIF KO mice of both genders infected with *T. crassiceps* cysticerci harbor similar numbers of parasites, with no change in sex-hormone levels. However, in wild-type strains, the sex-associated susceptibility to infection is observed, concomitantly with the feminization process in the chronically infected mice [43]. These results suggest a role for both IL-6 and MIF genes in sex-associated susceptibility in murine *T. crassiceps* cysticercosis.

The importance of sex hormones driving the specific immune response during cysticercosis was assessed in male and female mice by administration of Fadrozole (a P450-aromatase inhibitor) to suppress the production of 17β-estradiol [44]. A reduction was found in parasite loads (~70%) in infected mice treated with Fadrozole. The protective effect of the P450-aromatase inhibitor was associated, in male mice, with a recovery of the specific cellular immune response. Interleukin-6 (IL-6) serum levels and its production by splenocytes were dramatically augmented, together with an increase in its expression in the testes of infected male mice. Fadrozole treatment returned these levels to baseline values. These results suggest that P450-ase and IL-6 are key molecules in the feminization undergone by infected male mice and in regulating parasite loads. Fadrozole treatment appears to be a possible new therapeutic approach to control murine cysticercosis [44] and perhaps other parasites with active asexual reproduction in intermediate hosts.

Furthermore, it has also been demonstrated that administration of Tamoxifen (an anti-estrogen) produced an 80% parasite load reduction in female mice, and had a weaker effect of 50% in male mice. This protective effect was associated in both sexes with an increase in the mRNA levels of IL-2 (a cytokine associated to protection against cysticerci) and IL-4 (innocuous against infection). Tamoxifen treatment modified 17-β estradiol production in females, while serum testosterone was not affected. However, the expression of the two types of estrogen receptor (ER), ER-α and ER-β, in the spleen of infected mice of both sexes, was decreased by which is an anti-estrogen Tamoxifen treatment [45]. The *in vitro* treatment of

T. crassiceps with Tamoxifen, reduced reproduction and induced loss of motility in the parasite. These results indicate that Tamoxifen treatment is a new therapeutic possibility to treat cysticercosis, since it can act on both sides of the host-parasite relationship: increasing the cellular immune response protective against the parasite and acting directly upon the parasite, reducing its reproduction and increasing its mortality [45]. With all this information, we have postulated a flowchart that includes all known effects of sex steroids on the hosts' immune system, the molecules involved, and the impact upon cysticerci establishment, growth and reproduction in an immunocompetent host.

Another steroid that was recently tested and implicated in the regulation of the parasite loads during murine cysticercosis is progesterone (P_4). P_4 treatment has a dual effect: if mice of both sexes are non-gonadectomized (intact), P_4 treatment increased parasite loads, possibly through manipulation of the specific cellular immune response, as well as the steroid's promotion of parasite reproduction [46]. However, if mice are gonadectomized, P_4 completely decreases parasite loads, an impressive and unprecedented cysticidal effect, the likes of which are absent from other preventive or therapeutic measures [47]. These two experiments suggests that, in intact hosts, progesterone is metabolized to estradiol, that is permissive for parasite reproduction, while in castrated animals, there is an active metabolism of progesterone in the adrenal glands to androgens, resulting in a toxic effect in the parasite growth [43, 44]. The major steroid produced by the adrenal gland is the androgen (DHEA). So, another set of experiments showed the effect of DHEA on male and female infected mice. DHEA treatment reduced parasite loads by 70 and 80%, respectively. In contrast with the common assumption of DHEA as an immunostimulatory hormone, the immune response of our mice was not affected by DHEA treatment [48]. *In vitro*, treatment of *T. crassiceps* cysticerci with DHEA induced 80% reduction in parasite reproduction, which may partially explain the reduction of parasite loads observed *in vivo,* a partial effect suggesting the involvement of other unknown factors in the *in vivo* regulation of parasite loads [48].

Taenia Solium and Porcine Cysticercosis

As described for the mouse model of cysticercosis (CC), host's biological factors such as genetic background, the innate and acquired immunity, and gender can lead to resistance and/or susceptibility to cysticercosis/taeniosis by *Taenia solium*. It has been shown that sexual hormones play an important role in porcine CC. For instance, in castrated male pigs the prevalence of naturally acquired CC increased by 30%, while in pregnant sows the prevalence doubled, compared to non-castrated males and non-pregnant sows [49].

Another interesting finding, was found in experiments designed to explore the hormonal profiles of sex steroids and DHEA in serum of boars that had naturally acquired CC. A significant reduction in the T4 levels was observed, a change that was independent of the heterogeneous genetic background and wide age range. These findings suggest that sex steroids can be associated to *T. solium* susceptibility and transmission dynamics of this parasite under natural conditions [50].

Interestingly, sex steroids are not the only hormones that can be useful to this parasite. It has been recently described that the *in vitro* culture of *T. crassiceps* with insulin stimulates parasite reproduction two-fold and increases the average bud diameter. However, this hormone had no effect on *T. solium* cysticerci cultures [51]. Conversely, hamsters treated with P4 and experimentally infected with *T. solium* showed an 80% reduction of anchored-*T. solium* tapeworms, a reduced growth of these parasites and down-regulation of progesterone receptor (PR) expression in 50% of the duodenum associated tapeworms. Immune response of P4 treated hamsters showed an increase in IL-4, IL-6 and TNF-α cytokines and an exacerbated inflammatory infiltrate located along the lamina propria, compared to infected non-progesterone treated controls [52]. These results clearly support the fact that P4 protects against the establishment of the *T. solium* adult tapeworm by improving the immune system. The studies in mice and pigs have already been scaled to the natural human disease. A recent study on human neurocisticercosis, caused by *T. solium* larvae infiltration in the central nervous system (CNC) demonstrated a strong correlation between the endocrine and immune systems, gender and age during clinical manifestation and susceptibility to the disease. Cardenas *et al.*, designed a clinical study to evaluate the hormonal changes associated with NCC and their relationships. Since the proper diagnosis of the disease was fundamental in this study, a precise clinical and radiological description of the disease and a complete hormonal and immunological profile was performed in 50 patients and 22 healthy subjects.

Patients had lower DHEA levels compared to healthy subjects. Concerning gender, male patients showed a clear decrease in 17β-estradiol serum levels and high levels of Luteinizing Hormone (LH), while female patients with clinically severe disease showed lower levels of progesterone and androstenedione. Higher concentrations of follicle stimulating hormone (FSH) and lower concentrations of testosterone (similar to those reported previously during murine cysticercosis) were found in male patients with severe disease, when compared to the less clinically severe patients. Significant correlations were found between E2 and IL-10 in male patients, and between DHEA and IL-1β, and androstenedione and IL-17 in female patients, suggesting a possible immunoendocrine interaction. The study by Cardenas *et al.*, in neurocysticercotic patients constitutes the first demonstration that the presence of *T. solium* larvae in the central nervous system, can modify the host environment through the induction of endocrine and immunological changes. As the authors point out, these results provide a stimulating background to analyze the repercussions of hormonal changes during the course of the disease and on patient reproductive health [53]. Taken together, the above-presented evidence opens up the possibility of using hormone analogues, as novel anti-cysticercotic agents.

Trichinella Spiralis and the Pituitary Hormones

In the case of *Trichinella spiralis*, the influence of anterior pituitary hormones on the gastrointestinal tract of humans and animals has been previously reported. Hypophysectomy (HYPOX) in the rat causes atrophy of the intestinal mucosa, and reduction of gastric secretion and intestinal absorption, as well as increased susceptibility to bacterial and viral infections. Recent results from our group indicate that 5 days post infection, neurointermediate pituitary lobectomy (NIL) reduces the number of intestinally recovered *T. spiralis* larvae. Using semi-quantitative inmunofluorescent laser confocal microscopy, we observed that the mean intensity of all tested Th1 cytokines was markedly diminished, even in the duodenum of infected controls. In contrast, a high level of expression of these cytokines was noted in the NIL infected hamsters. Likewise, a significant decrease in the fluorescence intensity of Th2 cytokines (with the exception of IL-4) was apparent in the duodenum of control and sham infected hamsters, compared to animals with NIL surgeries, which showed an increase in the expression of IL-5 and IL-13. Histology of duodenal mucosa from NIL hamsters showed an exacerbated inflammatory infiltrate located along the lamina propria, which was related to the presence of the parasite. We conclude that hormones from each pituitary lobe affect the gastrointestinal immune responses to *T. spiralis* through various mechanisms [54].

CONCLUDING REMARKS

Until some years ago, the immune system was perceived as a system isolated from other body systems. The present review makes it evident that the immune and neuroendocrine systems share numerous ligands and receptors, which results in constant bidirectional communication. In fact, it has been postulated that an important function of the immune system is to serve as a sensory organ for cognoscitive stimuli that pass unnoticed to the nervous system, as could be infectious agents, such as parasites. Our present proposal is to reintegrate an important system to the physiological context of the whole organism. This will doubtlessly lead to an improved understanding of physiology, and generate changes in modern medical practice. For further understanding of the bidirectional communication process between the immune and neuroendocrine systems, it will be necessary to continue the search for ligands and receptors common to both systems, and to examine, in depth, the similarities and differences in their functional regulation. In addition, it will also constitute a challenge for physiologists to integrate this information to the context of the whole organism during helminth infections. On the other hand, new information about immunoneuroendocrine interactions in infected hosts will help to design novel therapies for the treatment and diagnosis of human diseases of apparently immune or endocrine origin. We have documented here that a complex interactive network involving the immune, endocrine and nervous systems, is in control of the parasite growth, reproduction and establishment. If such a complex management of parasite loads, as we shown here, between different hosts and worms, extends to other parasitic diseases in mammals, as current research seems to indicate, their means of exploration, greater understanding and forms of control must be reviewed and approached with designs matching in complexity and plasticity to that of the infections. The evidence presented above illustrates the complexity and importance of neuroimmunoendocrine interactions during cysticercosis and provides clues to the many other possible mechanisms of parasite establishment, growth and reproduction in an immunocompetent host. Further, strong neuroimmunoendocrine interactions may have implications in the control of transmission and treatment of this parasitic disease in porcines and humans. Of practical importance, the complexity of the cysticerci-host relationship suggests that all physiological factors (*i.e.*, sex, age) should be taken into account in the design of vaccines and new drugs.

ACKNOWLEDGEMENTS

Financial support: Grant 176803 from Consejo Nacional de Ciencia y Tecnología (CONACYT) de México and grant # IN-214011 from Programa de Apoyo a Proyectos de Investigación e Inovación Tecnológica (PAPIIT) from Dirección General de Asuntos del Personal Académico (DGAPA), UNAM; both J M-M. and Karen E. Nava Castro have Post-Doctoral fellowships from CONACyT.

CONFLICT OF INTEREST

The authors confirm that this chapter contents have no conflict of interest.

REFERENCES

[1] Cole TJ, Beckage NE, Tan FF, Srinivasan A, Ramaswamy SB. Parasitoid-host endocrine relations: self-reliance or co-optation? Insect Biochem Mol Biol. 2002;32(12):1673-9. Epub 2002/11/14.
[2] Chikanza IC, Grossman AB. Reciprocal interactions between the neuroendocrine and immune systems during inflammation. Rheum Dis Clin North Am. 2000;26(4):693-711. Epub 2000/11/21.
[3] Chrousos GP. The hypothalamic-pituitary-adrenal axis and immune-mediated inflammation. N Engl J Med. 1995;332(20):1351-62. Epub 1995/05/18.
[4] Da Silva JA. Sex hormones and glucocorticoids: interactions with the immune system. Ann N Y Acad Sci. 1999;876102-17; discussion 17-8. Epub 1999/07/23.
[5] Escobedo G, Larralde C, Chavarria A, Cerbon MA, Morales-Montor J. Molecular mechanisms involved in the differential effects of sex steroids on the reproduction and infectivity of Taenia crassiceps. J Parasitol. 2004;90(6):1235-44. Epub 2005/02/18.
[6] de Mendonca RL, Escriva H, Bouton D, Laudet V, Pierce RJ. Hormones and nuclear receptors in schistosome development. Parasitol Today. 2000;16(6):233-40. Epub 2000/05/29.
[7] de Souza EM, Rivera MT, Araujo-Jorge TC, de Castro SL. Modulation induced by estradiol in the acute phase of Trypanosoma cruzi infection in mice. Parasitol Res. 2001;87(7):513-20. Epub 2001/08/04.

[8] Escobedo G, Roberts CW, Carrero JC, Morales-Montor J. Parasite regulation by host hormones: an old mechanism of host exploitation? Trends Parasitol. 2005;21(12):588-93. Epub 2005/10/21.

[9] Gay-Andrieu F, Cozon GJ, Ferrandiz J, Peyron F. Progesterone fails to modulate Toxoplasma gondii replication in the RAW 264.7 murine macrophage cell line. Parasite Immunol. 2002;24(4):173-8. Epub 2002/05/16.

[10] Gomez Y, Valdez RA, Larralde C, Romano MC. Sex steroids and parasitism: Taenia crassiceps cisticercus metabolizes exogenous androstenedione to testosterone *in vitro*. J Steroid Biochem Mol Biol. 2000;74(3):143-7. Epub 2000/11/22.

[11] Hernandez-Bello R, Ramirez-Nieto R, Muniz-Hernandez S, Nava-Castro K, Pavon L, Sanchez-Acosta AG, Morales-Montor J. Sex steroids effects on the molting process of the helminth human parasite Trichinella spiralis. J Biomed Biotechnol. 2011;2011625380. Epub 2011/12/14.

[12] Huerta L, Terrazas LI, Sciutto E, Larralde C. Immunological mediation of gonadal effects on experimental murine cysticercosis caused by Taenia crassiceps metacestodes. J Parasitol. 1992;78(3):471-6. Epub 1992/06/01.

[13] Liu L, Benten WP, Wang L, Hao X, Li Q, Zhang H, Guo D, Wang Y, Wunderlich F, Qiao Z. Modulation of Leishmania donovani infection and cell viability by testosterone in bone marrow-derived macrophages: signaling *via* surface binding sites. Steroids. 2005;70(9):604-14. Epub 2005/06/21.

[14] Nava-Castro K, Hernandez-Bello R, Muniz-Hernandez S, Camacho-Arroyo I, Morales-Montor J. Sex steroids, immune system, and parasitic infections: facts and hypotheses. Ann N Y Acad Sci. 2012;126216-26. Epub 2012/07/25.

[15] Hernandez-Bello R, Escobedo G, Guzman C, Ibarra-Coronado EG, Lopez-Griego L, Morales-Montor J. Immunoendocrine host-parasite interactions during helminth infections: from the basic knowledge to its possible therapeutic applications. Parasite Immunol. 2010;32(9-10):633-43. Epub 2010/08/10.

[16] Escobedo G, Lopez-Griego L, Morales-Montor J. Neuroimmunoendocrine modulation in the host by helminth parasites: a novel form of host-parasite coevolution? Neuroimmunomodulation. 2009;16(2):78-87. Epub 2009/02/13.

[17] Hoberg EP. Phylogeny of Taenia: Species definitions and origins of human parasites. Parasitol Int. 2006;55 SupplS23-30. Epub 2005/12/24.

[18] Nava-Castro K, Muñiz-Hernández S, Hernández-Bello R, Morales-Montor J. The neuroimmunoendocrine network during worm helminth infections. International Survival Journa. 2011;8(1):142-52.

[19] Locksley RM. Exploitation of immune and other defence mechanisms by parasites: an overview. Parasitology. 1997;115 SupplS5-7. Epub 1997/01/01.

[20] Damian RT. Parasite immune evasion and exploitation: reflections and projections. Parasitology. 1997;115 SupplS169-75. Epub 1997/01/01.

[21] Arteaga M, Chavarria A, Morales Montor J. [Immunoneuroendocrine communication network and homeostasis regulation: the use of hormones and neurohormones as immunotherapy]. Rev Invest Clin. 2002;54(6):542-9. Epub 2003/04/11. La red de comunicacion neuroinmunoendocrina y la regulacion de la homeostasis: el uso de hormonas y neurohormonas como inmunoterapia.

[22] Klein SL. The effects of hormones on sex differences in infection: from genes to behavior. Neurosci Biobehav Rev. 2000;24(6):627-38. Epub 2000/08/15.

[23] Hoby S, Schwarzenberger F, Doherr MG, Robert N, Walzer C. Steroid hormone related male biased parasitism in chamois, Rupicapra rupicapra rupicapra. Vet Parasitol. 2006;138(3-4):337-48. Epub 2006/02/25.

[24] Hepworth MR, Hardman MJ, Grencis RK. The role of sex hormones in the development of Th2 immunity in a gender-biased model of Trichuris muris infection. Eur J Immunol. 2010;40(2):406-16. Epub 2009/12/02.

[25] McDermott JR, Leslie FC, D'Amato M, Thompson DG, Grencis RK, McLaughlin JT. Immune control of food intake: enteroendocrine cells are regulated by CD4+ T lymphocytes during small intestinal inflammation. Gut. 2006;55(4):492-7. Epub 2005/11/22.

[26] Hildreth MB, Granholm NH. Effect of mouse strain variations and cortisone treatment on the establishment and growth of primary Echinococcus multilocularis hydatid cysts. J Parasitol. 2003;89(3):493-5. Epub 2003/07/26.

[27] Barnard CJ, Behnke JM, Gage AR, Brown H, Smithurst PR. The role of parasite-induced immunodepression, rank and social environment in the modulation of behaviour and hormone concentration in male laboratory mice (Mus musculus). Proc Biol Sci. 1998;265(1397):693-701. Epub 1998/06/03.

[28] Kurtis JD, Friedman JF, Leenstra T, Langdon GC, Wu HW, Manalo DL, Su L, Jiz M, Jarilla B, Pablo AO, McGarvey ST, Olveda RM, Acosta LP. Pubertal development predicts resistance to infection and reinfection with Schistosoma japonicum. Clin Infect Dis. 2006;42(12):1692-8. Epub 2006/05/18.

[29] Watanabe K, Hamano S, Noda K, Koga M, Tada I. Strongyloides ratti: additive effect of testosterone implantation and carbon injection on the susceptibility of female mice. Parasitol Res. 1999;85(7):522-6. Epub 1999/06/26.

[30] Morales-Montor J, Mohamed F, Damian RT. Schistosoma mansoni: the effect of adrenalectomy on the murine model. Microbes Infect. 2004;6(5):475-80. Epub 2004/04/28.

[31] Abebe F, Birkeland KI, Gaarder PI, Petros B, Gundersen SG. The relationships between dehydroepiandrosterone sulphate (DHEAS), the intensity of Schistosoma mansoni infection and parasite-specific antibody responses. A cross-sectional study in residents of endemic communities in north-east Ethiopia. APMIS. 2003;111(2):319-28. Epub 2003/04/30.

[32] Fulford AJ, Webster M, Ouma JH, Kimani G, Dunne DW. Puberty and Age-related Changes in Susceptibility to Schistosome Infection. Parasitol Today. 1998;14(1):23-6. Epub 2006/10/17.

[33] Larralde C, Morales J, Terrazas I, Govezensky T, Romano MC. Sex hormone changes induced by the parasite lead to feminization of the male host in murine Taenia crassiceps cysticercosis. J Steroid Biochem Mol Biol. 1995;52(6):575-80. Epub 1995/06/01.

[34] Terrazas LI, Bojalil R, Govezensky T, Larralde C. Shift from an early protective Th1-type immune response to a late permissive Th2-type response in murine cysticercosis (Taenia crassiceps). J Parasitol. 1998;84(1):74-81. Epub 1998/03/06.

[35] Terrazas LI, Bojalil R, Govezensky T, Larralde C. A role for 17-beta-estradiol in immunoendocrine regulation of murine cysticercosis (Taenia crassiceps). J Parasitol. 1994;80(4):563-8. Epub 1994/08/01.

[36] Morales-Montor J, Gamboa-Dominguez A, Rodriguez-Dorantes M, Cerbon MA. Tissue damage in the male murine reproductive system during experimental Taenia crassiceps cysticercosis. J Parasitol. 1999;85(5):887-90. Epub 1999/11/30.

[37] Morales-Montor J, Rodriguez-Dorantes M, Cerbon MA. Modified expression of steroid 5 alpha-reductase as well as aromatase, but not cholesterol side-chain cleavage enzyme, in the reproductive system of male mice during (Taenia crassiceps) cysticercosis. Parasitol Res. 1999;85(5):393-8. Epub 1999/05/05.

[38] Morales-Montor J, Rodriguez-Dorantes M, Mendoza-Rodriguez CA, Camacho-Arroyo I, Cerbon MA. Differential expression of the estrogen-regulated proto-oncogenes c-fos, c-jun, and bcl-2 and of the tumor-suppressor p53 gene in the male mouse chronically infected with Taenia crassiceps cysticerci. Parasitol Res. 1998;84(8):616-22. Epub 1998/09/25.

[39] Bojalil R, Terrazas LI, Govezensky T, Sciutto E, Larralde C. Thymus-related cellular immune mechanisms in sex-associated resistance to experimental murine cysticercosis (Taenia crassiceps). J Parasitol. 1993;79(3):384-9. Epub 1993/06/01.

[40] Terrazas LI, Cruz M, Rodriguez-Sosa M, Bojalil R, Garcia-Tamayo F, Larralde C. Th1-type cytokines improve resistance to murine cysticercosis caused by Taenia crassiceps. Parasitol Res. 1999;85(2):135-41. Epub 1999/02/06.

[41] Morales-Montor J, Baig S, Hallal-Calleros C, Damian RT. Taenia crassiceps: androgen reconstitution of the host leads to protection during cysticercosis. Exp Parasitol. 2002;100(4):209-16. Epub 2002/07/20.

[42] Morales-Montor J, Baig S, Mitchell R, Deway K, Hallal-Calleros C, Damian RT. Immunoendocrine interactions during chronic cysticercosis determine male mouse feminization: role of IL-6. J Immunol. 2001;167(8):4527-33. Epub 2001/10/10.

[43] Morales-Montor J, Baig S, Kabbani A, Damian RT. Do interleukin-6 and macrophage-migration inhibitory factor play a role during sex-associated susceptibility in murine cysticercosis? Parasitol Res. 2002;88(10):901-4. Epub 2002/09/05.

[44] Morales-Montor J, Hallal-Calleros C, Romano MC, Damian RT. Inhibition of p-450 aromatase prevents feminisation and induces protection during cysticercosis. Int J Parasitol. 2002;32(11):1379-87. Epub 2002/09/28.

[45] Vargas-Villavicencio JA, Larralde C, De Leon-Nava MA, Escobedo G, Morales-Montor J. Tamoxifen treatment induces protection in murine cysticercosis. J Parasitol. 2007;93(6):1512-7. Epub 2008/03/05.

[46] Vargas-Villavicencio JA, Larralde C, De Leon-Nava MA, Morales-Montor J. Regulation of the immune response to cestode infection by progesterone is due to its metabolism to estradiol. Microbes Infect. 2005;7(3):485-93. Epub 2005/04/05.

[47] Vargas-Villavicencio JA, Larralde C, Morales-Montor J. Gonadectomy and progesterone treatment induce protection in murine cysticercosis. Parasite Immunol. 2006;28(12):667-74. Epub 2006/11/14.

[48] Vargas-Villavicencio JA, Larralde C, Morales-Montor J. Treatment with dehydroepiandrosterone *in vivo* and *in vitro* inhibits reproduction, growth and viability of Taenia crassiceps metacestodes. Int J Parasitol. 2008;38(7):775-81. Epub 2007/12/18.

[49] Morales J, Velasco T, Tovar V, Fragoso G, Fleury A, Beltran C, Villalobos N, Aluja A, Rodarte LF, Sciutto E, Larralde C. Castration and pregnancy of rural pigs significantly increase the prevalence of naturally acquired Taenia solium cysticercosis. Vet Parasitol. 2002;108(1):41-8. Epub 2002/08/23.

[50] Pena N, Morales J, Morales-Montor J, Vargas-Villavicencio A, Fleury A, Zarco L, de Aluja AS, Larralde C, Fragoso G, Sciutto E. Impact of naturally acquired Taenia solium cysticercosis on the hormonal levels of free ranging boars. Vet Parasitol. 2007;149(1-2):134-7. Epub 2007/08/25.

[51] Escobedo G, Romano MC, Morales-Montor J. Differential *in vitro* effects of insulin on *Taenia crassiceps* and *Taenia solium* cysticerci. J Helminthol. 2009;83(4):403-12. Epub 2009/06/25.

[52] Escobedo G, Camacho-Arroyo I, Nava-Luna P, Olivos A, Perez-Torres A, Leon-Cabrera S, Carrero JC, Morales-Montor J. Progesterone induces mucosal immunity in a rodent model of human taeniosis by Taenia solium. International journal of biological sciences. 2011;7(9):1443-56. Epub 2011/11/24.

[53] Cardenas G, Valdez R, Saenz B, Bottasso O, Fragoso G, Sciutto E, Romano MC, Fleury A. Impact of Taenia solium neurocysticercosis upon endocrine status and its relation with immuno-inflammatory parameters. Int J Parasitol. 2012;42(2):171-6. Epub 2012/01/12.

[54] Hernandez-Cervantes R, Quintanar-Stephano A, López-Salazar V, López-Griego L, Hernández-Bello R, Carrero JC, Nava-Castro K, Morales-Montor J. Regulation of intestinal immune response by selective removal of the anterior, posterior, or entire pituitary gland in *Trichinella spiralis* infected golden hamsters. PLoS One. 2013;8(3):e59486. doi: 10.1371/journal.pone.0059486. Epub 2013 Mar 15

CHAPTER 2

The Immune Response During Toxocariosis by *Toxocara Canis*

Fernando Alba-Hurtado[1], Lorena Chávez-Guitrón[1], Victor Hugo del Río-Araiza[2], Karen Nava-Castro[3] and Jorge Morales-Montor[2,*]

[1]*Department of Parasitology, Autonomous National University of Mexico, Mexico City, Mexico;* [2]*Department of Immunology, Institute of Biomedical Investigations, Autonomous National University of Mexico, AP 70228, México DF 04510, México and* [3]*Faculty of Chemistry, Department of Biology, Autonomous National University of Mexico, México DF 04510, México*

Abstract: *Toxocara canis* is a nematode with a biological cycle that includes a definitive canine host and diverse paratenic hosts. These hosts include humans, rats, rabbits, birds, and pigs. This parasite is the causal agent for toxocariosis, which is an important parasitic infection in tropical and subtropical regions. Infection of BALB/c mice with *T. canis* elicited a Th2 response; however, this infection did not significantly alter the Th1 immune response. An appropriate animal model must primarily imitate the human host, the parasite's responses to the human host or the way that both the host and parasite interact. The knowledge of the immunological response in toxocariosis is relevant for understanding the protective mechanisms developed by the host against the parasite and the immune modulation effect on these mechanisms by the larvae. These parasite-host interactions could culminate in the success of the infection, the development of the disease, the destruction of the parasite or the interruption of its pathogenic mechanisms. This knowledge allows to design the methods of immunodiagnosis based on the detection of specific antibodies against parasite antigens and/or the detection of the parasites' antigens. Finally, the identification of the protective immune response mechanisms could serve in the development of strategies for the prevention, treatment and more adequate management of patients. In this chapter, we review certain aspects of the immunological responses that participate in the infection and in the disease, the relevant aspects of the humoral immunological response for the design of immunodiagnostic methods and for the development of vaccines.

Keywords: Toxocariosis, Toxocara canis, helminth, nematode, worm, immunity, immune response, immunoparasitology, Th1, Th2, cytokines, drug design, immunodiagnosis, epidemiology.

---

*Corresponding author **Jorge Morales-Montor:** Department of Immunology, Institute of Biomedical Research, U.N.A.M., AP 70228, México D.F. 04510; Tel: (525)622-3854; Fax: (525)622-3369; E-mails: jmontor66@biomedicas.unam.mx pr jmontor66@hotmail.com

Emilio Jirillo, Thea Magrone and Giuseppe Miragliotta (Eds)
All rights reserved-© 2014 Bentham Science Publishers

INTRODUCTION

Toxocariosis is a disease that is caused by the presence and action of the nematode parasite *Toxocara canis*. The adult parasite is in the small intestine of the dog, and its larvae may affect many animals that act as paratenic hosts, such as humans [1]. Other hosts that carry the adult parasite are foxes (*Alopex lagopus* and *Vulpes vulpes*), coyotes (*Canis latrans*) and wolves (*Canis lupus*) [2-5]. *T. canis* is a white colour nematode, dimorphic, up to 4 to 10 cm long in males and up to 18 cm long in females. *T. canis* has three well-developed lips at the anterior end, one dorsal and two sub-ventral ones, with two papillae. The internal surface of each lip has a dentigerous ridge or small teeth. *T. canis* has cervical alae that provide *T. canis* with arrow point aspects. The posterior end of the male ends in a curve towards its ventral portion, with two small equal spicules of 0.75 to 0.95 mm in length and a tapering end in appendage form. In females, the vulva opens in the medial region of the body and produces many eggs, which are not embryonated at the time of laying [6-9]. Eggs are brown, sub-spherical, 75 to 90 µm in size and have three layers. The outer layer is extremely fine and has slits that appear to be perforations and that are known as pits [6].

BIOLOGICAL CYCLE

Toxocariosis, which is caused by *T. canis*, is one of the main parasitic diseases of dogs. Its geographical distribution is worldwide, and due to its great incidence and pathogenicity in humans, toxocariosis is considered an important public health problem [9, 22]. The relations between this parasite and its hosts are extremely complex, although the biological cycle of *T. canis* is simple [10, 11]. In normal conditions, the development of the infecting larvae requires 9 to 11 days at 24°C and 3 to 5 days at 30°C, with atmospheric oxygen and relative humidity of 75% [12-14]. Infection occurs when dogs, humans or other susceptible hosts ingest the eggs with larvae. Once inside, these eggs hatch in the duodenum, and the second larval stage penetrates the intestinal wall. Then, the larvae enter the lymphatic flow or capillaries and arrive at the liver two days later through the portal vein. On the fourth day, the larvae reach the lungs, travelling through the cava vein and the right heart and pulmonary arteries. From this point, the migration route and larvae development vary according to the age of the dog [13]. In adult dogs, the second stage larvae that arrive at the lung, return to the heart and are distributed throughout the entire body, preferring striated muscles, liver, lungs and kidneys, where the larvae remain in a latent stage [9, 12, 15]. In contrast, in dog foetuses, the larvae leave lung capillaries, penetrate alveoli and migrate through the respiratory tract until the larvae reach the pharynx (tracheal migration), from which the larvae are swallowed. The larvae live in the stomach until the tenth day post-infection (p.i.), when the larvae travel to the duodenum, where the larvae become adults in 19-27 days p.i. At this time, the parasites are sexually mature, and males and females copulate, which results in the production of fertile eggs between 4 and 5 weeks p.i. [9, 13]. When the larvae reach the livers of foetuses, the larvae molt and transform into third stage larvae. When the pups are born, these larvae are in the lungs and remain there during the first week of life. Molting into the fourth stage occurs during the first week, when the larvae are in the lungs or later, when the larvae are in the stomach. Towards the end of the second week, the larvae molt into the fifth stage. Then, the larvae have a rapid growth period, and adult forms may be found at the end of the third week. A latency period of prenatal infections oscillates between 23 and 40 days after birth [9, 16]. Thus far, only second stage somatic larvae have been mentioned in adult dogs (acquired by the ingestion of larval eggs). These dogs rarely have adult parasites in their intestine. Nevertheless, after the pups are born, the somatic reactivated larvae reach the intestine of the bitches, which normally are exempt of adult parasites. The parasites mature 25 to 26 days post-partum and persist during an average of 60 days before spontaneous expulsion [11, 13, 17]. Interestingly, in addition to having post-natal infections, puppies usually also have prenatal infections. Perhaps under the influence of hormones of the gestating females, the somatic larvae are reactivated and penetrate the foetus between 42 to 43 gestation days [11, 13, 18]. Some studies have found that adult worms affect pups younger than six months two-fold more than adult dogs [10]. Not all somatic larvae are reactivated during the first gestation. Bitches that no longer ingest larval eggs are capable of contaminating their pups during three consecutive gestations [9]. The reactivation of somatic larvae continues to occur in the lactating bitch, and the larvae gain access to the mammary gland, being eliminated through milk and infesting the litter. The postnatal infestation of puppies during lactation is quantitatively equal to or more pronounced than the prenatal *in utero* infestation

[19]. Paratenic hosts, including humans, are infected by the ingestion of larval eggs of *T. canis*; the larvae invade lung alveoli and migrate to diverse organs, such as liver, other lung parts, brain and eye, where the larvae remain in a latent state during long periods [9, 13, 20, 21].

EPIDEMIOLOGY

Infection by *Toxocara* is present in almost all litters of dogs and cats, which daily eliminate an enormous amount of eggs in faeces and accumulate in the environment. When the eggs are protected from direct sunlight and from desiccation, they develop until reaching the infective phase in close to three weeks and persist viable in soil many months. Thus, the soil of zones where the dogs and cats with toxocariosis defecate is a constant source of infection. In addition, due to the action of precipitation, it is possible for the eggs to be transported to distant sites where great concentrations occur. A few milligrams of soil from the surface of these sites may contain hundreds of infective eggs, making it possible for a child to ingest dirt with thousands of these infective eggs, and older children or adults may acquire slight infestations by ingesting imperceptible amounts of highly contaminated material. The examination of the soil in parks and in game fields of different cities has demonstrated the presence of infective eggs of *T. canis*, constituting an infection source for children and contributing to high parasitosis indices in dogs, cats and other hosts. A potential risk is found not only in contaminated faeces and soil but also in the eggs that have adhered to the hair of dogs [23, 24]. This source of infection should not be underestimated because many pets share a home and bed with their owners.

The high incidence of persons with anti-*Toxocara* antibodies in different parts of the world varies between 2.6 to 81.5%, indicating the high degree of infestation by this parasite. Nevertheless, most individuals do not show clinical manifestations, and these manifestations only appear when many eggs are ingested or when the larvae are in critical places, such as the brain or eyes [25-27].

ANTIGENS

Many of the molecules that form the *T. canis* body are similar to the molecules of its host; therefore, these molecules are not recognised as foreign. However, other molecules are recognised as foreign and are capable of eliciting an immune response. This parasite has two types of antigens: the somatic antigens and the secretion and excretion antigens (TES-Ag).

Somatic antigens are molecules that form part of the body of the nematode, and most of these antigens have immunological cross-reactions with antigens of other helminths; therefore, these antigens have limited diagnostic importance [28-30]. Nevertheless, any antigen that has protection value belongs to this group. Certain antigens remain during the entire life of the nematode; however, there are other antigens that are specific to each life cycle stage [31].

TES-Ags are molecules produced and eliminated by the parasite. The most studied TES-Ags are produced by second stage larvae. In 1975, De Savigni developed a method to obtain TES-Ags from second stage larvae. The chemical analysis of TES-Ags has demonstrated that these antigens are a complex glycoprotein mixture. The most frequently found proteins joined to TES-Ags are N-acetylgalactosamine and galactose, whereas other proteins, such as arabinol, mannose, N-acetylglucosamine, glucose, fucosa and xylose, are not as frequent [32]. These carbohydrates are present in different proportions in some or all TES-Ags, forming epitopes that are linked to the protein complex of the antigen in either a strong or a weak manner. The immunological response is primarily directed towards glycosylated complexes of the antigens [33]. Up to 15 protein bands have been detected in TES-Ags, as determined by SDS-PAGE gels; the most abundant bands are 32, 55, 70, 120 and 400 kDa. Studies using monoclonal antibodies have established that the two main sites where TES-Ags are produced are in the larval esophageal glands and in a long branch of secreting column cells present in the pores of the cuticle. The excretion is performed through the cuticle by cuticular pores and by the oral pathway [34]. Antigens of molecular weights of 32, 70 and 120 kDa are linked to the cuticles of *T. canis* larvae. TES-Ags are released from the larvae when granulocytes of antibodies adhere to the TES-Ags. Furthermore, TES-Ags are constantly secreted trough the mouth and excretion pores of the parasite. Therefore, it has been proposed that TES-Ags are an immune evasion mechanism of the parasite because these antigens are the proteins against which an immune response is mounted [35].

In culture, other larval secreted molecules have been detected. Some of these molecules include TES-26/PEB-1 (homologous to a testicular protein of mammals), some lipids (however, no immunological response is mounted against these molecules, and its biological role has not yet been detected) and enzymes, such as superoxide dismutase, acetylcholinesterase and metallo-proteases. Likewise, mucins and lectins are secreted [36]. The number and types of TES-Ags recognised by western blot varies depending on the host. Rabbits frequently recognise nine antigens [37]; pigs, two [38]; humans, seven [39]; mice, four [40]; dogs, five [26]; and gerbils, eight [41]. The above suggests that TES-Ag immune dominance varies for each host species. Moreover, it has been experimentally demonstrated that there is a sequential recognition of these antigens. For instance, the sera of experimentally infected gerbils only recognised one antigen on day 20 p.i., whereas on day 40 p.i., four were recognised, and finally on day 130 p.i., eight antigens were recognised [41].

Immune Response to *T. Canis*

Infection by *T. canis* produces a series of events that may be modified by different factors, by the host and by the parasite. The type of mounted immune response in dogs (definitive host) differs from that mounted by paratenic hosts (including humans). There is also variation depending on the host's age and its physiological status, such as pregnancy and lactation, among others [11, 42]. For instance, in the murine model, infection with *T. canis* leads to persistent pulmonary inflammation, eosinophilia, an increase in the levels of circulating IgE levels, with airway hyperreactivity and, mainly, the production of Th2 cytokines.

When *T. canis* larvae enter any host, the larvae activate an innate immunological response characterised by leukocytosis, which has been observed between days 5 and 20 p.i. [41, 43, 44]. This increase is the result of a non-specific rise in lymphopoiesis and a total increase in neutrophils, lymphocytes, basophiles and monocytes in blood. The only cells that proportionally increase in blood and in tissues are eosinophils [1, 45, 46]. Some *T. canis* antigens have mitogenic activity on lymphocytes and induce an increase in lymphoid tissue and cell activity and in the size of the spleen in experimental models [47]. Notably, during acute inflammation, necrotic tissue produces a non-specific factor that induces leukocytosis [48]. Larvae that first enter the host are attacked by polymorphonuclear cells and macrophages that non-specifically attack the larvae cuticles. Nevertheless, the cuticle allows the larvae to resist the cytotoxic mechanisms of these cells. In contrast, the larvae also have the capability of activating a complementary response by an alternative route.

During larval migration within the host, the larvae induce an adaptive immune response and an increase in CD4 and CD8 lymphocytes. Then, *Toxocara* antigens stimulate macrophages to produce IL-6, which promotes the development of the Th2 type response, increasing IL-4, IL-5, IL-6, IL-10 and IL-13 [49-52]. In turn, the IL-4 increase stimulates the proliferation and maturation of B cells, the isotype variation from IgM to IgE and the production of specific IgG antibodies [53]. The IL-4 increase also contributes to the stimulation of mast cells, which increases the inflammatory response when mast cells degranulate. Likewise, this increase induces macrophages to produce IL-1, which stimulates B cells and a Th2 type response. In turn, the IL-5 increase stimulates eosinophil production, which is responsible for tissue and blood eosinophilia that is characteristic of this infection [54].

Many studies have shown that the TES-Ags predominantly stimulate a Th2 type response and an increase in IFN-γ levels in the plasma of infected mice, characteristic of the Th1 response [55]. IFN-γ acts on B, T, NK cells and macrophages and is the key mediator of immune responses mediated by cells. IFN-γ associates with IL-13 (which is a fibrogenic cytokine) through the regulation of TGF-β production in pulmonary inflammatory processes [56, 57]. The association of IFN-γ and IL-13 contributes to the formation of eosinophilic granulomas in other pathologies, such as pathogen-induced diseases (schistosomiasis) or autoimmune diseases (asthma, ulcerative colitis), which are also a characteristic when *T. canis* larvae persist for long periods in tissues [58-60].

At the same time that pro-inflammatory processes are activated, regulatory T cells (Treg) are also activated and produce IL-10 in *Toxocara* infection models [61, 62]. This cytokine is an immunosuppressant and anti-inflammatory cytokine that inhibits the granulomatous response to the parasite. IL-10 regulates inflammation and fibrosis by directly acting on fibroblasts, reducing the production of collagen

[63, 64]. This regulatory effect is apparently responsible for the control of the exaggerated immune response in the host when the *T. canis* larvae migrate through the entire organism. Likewise, the high number of eosinophils may cause the activation of Tregs, which then induces the production of IL-10 [60]. This same regulatory effect of infection by other helminth parasites has been proposed as a protection against atopic allergic reactions in skin [65, 66].

At the intestinal level in the definitive host, there is most likely a similar effect as with other helminths. The presence and harm produced by the parasite on the intestinal epithelium induces the production of alarmins (IL-25, IL-33 and thymic stromal lymphoprotein) by intestinal epithelium cells. In turn, these alarmins stimulate nuocytes to produce IL-4, IL-9 and IL-13, thus contributing to a direct Th2 type response. IL-13 has an effect on the goblet cells, and these cells produce much mucus, which contributes to the elimination of the parasites [49]. Interestingly, no correlation has been found between the levels of serum or of local antibodies (IgA and IgM) and the presence of adult worms in the intestine of the host [67, 68]. Moreover, Foxp3$^+$ cells increase in the intestinal wall of dogs when nematode intestinal infections occurs [69], suggesting that mucosal tolerance is involved in the persistence of the infection.

Humoral Immune Response

Infection by *T. canis* induces the production of antibodies against the parasite. In canine toxocariosis, specific IgM and IgG antibody titers are maintained for several months after contact with the parasite. The antibody titers are not correlated with adult parasite loads in the intestine; however, these titers are related to the amount of circulating antigens [67]. In paratenic hosts (including humans), antibody production at the beginning is similar to that in definitive hosts; however, the antibodies of the IgM isotype decrease during 10 days p.i., whereas antibodies of the IgG isotype progressively increase until day 30 p.i., and these levels remain constant for several months. Clinical studies show that patients with symptoms of visceral migrans larvae or ocular migrans larvae have higher amounts of antibodies of the IgG1 subclass, which are specific to *T. canis*, when compared with IgG2, IgG3 and IgG4 subclasses of antibodies. The total amount of IgE antibodies is also increased [70].

Eosinophilia

Generalised eosinophilia is one of the most evident signs of *T. canis* infection in both experimental hosts and humans. The characteristics of this eosinophilia varies between the different host species. In mice and gerbils, two peaks are produced during the first 40 days p.i. [41, 71], whereas in humans, eosinophilia persists over a year [72, 73], and in dogs, eosinophilia begins at 7 days p.i. and disappears at 42 days [74]. In prenatally infected pups, a peak of eosinophils is observed at 7 days after birth and slowly declines as eggs begin to be eliminated in faeces until reaching physiological levels at 42 days after birth [75]. These data indicate that the course of eosinophilia in prenatally infected pups is comparable to that in adult dogs.

Eosinophilia may be induced with few larvae and is dependent on IL-5. In experimental models of the infection, the administration of antibodies against IL-5 suppresses the increase in blood eosinophils [73, 76]. During experimental toxocariosis, CD4+ type 2 lymphocytes (Th2) are the main producers of IL-5 because when anti-CD4 antibodies are applied in murine models, one of the eosinophilia peaks is reduced. T CD4- and CD8- lymphocytes (double negatives) present in the skin, thymus, small intestine, liver, bone marrow and lung produce small amounts of IL-5, thus amplifying the eosinopoietic stimuli [46, 77].

In general, the role of eosinophils in the defence against infections by helminths has generated controversies. The results obtained *in vitro* indicate that these cells may have a toxic effect on certain parasites [78, 79] and that eosinophilia has been associated with the elimination of other nematodes, such as *Haemonchus contortus* [80]. However, in infections by *T. canis*, eosinophils increase during infection, surround the larvae in tissues and apparently do not produce serious harm to the larvae. *In vitro*, larvae incubation with cell populations enriched with eosinophils and with hyperimmune serum causes fixation to the larvae cuticle and the degranulation of eosinophils; however this incubation does not affect motility or viability of the larvae [81].

Consequences to the Host of Hyperimmune Activation During Infection: *Toxocara Canis* and Asthma

Asthma is a chronic inflammatory disease of the lower respiratory tract that is characterised by an increase in IgE, eosinophilic-induced inflammation, mucus hypersecretion, and bronchial hyper-reactivity after exposure to allergens. This disease is the result of a Th2 type response to aerial allergens [82]. During this disease, there is an increase in IL-4, IL-5 and IL-13 that mediates the synthesis of IgE, inflammatory cells, eosinophil degranulation and hyperactivity of the respiratory tract [83]. Some studies related *Toxocara* seroprevalence with allergic manifestations, including asthma. Nevertheless, there are other studies where this relation was not found. The reason behind this contradiction may be due to the differences in the way these studies were performed [58, 84-86]. Among these differences are the type of serological assay used in each study, the different criteria used to determine seropositivity, and the age and gender of the population under study. It is accepted that infection by *Toxocara* larvae is related to the onset of asthma [87], although some researchers have suggested that the parasitic infections by helminths reduce the risk of having allergies due to their immunosuppressant properties [88]. Nevertheless, the adaptation of the parasites to their hosts must be considered in the specific case of *T. canis* because this parasite is best adapted to its definitive host than to its paratenic hosts, such as humans, who respond more vigorously against the parasite, therefore producing a more serious pathogenicity [42].

In experimental models, *T. canis* larvae migrate to different tissues, including the lungs. Then, the larvae induce a Th2 type immune response in the lungs, together with an increase in eosinophils, macrophages, lymphocytes and IgE. Most of the larvae migrate from the lungs to other organs, although some remain trapped in the lungs within well-formed granulomas, and lung inflammation may remain up to three months [58, 89-91]. Likewise, some larvae may continue migrating and return to the lungs in such a manner that there can simultaneously be chronic and acute lesions (Fig. **1**). The type of cell infiltrate observed in the lung tissue of mice experimentally infected with *T. canis* is similar to that observed in experimental models in mice with allergic asthma produced by sensitisation with ovalbumin [92, 93].

As has been mentioned, *T. canis* infection triggers a Th2 type response, which is characterised by the production of IL-4, IL-5, IL-13 and by the infiltration of eosinophils, macrophages and mast cells. The presence of live or dead larvae and the circulation of parasite antigens have a mitogenic activity on lymphocytes, thus, this type of immune response remains for long periods. Additionally, the non-specific IgE against *T. canis* is increased. In allergic individuals, the amount of specific allergen-induced IgE is increased. When the allergen penetrates the airways, IgE reacts to the allergen and joins high and low affinity receptors of mast cells, eosinophils and macrophages, which secrete mediators involved in the early asthmatic response (platelet activation factor and leukotriene C_4) and late response (prostaglandin and leukotriene C_4). Based on this model (Fig. **2**), the induced immune response after *T. canis* infection may trigger allergic manifestations in individuals who are allergic or that have genetic predisposition to allergies [87, 94].

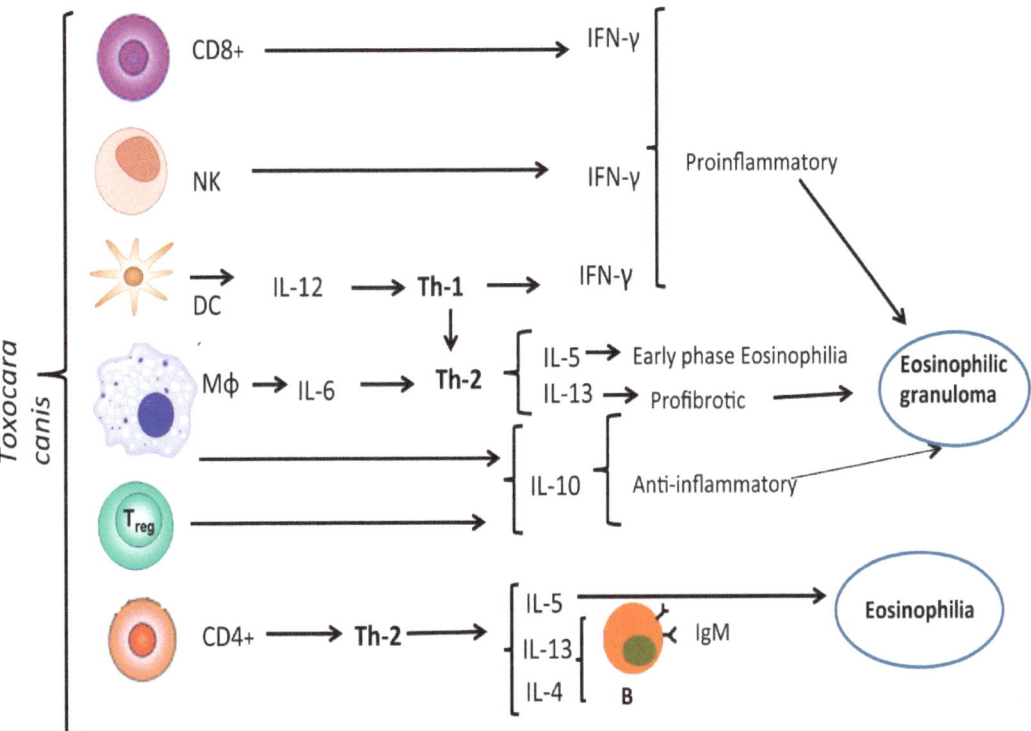

Figure 1: Scheme that shows the immune response to *T. canis* infection. The parasite can stimulate either the innate or adaptative response, presenting helminth-specific antigens to T cells. The mechanism includes macrophage (Mφ) activation, which causes Th2 polarisation *via* IL-6 secretion. Simultaneously, CD4+, CD8+, NK, DC and Tregs can be activated by TES-Ags to polarise local and systemic responses and/or to modulate effector responses. The host response includes anti-inflammatory, proinflammatory and profibrotic activities to localise and to eliminate the parasite.

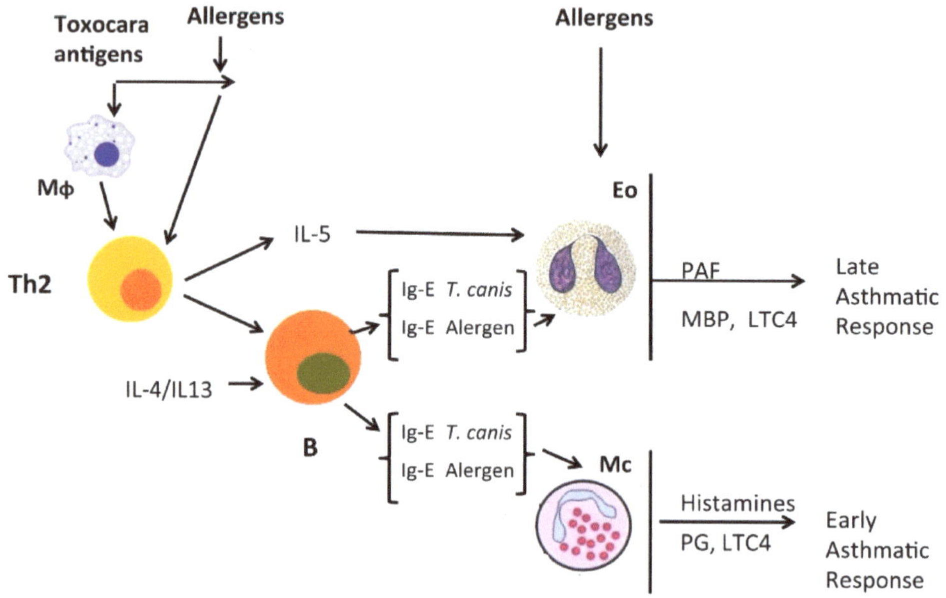

Figure 2: Proposed mechanism underlining the association between *Toxocara* infection and allergic asthma. Allergen stimuli result in the induction of T-helper 2 (Th2) cells producing cytokines such as IL-4, IL-13, and IL-5. Due to larval migration and to the Th2 response, macrophage (Mo) and eosinophil (Eo) infiltration, in addition to increase levels of IgE against the parasite and the allergen, is induced. After allergen challenge, IgE will interact with specific allergens and bind to high and low affinity receptors on mast cells (Mc) and on eosinophils, which secrete several mediators involved in the induction of the early and late asthmatic responses (platelet activation factor (PAF), leukotriene C4 (LTC4)).

Evasion of the Immune Response

Parasites are arguably the most highly evolved infectious organisms and, consequently, have developed mechanisms to facilitate their survival within the host. These mechanisms can be roughly grouped into two types. The first mechanism is to evade the immune response by evolving strategies such as antigenic variation and molecular mimicry or by affecting antigen processing and presentation. In the second mechanism, the parasite actually exploits a host system to its benefit and, thus, obtains an advantage in growth or in reproduction. Mechanisms such as fabulation provide parasites with a dual benefit: first, obtaining amino acids for metabolism, and second by preventing the surface-bound antibody from interfering with parasite–host-cell interactions. A striking example of the exploitation of host molecules is the ability of several *Schistosoma* species to use host-synthesised cytokines as indirect growth factors. Additional evidence suggests that the binding of host immunoglobulin by schistosome surface paramyosin may lead to immune evasion through molecular masquerade while interfering with Fc interactions with leukocyte surface receptors.

After a *T. canis* infection, the infected organism displaces elements of the innate and adaptive immune responses to eliminate the parasite. Likewise, the parasite attempts to survive and to elude the immune host response, thus establishing an equilibrium between the parasite and the host. The type of response to the parasite varies between the different tissues; the inflammatory response in the lungs is constant for several months, whereas in other tissues, such as muscle and brain, the inflammatory response is less, and the larvae may be maintained in a state of hypobiosis [25].

T. canis externally presents a complex glycoprotein layer called the cuticle. The cuticle is the first surface of the parasite that is exposed to its host, and the events that occur at this surface are essential for the recognition and for the evasion of the parasite. The cuticle of the *T. canis* larvae is formed by keratin covered with a glycocalyx rich in carbohydrates that form a downy anionic cover of approximately 10 μm in thickness [34]. The external layer of the cuticle is called the epicuticle, which is a dense layer of granular material that is eliminated from the surface of the larvae whenever inflammatory cells or antibodies attack it. Electron microscopy studies have demonstrated that when *T. canis* larvae are incubated with immune sera or with eosinophils, the epicuticle condenses, and the densest portion separates from the surface, along with antibodies and eosinophils, without serious harm to the larvae, which can survive for a long time. The above finding demonstrates that this layer protects larvae from some mechanisms of the immune response by the host [95].

Some of the surface glycoproteins of the larvae are continuously secreted and form part of the TES-Ags. This capacity of the larvae allows them to eliminate antibodies joined to their surface or to leave antigens in the tissues the larvae traverse while migrating, and antibodies or cells are joined to these antigens once larvae are no longer there [25]. Likewise, the TES-Ag link with C3, therefore blocking the classic and the alternate complement pathway [96].

Additionally, the TES-Ags apparently may modulate the systemic immune response of its host. For example, TES-32 (Tc-CTL-1) is a lectin highly similar to mammal lectins and to *Caenorhabditis elegans* lectins. Lectins are proteins that join with high specificity to carbohydrates. Among the lectins, N-acetyl-galactosamine and L-lactose are present in the microorganisms; these lectins are mediators for key events in the immune response to infection, beginning with the inflammatory affluence to the site where the parasite is found (Fig. **3**). Therefore, the liberation of parasitic origin lectins with receptors similar to the host's receptors may block this process. Thus, *T. canis* may interfere with the extravasation of leukocytes in the infection sites [97, 98].

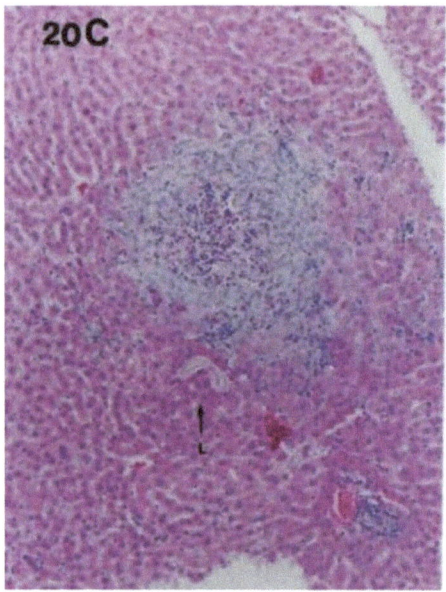

Figure 3: Liver histological view; gerbil inoculated with *T. canis* larvae and sacrificed 40 days p.i. A chronic lesion is shown with neutrophils and eosinophils at middle, surrounded by fibrocytes and collagen. In the outer zone, there is a neutrophil and lymphocyte infiltrate; out of the inflammatory zone and away from the immune response, an apparently intact larva can be observed.

Another evasion of the immune response mechanism is the capability of larvae to traverse the fibrotic tissue of granulomas and to migrate to form other granulomas. It is common to cut open granulomas where there is no evidence of the larva that served as a nest for the inflammatory reaction with eosinophilia (Fig. **4**) [25].

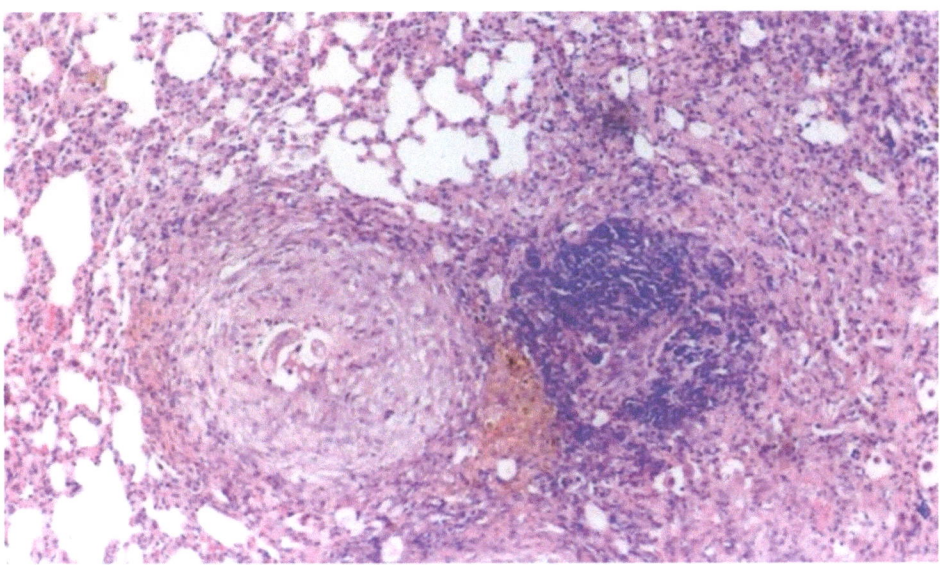

Figure 4: Lung histological view; gerbil inoculated with *T. canis* larvae and sacrificed 40 days p.i. A chronic granuloma is shown. The outer zone is primarily composed of fibrocytes and collagen, and the inner zone has eosinophils and a larva in the middle. Behind the larva, an acute lesion with an infiltrate of neutrophils, eosinophils and some macrophages can be observed.

Immunodiagnosis

Pups eliminate eggs in faeces, and therefore, conventional coproparasitoscopy examinations are efficient for diagnosis (Faust technique). Adult dogs and paratenic hosts (including humans) do not develop adult worms; these hosts only have somatic larva in tissues and do not eliminate eggs in faecal matter. Biopsies and histopathology processing may detect larvae in tissues with high specificity [99]; however, due to the invasiveness and scant sensitivity of this technique, this method is infrequently applied. Therefore, current diagnosis is based on the detection of specific antibodies by serological assays.

Different immunological techniques have been used, such as radial double diffusion [100], intradermal reactions [101], capillary tube precipitation [102], immunofluorescence [103], counter-immune electrophoresis [104] and hemagglutination [105], for the diagnosis of toxocariosis in humans and in other paratenic hosts. Currently, due to their high specificity and sensitivity, the two most used techniques are ELISA and Western blot [106, 107]. In the past, soluble antigens of adult *T. canis* or from the rupture of larval eggs were used for immunodiagnosis; however, TES-Ags are currently used more due to their higher specificity.

The ELISA test using *T. canis* larvae secretions and excretions detects total immunoglobulins in serum, although total immunoglobulins can also be detected in other body fluids, such as the vitreous humour and cerebrospinal liquid [108-110]. The sensibility of this technique varies with the degree of infection; in general, the level of sensibility is considered to range from 80 to 95%, and specificity ranges from 90 to 95% [111, 112]. Some authors suggest that the sera of the patients should be previously incubated with extracts of *Ascaris suum* to increase the specificity of the ELISA test [113]. The existence of commercial ELISA kits for immunodiagnostics of toxocariosis has facilitated diagnosis.

Confirmation is achieved by the Western blot technique; using this technique, two TES-Ag patterns have been determined that are recognised by human sera. These patterns were named Low Molecular Weight (LMW) and High Molecular Weight (HMW). The HMW pattern forms 200, 147 and 132 kDa bands. These antigens may have cross-reacted with other helminth antigens, such as those antigens from *Strongyloides*, *sp. Fasciola hepatica*, *Ascaris suum*, *Toxascaris leonina*, *Schistosoma sp.* and *Onchocerca sp.* [107, 114-116]. LMW antigens are formed by 24, 28, 30 and 35 kDa bands and are considered to be specific; therefore, these antigens do not cross-react with other helminth antigens [107].

In cases of ocular larva migrans, serology may not be conclusive because the serum antibodies are present at low levels or may even be absent. Therefore, ELISA or Western blot may be performed with specific anti-*Toxocara* antibodies produced locally in the eye for diagnosis confirmation [117-119].

CONCLUDING REMARKS

The above-presented evidence illustrates the importance of the immune response and its interactions between *T. canis* and its hosts, and provides possible new mechanisms for parasite establishment, growth and reproduction in an immunocompetent host. The above evidence strongly suggests an important role for Th1 and Th2 immune responses during toxocariosis in all models of the disease, in mice and rats, as well as natural infections in humans. Possible interactions between the host immune system and the *Toxocara* parasite affect the final disease outcome, although these interactions have not been well characterised during acute or chronic toxocariosis. These host-immune interactions during toxocariosis may have implications in the transmission control and treatment of this worldwide parasitic disease in humans. In practical matters, the complexity of the *Toxocara* parasite relation suggests that all immunological factors (*i.e.*, innate immunity, humoral, and cellular developmental stage) should be considered in the design of vaccines and of new drugs. Interventions aimed at the immunological network appear to be possible new therapeutic approaches to control toxocariosis in its final host and perhaps other infections.

ACKNOWLEDGEMENTS

Declared none.

CONFLICT OF INTEREST

The authors confirm that this chapter contents have no conflict of interest.

REFERENCES

[1] Strube C, Heuer L, Janecek E. *Toxocara* spp. infections in paratenic hosts. Veterinary parasitology. 2012. Epub 2013/01/15.
[2] Dubey JP. Patent Toxocara canis infection in ascarid-naive dogs. The Journal of parasitology. 1978;64(6):1021-3. Epub 1978/12/01.
[3] Guberti V, Stancampiano L, Francisci F. Intestinal helminth parasite community in wolves (Canis lupus) in Italy. Parassitologia. 1993;35(1-3):59-65. Epub 1993/12/01.
[4] Richards DT, Harris S, Lewis JW. Epidemiological studies on intestinal helminth parasites of rural and urban red foxes (Vulpes vulpes) in the United Kingdom. Veterinary parasitology. 1995;59(1):39-51. Epub 1995/08/01.
[5] Skirnisson K, Eydal M, Gunnarsson E, Hersteinsson P. Parasites of the arctic fox (Alopex lagopus) in Iceland. Journal of wildlife diseases. 1993;29(3):440-6. Epub 1993/07/01.
[6] Alba HF, Flores-Alatorre L, Cuéllar OJ, Martínez LJP, editors. Desarrollo de un nuevo modelo de toxocariosis ocular. Memorias del XXV Congreso Nacional de Microbiología; 1994; Ciudad Obregón, Son. México.
[7] Dunn AM. Helmintología Veterinaria. 2a. Edición ed1893.
[8] Quiroz RH. Parasitología y Enfermedades Parasitarias de Animales Domésticos: Edit. Limusa; 1984.
[9] Soulsby IJL. Helminths, Arthropods and Protozoa of Domesticated Animals. USA: Lea &Febiger; 1982.

[10] Alba-Hurtado F. Toxocara canis, un problema de salud pública. Av Med Vet. 1991;10:191-7.
[11] Schnieder T, Laabs EM, Welz C. Larval development of Toxocara canis in dogs. Veterinary parasitology. 2011;175(3-4):193-206. Epub 2010/11/26.
[12] Beaver PC, Juns RC, Cupp EW. Parasitología Clínica. 2a. Ed. ed. Barcelona, España: Salvat; 1986.
[13] Olsen OW. Animal Parasites. Baltimore, Maryland, USA: Park Press; 1974.
[14] Olsen OW. Animal Parasites, their life style and ecology. 3rd. Edition ed. USA: Universal Park Press; 1979.
[15] Sprent JF. Observations on the development of Toxocara canis (Werner, 1782) in the dog. Parasitology. 1958;48(1-2):184-209. Epub 1958/05/01.
[16] Kirk RW. Práctica clínica canina en pequeñas especies. 4a. Edición ed. México, D.F.: Edit. Interamericana; 1984.
[17] Shrand H. Visceral Larva Migrans. Toxocara Canis Infection. Lancet. 1964;1(7347):1357-9. Epub 1964/06/20.
[18] Douglas JR, Beker NR. The chronology of experimental intrauterine infection with Toxocara canis (Werner, 1782) in the dog. J Parasitol. 1959;45:43-4.
[19] Martinez AA. Toxocariosis canina. Av Med Vet. 1989;6:272-6.
[20] Carvalho EA, Rocha RL. Toxocariosis: visceral larva migrans in children. Jornal de pediatria. 2011;87(2):100-10. Epub 2011/04/20.
[21] Cypess RH. Visceral larva migrans in Parasitic zoonoses1982.
[22] Schantz MP, Glickman LT. Toxocara visceral larva migrans. New Engl J Med. 1978;298:436-8.
[23] Roddie G, Stafford P, Holland C, Wolfe A. Contamination of dog hair with eggs of Toxocara canis. Veterinary parasitology. 2008;152(1-2):85-93. Epub 2008/02/05.
[24] Wolfe A, Wright IP. Human toxocariosis and direct contact with dogs. The Veterinary record. 2003;152(14):419-22. Epub 2003/04/24.
[25] Alba-Hurtado F. Evaluación de un modelo de Toxocariosis Ocular y Sistémica empleando Jerbos (Merionesunguiculatus). México: Universidad Nacional Autónoma de México; 1999.
[26] Munoz-Guzman MA, Alba-Hurtado F. Antígenos de secreción-excreción de Toxocara canis reconocidos por cachorros del área metropolitana de la Ciudad de México. Vet Méx. 2010;41:59-64.
[27] Smith H, R. N. Diagnostic limitations an future trends in the serodiagnosis of human toxocariosis. In: C.V. H, H.V. S, editors. Toxocara: the enigmatic parasite. Trowbridge, UK: Cromwell Press; 2006. p. 89-112.
[28] Glickman KW, Grieve RB, Schantz PM. Immunodiganosis of parasitic diseases: Academic Press, N.Y.; 1986.
[29] Peixoto PL, Nascimento E, Cançado GGL, Miranda RRCd, Rocha RL, Araújo RN, *et al.* Identification of candidate antigens from adult stages of Toxocara canis for the serodiagnosis of human toxocariosis. Memórias do Instituto Oswaldo Cruz. 2011;106:200-6.
[30] Smith HV, Quinn R, Bruce RG, Girdwood RW. Development of the serological response in rabbits infected with Toxocara canis and Toxascaris leonina. Transactions of the Royal Society of Tropical Medicine and Hygiene. 1982;76(1):89-94. Epub 1982/01/01.
[31] Fillaux J, Magnaval JF. Laboratory diagnosis of human toxocariosis. Veterinary Parasitology. 2013(0).
[32] Meghji M, Maizels RM. Biochemical properties of larval excretory-secretory glycoproteins of the parasitic nematode Toxocara canis. Molecular and biochemical parasitology. 1986;18(2):155-70. Epub 1986/02/01.

[33] Maizels RM, Kennedy MW, Meghji M, Robertson BD, Smith HV. Shared carbohydrate epitopes on distinct surface and secreted antigens of the parasitic nematode Toxocara canis. J Immunol. 1987;139(1):207-14. Epub 1987/07/01.

[34] Page AP, Rudin W, Fluri E, Blaxter ML, Maizels RM. Toxocara canis: a labile antigenic surface coat overlying the epicuticle of infective larvae. Experimental parasitology. 1992;75(1):72-86. Epub 1992/08/01.

[35] Maizels RM, de Savigny D, Ogilvie BM. Characterization of surface and excretory-secretory antigens of Toxocara canis infective larvae. Parasite immunology. 1984;6(1):23-37. Epub 1984/01/01.

[36] Niedfeld G, Pezzani B, Minvielle M, Basualdo Farjat JA. Presence of lipids in the secretory/excretory product from Toxocara canis. Veterinary parasitology. 1993;51(1-2):155-8. Epub 1993/12/01.

[37] Morales OL, Lopez MC, Nicholls RS, Agudelo C. Identification of toxocara canis antigens by Western blot in experimentally infected rabbits. Revista do Instituto de Medicina Tropical de Sao Paulo. 2002;44(4):213-6. Epub 2002/09/10.

[38] Sommerfelt IE, Santillan G, Lopez C, Ribicich M, Franco AJ. Immunological and hematological response in experimental Toxocara canis-infected pigs. Veterinary parasitology. 2001;96(2):127-34. Epub 2001/03/07.

[39] Magnaval JF, Glickman LT, Dorchies P, Morassin B. Highlights of human toxocariosis. The Korean journal of parasitology. 2001;39(1):1-11. Epub 2001/04/17.

[40] Sarimehmetoglu HO, Burgu A, Aycicek H, Gonenc B, Tanyuksel M, Kara M. Application of western blotting procedure for the immunodiagnosis of visceral larva migrans in mice by using excretory/secretory antigens. DTW Deutsche tierarztliche Wochenschrift. 2001;108(9):390-2. Epub 2001/10/16.

[41] Alba-Hurtado F, Munoz-Guzman MA, Valdivia-Anda G, Tortora JL, Ortega-Pierres MG. Toxocara canis: larval migration dynamics, detection of antibody reactivity to larval excretory-secretory antigens and clinical findings during experimental infection of gerbils (Meriones unguiculatus). Experimental parasitology. 2009;122(1):1-5. Epub 2009/06/24.

[42] Maizels RM. Toxocara canis: Molecular basis of immune recognition and evasion. Veterinary parasitology. 2012. Epub 2013/01/29.

[43] Glickman LT, Summers BA. Experimental Toxocara canis infection in cynomolgus macaques (Macaca fascicularis). American journal of veterinary research. 1983;44(12):2347-54. Epub 1983/12/01.

[44] Tomimura T, Yokota M, Takiguchi H. Experimental visceral larva migrans in monkeys. I. Clinical, hematological, biochemical and gross pathological observations on monkeys inoculated with embryonated eggs of the dog ascarid, Toxocara canis. Nihon juigaku zasshi The Japanese journal of veterinary science. 1976;38(6):533-48. Epub 1976/12/01.

[45] Alba-Hurtado F, Diaz-Otero F, Valdivia G, Reyes R, Tsutsumi V, Acosta G. Cellular immune response of intracecally inoculated Mongolian gerbils with Entamoeba histolytica trophozoites. Revista latinoamericana de microbiologia. 1999;41(4):205-10. Epub 2000/08/10.

[46] Kusama Y, Takamoto M, Kasahara T, Takatsu K, Nariuchi H, Sugane K. Mechanisms of eosinophilia in BALB/c-nu/+ and congenitally athymic BALB/c-nu/nu mice infected with Toxocara canis. Immunology. 1995;84(3):461-8. Epub 1995/03/01.

[47] Wang MQ, Jiang HJ, Inoue H, Myozaki M, Yamashita U. B cell mitogenic activity of Toxocara canis adult worm antigen. Parasite immunology. 1995;17(12):609-15. Epub 1995/12/01.

[48] Sell S. Immunology, Immunopathology, Immunity. Stanford, Connecticut, USA: Ed. Appleton and Lange; 1996.

[49] Allen JE, Maizels RM. Diversity and dialogue in immunity to helminths. Nature reviews Immunology. 2011;11(6):375-88. Epub 2011/05/26.

[50] Finkelman FD, Shea-Donohue T, Morris SC, Gildea L, Strait R, Madden KB, et al. Interleukin-4- and interleukin-13-mediated host protection against intestinal nematode parasites. Immunological reviews. 2004;201:139-55. Epub 2004/09/14.

[51] Turner JD, Faulkner H, Kamgno J, Cormont F, Van Snick J, Else KJ, et al. Th2 cytokines are associated with reduced worm burdens in a human intestinal helminth infection. The Journal of infectious diseases. 2003;188(11):1768-75. Epub 2003/11/26.

[52] Valli JL, Williamson A, Sharif S, Rice J, Shewen PE. In vitro cytokine responses of peripheral blood mononuclear cells from healthy dogs to distemper virus, Malassezia and Toxocara. Veterinary immunology and immunopathology. 2010;134(3-4):218-29. Epub 2009/11/03.

[53] Tizard IR. Introducción a la Inmunología Veterinaria: Elsevier Saunders; 2009.

[54] Yamaguchi Y, Suda T, Suda J, Eguchi M, Miura Y, Harada N, et al. Purified interleukin 5 supports the terminal differentiation and proliferation of murine eosinophilic precursors. The Journal of experimental medicine. 1988;167(1):43-56. Epub 1988/01/01.

[55] Pecinali NR, Gomes RN, Amendoeira FC, Bastos AC, Martins MJ, Pegado CS, et al. Influence of murine Toxocara canis infection on plasma and bronchoalveolar lavage fluid eosinophil numbers and its correlation with cytokine levels. Veterinary parasitology. 2005;134(1-2):121-30. Epub 2005/09/20.

[56] Fichtner-Feigl S, Strober W, Kawakami K, Puri RK, Kitani A. IL-13 signaling through the IL-13[alpha]2 receptor is involved in induction of TGF-[beta]1 production and fibrosis. Nat Med. 2006;12(1):99-106.

[57] Munitz A, Brandt EB, Mingler M, Finkelman FD, Rothenberg ME. Distinct roles for IL-13 and IL-4 via IL-13 receptor alpha1 and the type II IL-4 receptor in asthma pathogenesis. Proceedings of the National Academy of Sciences of the United States of America. 2008;105(20):7240-5. Epub 2008/05/16.

[58] Buijs J, Lokhorst WH, Robinson J, Nijkamp FP. Toxocara canis-induced murine pulmonary inflammation: analysis of cells and proteins in lung tissue and bronchoalveolar lavage fluid. Parasite immunology. 1994;16(1):1-9. Epub 1994/01/01.

[59] Meeusen EN, Balic A. Do eosinophils have a role in the killing of helminth parasites? Parasitol Today. 2000;16(3):95-101. Epub 2000/02/26.

[60] Nagy D, Bede O, Danka J, Szenasi Z, Sipka S. Analysis of serum cytokine levels in children with chronic cough associated with Toxocara canis infection. Parasite immunology. 2012;34(12):581-8. Epub 2012/09/27.

[61] Aranzamendi C, Sofronic-Milosavljevic L, Pinelli E. Helminths: Immunoregulation and Inflammatory Diseases-Which Side Are Trichinella spp. and Toxocara spp. on? Journal of parasitology research. 2013;2013:329438. Epub 2013/02/01.

[62] Torina A, Caracappa S, Barera A, Dieli F, Sireci G, Genchi C, et al. Toxocara canis infection induces antigen-specific IL-10 and IFNgamma production in pregnant dogs and their puppies. Veterinary immunology and immunopathology. 2005;108(1-2):247-51. Epub 2005/09/08.

[63] Arai T, Abe K, Matsuoka H, Yoshida M, Mori M, Goya S, et al. Introduction of the interleukin-10 gene into mice inhibited bleomycin-induced lung injury in vivo. American journal of physiology Lung cellular and molecular physiology. 2000;278(5):L914-22. Epub 2000/04/27.

[64] Moore KW, de Waal Malefyt R, Coffman RL, O'Garra A. Interleukin-10 and the interleukin-10 receptor. Annual review of immunology. 2001;19:683-765. Epub 2001/03/13.

[65] Sugane K, Oshima T. Interrelationship of eosinophilia and IgE antibody production to larval ES antigen in Toxocara canis infected mice. Parasite immunology. 1984;6(5):409-20. Epub 1984/09/01.

[66] Yazdanbakhsh M, Kremsner PG, van Ree R. Allergy, parasites, and the hygiene hypothesis. Science. 2002;296(5567):490-4. Epub 2002/04/20.

[67] Matsumura K, Kazuta Y, Endo R, Tanaka K. The IgM antibody activities in relation to the parasitologic status of Toxocara canis in dogs. Zentralblatt fur Bakteriologie, Mikrobiologie und Hygiene 1 Abt Originale A, Medizinische Mikrobiologie, Infektionskrankheiten und Parasitologie = International journal of microbiology and hygiene A, Medical micro. 1983;255(2-3):402-5. Epub 1983/09/01.

[68] Matsumura K, Kazuta Y, Endo R, Tanaka K. Detection of circulating toxocaral antigens in dogs by sandwich enzyme-immunoassay. Immunology. 1984;51(3):609-13. Epub 1984/03/01.

[69] Junginger J, Schwittlick U, Lemensieck F, Nolte I, Hewicker-Trautwein M. Immunohistochemical investigation of Foxp3 expression in the intestine in healthy and diseased dogs. Veterinary research. 2012;43(1):23. Epub 2012/03/24.

[70] Kayes SG. Inflammatory and immunological responses to Toxocara canis. In: C.V. H, H.V. S, editors. Toxocara: the enigmatic parasite. Trowbridge, UK: Cromwell Press; 2006. p. 158-73.

[71] Sugane K, Oshima T. Eosinophilia, granuloma formation and migratory behaviour of larvae in the congenitally athymic mouse infected with Toxocara canis. Parasite immunology. 1982;4(5):307-18. Epub 1982/09/01.

[72] Beaver PC, Snyder CH, Carrera GM, Dent JH, Lafferty JW. Chronic eosinophilia due to visceral larva migrans; report of three cases. Pediatrics. 1952;9(1):7-19. Epub 1952/01/01.

[73] Limaye AP, Abrams JS, Silver JE, Ottesen EA, Nutman TB. Regulation of parasite-induced eosinophilia: selectively increased interleukin 5 production in helminth-infected patients. The Journal of experimental medicine. 1990;172(1):399-402. Epub 1990/07/01.

[74] Zimmermann U. Quantitative Intersuchungen über die Wandering und Streuung der Larven von Toxocara canis WERNER 1782 (Anisakidae) im definitiven Wirt (Beagle) nach fraktionierter Erstund Reinfektion. . Hannover, Germany: University of Veterinary Medicine; 1983.

[75] Voβmann MT. Klinische, hämatologische und serologische Befundebei Welpennachpränataler Infektion mit Toxocara canis WERNER 1789 (Anisakidae). Hannover, Hannover, Germany: University of Veterinary Medicine 1985.

[76] Coffman RL, Seymour BW, Hudak S, Jackson J, Rennick D. Antibody to interleukin-5 inhibits helminth-induced eosinophilia in mice. Science. 1989;245(4915):308-10. Epub 1989/07/21.

[77] Takamoto M, Kusama Y, Takatsu K, Nariuchi H, Sugane K. Occurrence of interleukin-5 production by CD4- CD8- (double-negative) T cells in lungs of both normal and congenitally athymic nude mice infected with Toxocara canis. Immunology. 1995;85(2):285-91. Epub 1995/06/01.

[78] Abbas AK, Lichtman AHH, Pillai S. Cellular and Molecular Immunology. 7th. Edition ed: Elsevier Saunders; 2011.

[79] Mahmoud AA, Warren KS. Algorithms in the diagnosis and management of exotic diseases. XX. Toxoplasmosis. The Journal of infectious diseases. 1977;135(3):493-6. Epub 1977/03/01.

[80] Alba-Hurtado F, Muñoz-Guzman M. Immune response associated with resistance to Heamonchosis in sheep. Biomed Res Int. 2013:11 pages.

[81]   Fattah DI, Maizels RM, McLaren DJ, Spry CJ. Toxocara canis: interaction of human blood eosinophils with the infective larvae. Experimental parasitology. 1986;61(3):421-31. Epub 1986/06/01.

[82]   Weiss ST. Parasites and asthma/allergy: what is the relationship? The Journal of allergy and clinical immunology. 2000;105(2 Pt 1):205-10. Epub 2000/02/12.

[83]   Holt PG, Macaubas C, Stumbles PA, Sly PD. The role of allergy in the development of asthma. Nature. 1999;402(6760 Suppl):B12-7. Epub 1999/12/10.

[84]   Chan PW, Anuar AK, Fong MY, Debruyne JA, Ibrahim J. Toxocara seroprevalence and childhood asthma among Malaysian children. Pediatrics international : official journal of the Japan Pediatric Society. 2001;43(4):350-3. Epub 2001/07/27.

[85]   Munoz-Guzman MA, del Rio-Navarro BE, Valdivia-Anda G, Alba-Hurtado F. The increase in seroprevalence to Toxocara canis in asthmatic children is related to cross-reaction with Ascaris suum antigens. Allergologia et immunopathologia. 2010;38(3):115-21. Epub 2010/03/17.

[86]   Sharghi N, Schantz PM, Caramico L, Ballas K, Teague BA, Hotez PJ. Environmental exposure to Toxocara as a possible risk factor for asthma: a clinic-based case-control study. Clinical infectious diseases : an official publication of the Infectious Diseases Society of America. 2001;32(7):E111-6. Epub 2001/03/27.

[87]   Cooper PJ. Toxocara canis infection: an important and neglected environmental risk factor for asthma? Clinical and experimental allergy : journal of the British Society for Allergy and Clinical Immunology. 2008;38(4):551-3. Epub 2008/02/05.

[88]   Maizels RM. Infections and allergy - helminths, hygiene and host immune regulation. Current opinion in immunology. 2005;17(6):656-61. Epub 2005/10/06.

[89]   Akuthota P, Weller PF. Eosinophilic pneumonias. Clinical microbiology reviews. 2012;25(4):649-60. Epub 2012/10/05.

[90]   Kayes SG. Human toxocariosis and the visceral larva migrans syndrome: correlative immunopathology. Chemical immunology. 1997;66:99-124. Epub 1997/01/01.

[91]   Pinelli E, Brandes S, Dormans J, Fonville M, Hamilton CM, der Giessen J. Toxocara canis: effect of inoculum size on pulmonary pathology and cytokine expression in BALB/c mice. Experimental parasitology. 2007;115(1):76-82. Epub 2006/08/16.

[92]   Hessel EM, Van Oosterhout AJ, Hofstra CL, De Bie JJ, Garssen J, Van Loveren H, *et al.* Bronchoconstriction and airway hyperresponsiveness after ovalbumin inhalation in sensitized mice. European journal of pharmacology. 1995;293(4):401-12. Epub 1995/12/07.

[93]   Pinelli E, Dormans J, Fonville M, van der Giessen J. A comparative study of toxocariosis and allergic asthma in murine models. Journal of helminthology. 2001;75(2):137-40. Epub 2001/08/25.

[94]   Pinelli E, Aranzamendi C. Toxocara infection and its association with allergic manifestations. Endocrine, metabolic & immune disorders drug targets. 2012;12(1):33-44. Epub 2012/01/05.

[95]   Badley JE, Grieve RB, Rockey JH, Glickman LT. Immune-mediated adherence of eosinophils to Toxocara canis infective larvae: the role of excretory-secretory antigens. Parasite immunology. 1987;9(1):133-43. Epub 1987/01/01.

[96]   Maizels RM, Page AP. Surface associated glycoproteins from Toxocara canis larval parasites. Acta tropica. 1990;47(5-6):355-64. Epub 1990/07/01.

[97]   Loukas A, Hintz M, Linder D, Mullin NP, Parkinson J, Tetteh KK, *et al.* A family of secreted mucins from the parasitic nematode Toxocara canis bears diverse mucin domains but shares similar flanking six-cysteine repeat motifs. The Journal of biological chemistry. 2000;275(50):39600-7. Epub 2000/08/22.

[98] Loukas A, Mullin NP, Tetteh KK, Moens L, Maizels RM. A novel C-type lectin secreted by a tissue-dwelling parasitic nematode. Current biology : CB. 1999;9(15):825-8. Epub 1999/09/02.
[99] Parsons JC, Bowman DD, Grieve RB. Tissue localization of excretory-secretory antigens of larval Toxocara canis in acute and chronic murine toxocariosis. The American journal of tropical medicine and hygiene. 1986;35(5):974-81. Epub 1986/09/01.
[100] Cypess RH, Karol MH, Zidian JL, Glickman LT, Gitlin D. Larva-specific antibodies in patients with visceral larva migrans. The Journal of infectious diseases. 1977;135(4):633-40. Epub 1977/04/01.
[101] Collins RF, Ivey MH. Specificity and sensitivity of skin test reactions to extracts of Toxocara canis and Ascaris suum. I. Skin tests done on infected guinea pigs. The American journal of tropical medicine and hygiene. 1975;24(3):455-9. Epub 1975/05/01.
[102] Dafalla AA. The serodiagnosis of human toxocariosis by the capillary-tube precipitin test. Transactions of the Royal Society of Tropical Medicine and Hygiene. 1975;69(1):146-7. Epub 1975/01/01.
[103] Annen JM, Eckert J, Hess U. [Simple method for obtaining Toxocara canis antigen for the indirect immunofluorescence technic]. Acta tropica. 1975;32(1):37-47. Epub 1975/01/01. Eine einfache Methode zur Gewinnung von Toxocara canis-Antigen fur die indirekte Immunofluoreszenz-Technik.
[104] Enayat MS, Pezeshki M. The comparison of counterimmunoelectrophoresis with indirect haemagglutination test for detection of antibodies in experimentally infected guinea pigs with Toxocara canis. Journal of helminthology. 1977;51(2):143-8. Epub 1977/06/01.
[105] Krupp IM. Hemagglutination test for the detection of antibodies specific for Ascaris and Toxocara antigens in patients with suspected visceral larva migrans. The American journal of tropical medicine and hygiene. 1974;23(3):378-84. Epub 1974/05/01.
[106] Glickman L, Schantz P, Dombroske R, Cypess R. Evaluation of serodiagnostic tests for visceral larva migrans. The American journal of tropical medicine and hygiene. 1978;27(3):492-8. Epub 1978/05/01.
[107] Magnaval JF, Fabre R, Maurieres P, Charlet JP, de Larrard B. Application of the western blotting procedure for the immunodiagnosis of human toxocariosis. Parasitology research. 1991;77(8):697-702. Epub 1991/01/01.
[108] Alba-Hurtado F, Tortora PJ, Tsutsumi V, Ortega-Pierres MG. Histopathological investigation of experimental ocular toxocariosis in gerbils. International journal for parasitology. 2000;30(2):143-7. Epub 2000/03/08.
[109] Eberhardt O, Bialek R, Nagele T, Dichgans J. Eosinophilic meningomyelitis in toxocariosis: case report and review of the literature. Clinical neurology and neurosurgery. 2005;107(5):432-8. Epub 2005/07/19.
[110] Feldberg NT, Shields JA, Felerman JL. Antibody to Toxocara canis in the aqueous humor. Archives of Ophthalmology. 1981;99:1563-4.
[111] Despommier D. Toxocariosis: clinical aspects, epidemiology, medical ecology, and molecular aspects. Clinical microbiology reviews. 2003;16(2):265-72. Epub 2003/04/15.
[112] Smith H, Holland C, Taylor M, Magnaval JF, Schantz P, Maizels R. How common is human toxocariosis? Towards standardizing our knowledge. Trends in parasitology. 2009;25(4):182-8. Epub 2009/03/10.
[113] Lynch NR, Wilkes LK, Hodgen AN, Turner KJ. Specificity of Toxocara ELISA in tropical populations. Parasite immunology. 1988;10(3):323-37. Epub 1988/05/01.

[114] Cuellar C, Fenoy S, Guillen JL. Cross-reactions of sera from Toxascaris leonina and Ascaris suum infected mice with Toxocara canis, Toxascaris leonina and Ascaris suum antigens. International journal for parasitology. 1995;25(6):731-9. Epub 1995/06/01.
[115] Nicholas WL, Stewart AC, Mitchell GF. Antibody responses to Toxocara canis using sera from parasite-infected mice and protection from toxocariosis by immunisation with ES antigens. The Australian journal of experimental biology and medical science. 1984;62 (Pt 5):619-26. Epub 1984/10/01.
[116] Stevenson P, Jacobs DE. Toxocara infection in pigs. The use of indirect fluorescent antibody tests and an *in vitro* larval precipitate test for detecting specific antibodies. Journal of helminthology. 1977;51(2):149-54. Epub 1977/06/01.
[117] Benitez del Castillo JM, Herreros G, Guillen JL, Fenoy S, Banares A, Garcia J. Bilateral ocular toxocariosis demonstrated by aqueous humor enzyme-linked immunosorbent assay. American journal of ophthalmology. 1995;119(4):514-6. Epub 1995/04/01.
[118] de Visser L, Rothova A, de Boer JH, van Loon AM, Kerkhoff FT, Canninga-van Dijk MR, *et al*. Diagnosis of ocular toxocariosis by establishing intraocular antibody production. American journal of ophthalmology. 2008;145(2):369-74. Epub 2007/12/07.
[119] Magnaval JF, Malard L, Morassin B, Fabre R. Immunodiagnosis of ocular toxocariosis using Western-blot for the detection of specific anti-Toxocara IgG and CAP for the measurement of specific anti-Toxocara IgE. Journal of helminthology. 2002;76(4):335-9. Epub 2002/12/25.

CHAPTER 3

Mechanisms of Immune Modulation by *Fasciola Hepatica*: The Impact of Innate Immune Cells on the Developing Adaptive Immune Response

Sandra M. O'Neill[*] and Sheila Donnelly

School of Biotechnology, Faculty of Science and Health, Dublin, Ireland, and the i3 Institute, University of Technology Sydney, Ultimo, New South Wales, Australia

Abstract: *Fasciola (F.) hepatica* lives for prolonged periods within its host due to its ability to modulate host immune responses. Unlike other helminths, within hours post-infection it drives antigen specific Th2/Treg responses. This polarisation of the host immune response continues throughout all developmental stages within the definitive host. Central to the parasite's ability to produce such an immune outcome is the secretion of a plethora of molecules that interact with innate immune cells impairing their ability to promote Th1/Th17 responses. This firmly establishes *F. hepatica* as an important model to examine the anti-inflammatory properties of helminths. In this chapter, we specifically examine the communication between the secreted and shed molecules from *F. hepatica* and dendritic cells, macrophages and mast cells. In particular, we aim to highlight the impact that this interaction has on the development of Th1/Th17 immune responses. This chapter examines the diverse range of *F. hepatica* molecules that utilise different immune mechanisms to achieve the same overall outcome, thus ensuring redundancy in the development of Th2/Treg immune responses associated with *F. hepatica* infection.

Keywords: *Fasciola hepatica*, Th1, Th2, Treg, dendritic cells, macrophages, mast cells, IL-4, IL-10, IL-5, excretory-secretory molecules, tegumental antigens, cathepsin L, peroxredoxin, human defence molecule, sigma Class Glutathione transferase, immune modulatory molecules.

INTRODUCTION

Fasciola hepatica while an important zoonotic helminth in humans and animals is a unique model to study helminth immunity. Like other helminth parasites, *F.*

---

*Corresponding author **Sandra M. O'Neill**: School of Biotechnology, Faculty of Science and Health, Dublin, Ireland, and the i3 Institute, University of Technology Sydney, Ultimo, New South Wales, Australia; Tel: 003531-7005455; Fax: 003531-7005412; E-mail: sandra.oneill@dcu.ie

Emilio Jirillo, Thea Magrone and Giuseppe Miragliotta (Eds)
All rights reserved-© 2014 Bentham Science Publishers

hepatica promotes a polarised switch in the phenotype of host immune responses towards a Th2/regulatory phenotype. However, unlike other helminths, this switch occurs only hours after ingestion of *F. hepatica* metacercaraie. An immediate suppression of antigen specific Th1 immune responses is maintained throughout infection, while Th2/Treg immune responses are simultaneously promoted and magnified as infection progresses. This significantly contrasts with most other helminth infections where the phenotype of immune response varies as the worm develops from juvenile to adult within the definitive host [1]. For example during *Schistosoma* infection a Th1 immune response is observed in the first six weeks post infection and this response switches to a dominant Th2 and then **T-regulatory (Treg)** immune response once egg production by the adult worm ensues [2].

It is known that helminth secreted molecules can mimic the immune response to infection and due to the size of the *F. hepatica* worms it is easy to obtain large quantities of native parasite material. Since the major native molecules can be easily isolated and characterized, significant strides have been made in understanding the interaction of these molecules with host immune cells [2-5]. Many of these immune modulatory molecules are expressed at all stages of infection highlighting their importance to parasite survival within the host. In addition, some molecules are only produced at specific developmental stages, we have found that they share immune-modulatory properties with other stage-specific molecules. This redundancy ensures an uninterrupted suppression of host Th1 immune responses and thus a prolonged prevention of parasite expulsion [6, 7]. These molecules are also common to most helminths and thus likely represent a shared mechanism of immune modulation.

It is clear from studies in laboratory models and livestock that Th1 immune responses are required for immune protection and since many *F. hepatica* molecules are available in native and recombinant form a number of vaccine candidates that confer good Th1 mediated protection in sheep and cattle have been developed [8]. Since the innate immunity is critical to the development of adaptive immune responses that promote parasite specific and protective immune responses in this chapter we will examine recent studies on the interaction of helminth infection and its antigens on innate immune cells and their impact on the development of adaptive immunity.

The Liver Fluke – *Fasciola hepatica*

Fasciolosis is a liver disease caused by *F. hepatica*, a trematode worm commonly known as liver fluke. It inhabits primarily temperate zones, infecting mainly agricultural animals, including cattle and sheep. Fasciolosis is a major food-borne zoonosis found globally with no continent being free from infection. The World Health Organisation has designated fasciolosis as a neglected tropical disease [9] with approximately 2.4 million people infected worldwide and 180 million people at risk of infection [8, 10]. The risk of human infection increases in regions where people and animals live in close proximity such as Bolivia, Peru, Iran, Cuba and Egypt [10, 11].

Fasciola infection in the primary host begins following ingestion of metacercariae deposited on aquatic plants or immersed on surface water. Upon being exposed to the acidic environment of the gut, the juvenile worms excyst, penetrate the intestinal wall and migrates through the peritoneal cavity towards the liver parenchyma. After several weeks of feeding and migrating in the liver, the now adult worms reach the bile duct where fully mature flukes produce eggs (50,000 eggs per fluke, per day) and chronic disease ensues [12]. Mammalian hosts are commonly infected with 50 or more flukes [13]. In humans the severity of infection can vary from being asymptomatic to a severe and debilitating disease with extensive tissue damage and bile duct hyperplasia; however no fatalities have been reported [10]. In animals, symptoms manifest as weight loss, anaemia and hypoproteinemia and can lead to death, particularly in sheep. Reduction in milk and wool production contributes to the loss in productivity resulting in $3 billion to the global economy annually [8]. Infection increases susceptibility to secondary bacterial infections such as tuberculosis and salmonella [14] making *Fasciolosis* a great burden to the agricultural and medical sector.

F. hepatica Modulates Host Protective Immune Responses

Like other helminth parasites, during *F. hepatica* infection, cattle, sheep and mice exhibit potent antigen specific Th2 immune responses [15-18] that are characterised by the production of interleukin (IL)-4, IL-5, and absence of IFN-γ and IL-2 [2, 17]. Other factors associated with Th2 immune responses such as mastocytosis, hypereosinophila and IgE are also observed during *F. hepatica* infection. During the chronic stages of infection in both cattle and mice, regulatory T cells secreting IL-10 and TGFβ emerge [19, 20]. There is a dearth of studies on immune responses during human infections; however similar to studies in livestock and animal models evidence suggests that a polarised Th2/T_{reg} response exists, as high circulating IL-10 and reduced IFNγ are detected in chronically infected individuals [21]. The Th2 associated antibodies, IgG4 and IgE and hypereosinophilia are also observed [22, 23].

F. hepatica survives within its definitive host for prolonged periods of time; from 2-20 years in cattle and sheep respectively [8]. We (and others) have reported that the ability of *F. hepatica* to efficiently inhibit the development of host parasite-specific Th1 responses ensures its longevity within the host [18, 19, 24, 25]. Host immune protection to *F. hepatica* is mediated by parasite-specific Th1 type immune responses [15,16] as demonstrated in studies in cattle where IFNγ and high levels of *Fasciola*-specific IgG1 antibody are associated with immune protection [15, 16]. Experimentally it was shown that IL-4$^{-/-}$ mice, that cannot drive Th2 immune response, are less susceptible to *F. hepatica* infection with reduced liver damage compared to IFN-γ receptor deficient mice that exhibit polarised Th2 responses and are more susceptible to infection [18]. Furthermore, efficacy of vaccines against *F. hepatica* correlated with enhanced lymphocyte proliferation and IFN-γ expression in response to parasite antigen and production of the Th1 associated phenotype of antibody (IgG2a in mice – and IgG1 in cattle) [15, 16]. Th2/T_{reg} immune responses were shown to have a critical role in the suppression of parasite-specific Th1 immune response, however many *Fasciola* secreted molecules turn off innate immune cells capacity to differentiate CD4$^+$ cells into Th1/Th17 subsets.

F. hepatica Modulates the Adaptive Immune Response by Altering the Activity of Innate Immune Cells

The phenotype of innate immune responses determines the phenotype of adaptive immune response. While dendritic cells (DCs) are well characterised as the professional antigen presenting cells, macrophages and mast cells are also involved in polarising the T cell response to infection. While it is known that cross talk with other innate immune cells such as eosinophils, basophils and neutrophils is also important during helminth infection little is known about its influence on the development of the adaptive immune responses during *Fasciola* infection. Within the first few hours of infection with *F. hepatica*, innate immune cells are switched to phenotypes that are unable to support the development of Th1 adaptive immune responses and instead promote the developing Th2/T_{reg} response. For example, 24 hours after infection, mouse macrophages display enhanced expression of markers that are characteristic of a regulatory M2 phenotype [2]. In addition, DCs appear to lack surface markers of classical activation that are required to promote the differentiation of Th1 immune responses [19, 26-28].

Both the surface tegument and the secretions of *F. hepatica* contain the molecules most likely to manipulate the host's immune response as these are in a position to interact with immune cells [2, 25]. During its presence in the host, the parasite excretes and secretes a mixture of molecules (termed **FhES**) which originate in the parasite gut and are regularly expelled into the local host environment. The major components of FhES have been identified and extensively reviewed elsewhere [29]. In summary they are predominantly the enzymes involved in migration (cathepsin L1 and L2), acquisition of host nutrients (cathepsin L1 and L2, Cathepsin B, leucine aminopeptidase, fatty acid-binding protein), defence against reactive oxygen species (peroxiredoxin, glutathione transferase) and modulation of host immune responses (cathepsin L1 and L2, Cathepsin B, leucine aminopeptidase, fatty acid-binding protein, peroxiredoxin, glutathione transferase and human defence molecule). A second antigen source during *F. hepatica* infection is its unique glycocalyx **tegumental coat (FhTeg)** which has multiple functions such as absorption of exogenous nutrients, synthesis and secretion of various substances, osmoregulation and protection against host enzymes and bile [29]. As the parasite migrates through host tissue, FhTeg is shed every 2-3 hrs, thus playing an additional role in the modulation of host immune responses. While proteomic analysis has identified the proteins present in FhTeg, unlike FhES the immune modulatory role of individual molecules has yet to be fully examined [30]. In summary, the proteins identified included a mixture of excretory-secretory proteins (cathepsin L1 and L2, Cathepsin B, peroxiredoxin, leucine aminopeptidase, fatty acid-binding protein, glutathione transferase), membrane associated proteins, energy metabolism and cytoskeleton components [30, 31]. Recent studies have identified exosome-like vesicles within the tegument of *F. hepatica* and in the insoluble fraction of FhES. The proteome of these vesicles accounted for 52% of proteins currently identified in FhES, with analysis revealing a number of protease enzymes (like cathepsins and leucine aminopeptidase), in addition to detoxifying enzymes (such as heat-shock proteins, peroxiredoxin and fatty-acid binding proteins) [32]. While there has been no report on the impact these exosomes may have on host immune responses, it is quite likely that the parasite uses these vesicles as a mechanism of transporting immune-modulating proteins (such as cathepsin L1, peroxiredoxin, glutathione S-transferase) into host cells to alter their phenotype and biological activity as demonstrated for other human parasites [33].

We have shown that FhES can induce the production of a Th2 immune response in mice [2], while both FhES and FhTeg inhibit the development of Th1 immune responses [3, 25]. Innate immune cells are critical in driving these immune responses and recent studies examining the interactions of *F. hepatica* infection and molecules with innate immune cells have focused upon the following three main cells types: dendritic cells, macrophages and mast cells. These findings are summarised in Table **1** and each of these cell types will be discussed separately in detail.

Table 1: Modulation of Innate Immune cells by *Fasciola* antigens

F. Hepatica Antigen	Immune Modulatory Properties	References
Dendritic Cells		
Excretory-secretory products	Immature phenotype ↑ (increase) IL-10 Induces Th2/Treg immune responses Inhibits TLR activation of dendritic cells	[26]
Liver fluke homogenate	Immature phenotype ↑ IL-10, TGFβ Induces Th2/Treg immune responses Inhibits TLR activation of dendritic cells	[27]
Tegumental antigens	Immature phenotype	[25]

Table 1 Contd….

	Inhibits Th1 immune responses Inhibits phagocytosis Induces Mast cell migration Inhibits TLR and non-TLR activation of dendritic cells Inhibits NFκB and MAPKinases Induces SOCS	[28]
Cathepsin L	↑ CD40, IL-6, IL-12p40, MIP2 Suppresses IL-23 InhibitsTh17 cells Induces p38	[4]
Sigma class glutathione transferase	↑ CD40, IL-6, IL-12p40, MIP2 Suppresses IL-23 InhibitsTh17 cells Induces JNK, NFκB, ERK and IRF5 ↑ PGE2	[4] [5]
Macrophages		
Excretory-secretory products	Induces regulatory /M2 macrophages ↑ Fizz, Arginase and Relm1 ↑ IL-10, PGE2, TGFb Promotes Th2 immune responses Inhibits Th1 immune responses	[2]
Peroxredoxin	Induces regulatory /M2 macrophages ↑ Fizz, Arg and Relm1 ↑ IL-10, PGE2 Promotes Th2 immunity Inhibits Th1 immune responses	[3] [17]
Cathepsin L	Inhibits the activation of M1 macrophages Inhibits Th1 immune responses Prevents and cleaves the expression of TLR3 Inhibits MyD88 independent signalling Inhibits the releases of IL-6, IFNγ and IL-12	[38]
Human defense molecule	Inhibits vacuolar ATPase Prevents antigen degradation inhibiting antigen presentation Induces M2 macrophages	[6] [39]
Mast cells		
Tegumental antigens	Immature phenotype Inhibits Th1 immune responses Induces Mast cell migration Inhibits TLR activation of mast cells Inhibits NFκB and MAP Kinases Induces SOCS	[49] [50]

Dendritic Cells

During infection with *F. hepatica,* as juvenile flukes migrate through the peritoneal cavity, the absolute numbers of CD11c$^+$ DC populations are significantly increased [19] and display typical immature phenotypic characteristics of helminth infection, with lower expression of co-stimulatory markers (CD40, CD80 and CD86), MHC class II and enhanced expression of CCR5. These cells express enhanced levels of intracellular IL-10 and exhibit higher cell surface levels of **LAP (*Latency Associated Peptide*)** that binds *TGF-β1* forming a latent complex. Functionally, the DCs isolated from mice infected with *F. hepatica* suppress the secretion of antigen specific IL-17 and IFNγ from naïve DO11.10 OVA TCR Tg CD4$^+$ T cells. However, blocking IL-10 and TGF-β did not reverse this effect which suggests that cell-cell contact may be required and that the lack of MHC II and co-stimulatory molecules may be sufficient to have a negative effect on the development of T-cell responses during *F. hepatica* infection [19].

FhES and **whole parasite homogenate (FhLFH)** induce an immature DC phenotype *in vitro* with similar characteristics to that observed during natural infection. While FhES and FhLFH induce or promote IL-10 secretion from DCs, when injected *in vivo* they promote Th2/T$_{reg}$ immune responses. During infection these antigens also induce antigen specific Th2/T$_{reg}$ immune responses in the spleen and local lymph nodes and these responses can be mimicked by intraperitonally injection of these antigens [17, 26, 27]. When DCs are stimulated with FhTeg, the activated DCs do not secrete IL-10 or induce Th2/T$_{reg}$ immune responses suggesting that this antigen has different immune modulatory properties. FhTeg also impairs DC function by inhibiting its phagocytic capacity and its ability to prime T-cells [25].

FhES, FhLFH and FhTeg suppress TLR activated DCs maturation and function by inhibiting cytokine secretion and expression of co-stimulatory markers following TLR activation. Further studies on FhTeg demonstrate a suppression of NF-κB and the MAPKs p38, JNK and ERK, important signalling molecules in inflammatory processes [28] which could explain its modulatory effects. These findings correlate with other studies as *Schistosoma mansoni* egg antigens reduce

LPS-stimulated phosphorylation of p38, JNK and ERK in murine DCs [34] while *S. haematobium* and *Ascaris* lumbricoides infection suppresses LPS induced p38 phosphorylation, but not ERK activation of DCs [35,36]. FhTeg enhances expression of SOCS3 in DCs [28], a negative regulator of the TLR pathway. SOCS3 is a member of a family of inhibitory molecules that auto-regulation pathogen induced inflammatory responses [37]. It is likely that *F. hepatica* utilising these mechanisms to suppress Th1 immune responses to bystander infections.

Enzymes are secreted in large quantities into *F. hepatica* gut and are expelled from the parasite into the host environment. Peptidases are important as they degrade host proteins so they can be used for nutrients by *F. hepatica* [7]. They also serve an important role in modulating the host's immune response, by preventing the immune-mediated elimination of the parasite [38] while **glutathione transferase are important antioxidants that disarm host immune responses [4]**. *F. hepatica* **cysteine peptidases** (FhCL1) and **sigma class glutathione transferase (FhGST-S1)** but not mu class GST induce partial activation of DCs that secrete IL-6, IL-12p40 and MIP-2 and enhanced CD40 expression. In addition, FhCL1 and FhGST-S1 primed DCs secreted reduced levels of IL-23 in response to LPS activation and this correlates with attenuated IL-17 production from OVA-specific T-cells *in vivo*. These molecules therefore suppress immune responses associated with chronic inflammation. While these enzymes interacted with DCs in a TLR4 independent manner their subsequent intracellular signalling pathways diverge as rFhCL1 signals through p38 while FhGST-S1 induces the expression of JNK, p38, p-NF-κBp65 and IRF5. This suggests that while these molecules had similar function their mechanism were different ensuring redundancy [4]. FhGST-S1 also induces Prostaglandin E2 secretion from dendritic cells and macrophages, an important factor in the promotion of Th2/Treg immune responses [5].

Macrophages

For many helminth parasites, as infection progresses from acute to chronic stages, there is a correlative switch in macrophage phenotypes from M1 to M2 [39], which has been explained as a necessary functional switch from killing to repair to ultimately benefiting both the parasite and host [40, 41]. However, as quickly as 24 hours post oral infection with *F. hepatica* metacercariae, as juvenile flukes migrate through the intestinal epithelium, a suppression of M1-associated genetic markers (unpublished data) is observed in peritoneal macrophage while in tandem these cells display an increase in the expression in Fizz1. Within 3 days post infection the genetic profile of these cells are fully characteristic of M2 macrophages. Functionally, we have shown that these macrophages are hyporesponsive to Th-1 associated inflammatory ligands and are unable to support the differentiation of type 1 cells from naive $CD4^+$ T cells. In contrast, they effectively promote the polarisation of Th2 type immune responses [2]. Since helminth infection causes a switch from M1 to M2 phenotypes the parasite itself must dictate the phenotype of the immune response. Indeed, just like an infection, the intraperitoneal injection of FhES to mice replicates the activation of M2 macrophage and parasite-specific Th-2 immune responses and at the same time inhibits the ability of macrophages to drive inflammatory Th-1 responses [2, 17].

The most abundant protein within FhES has been identified as the **cysteine protease enzyme, FhCL1**, which represents approximately 80% of FhES [7]. Importantly, this is also the most predominant protein secreted by juvenile worms as they penetrate the intestinal epithelium. Given such abundance within FhES, it was surprising, that unlike FhES, intraperitoneal delivery of FhCL1 to mice did not induce the development of parasite-specific Th2 immune responses [42]. However, further investigation revealed that it is this enzyme that confers FhES with the ability to inhibit the activation of M1 macrophages. Intraperitoneally delivered FhCL1 in mice is taken up into the early endosomes of macrophages where it either cleaved or prevents expression of Toll-like Receptor 3 (TLR-3), thus preventing MyD88-independent and TRIF-dependent signalling pathways in macrophages. This modulation of macrophage activity by FhCL1 *in vivo* is thought to explain its protective effect in mice in a lethal model of septic shock by preventing the release of the inflammatory mediators, nitric oxide, IL-6, TNF and IL-12, from macrophages [28].

In contrast, mice injected with functionally recombinant **Peroxiredoxin (FhPrx)** exhibit increased populations of regulatory/M2 macrophages, as verified by the expression of the markers, Ym1 and Arg1 [2, 17]. The induction of these macrophage population was mimicked by FhPrx *in vivo* and also following incubation with peritoneal macrophages *in vitro*, indicating that FhPrx directly interacted with, and modulated the phenotype of, macrophage populations. Importantly, these FhPrx-activated M2-like macrophages promoted the differentiation of T-cells into a Th2 phenotype. Passive transfer of sheep anti-FhPrx antibodies into mice infected with *F. hepatica* blocked the development of parasite-specific Th2 responses demonstrating a critical role for FhPrx in the polarization of the host immune response [2, 6].

***F. hepatica*, helminth defence molecule (FhHDM-1)** also interacts with macrophages following intraperitoneal injection in mice. FhHDM-1 is cleaved by lysosomal cathepsin L, after endocytosis by macrophages. A C-terminal peptide containing a conserved amphipathic helix is released and this peptide inhibits vacuolar ATPase, a proton pump critical to maintaining the low pH of the endosome that is necessary for antigen degradation by proteolysis before peptides are translocated to MHC Class II. Blocking vATPase by the parasite will inhibit antigen presentation and impair cellular and humoral immune responses to parasite antigens [43]. Interestingly, it has been suggested that antigen presenting activity in macrophages is likely switched off as macrophages switch to an M2 phenotype associated with immune regulation and wound repair. Supporting this hypothesis, we have shown that peritoneal macrophages harvested from mice injected with FhHDM-1 display increased expression the typical markers of M2 macrophages such asYm1, Arg1 and Fizz1 (manuscript in preparation).

Mast Cells

Enhanced numbers of mast cell is a key feature of fasciolosis as mast cells are observed during natural infection at the site of infection in both cattle and sheep [44, 45]. Mastocytosis is also observed in laboratory models of *F. hepatica* infection, with increased mast cell numbers in rat gut mucosa [46] and mouse liver and peritoneal cavity. FhTeg but not FhES can significantly enhance mast cell numbers in the peritoneal cavity. However, FhTeg primed mast cells do not proliferate, suggesting that during infection the increase in mast cell populations is the result of cellular migration. *In vitro* evidence demonstrates that FhTeg activated DCs promote mast cell migration through the release of mast cell migratory chemokines, MIP2 (CXCL2) and MIP1α (CCL3) [47-49].

While mast cells are critical to the expulsion of gut helminths [50] its role in *Fasciola* infection is less clear. However, given the migratory pathway of the fluke where they burrow through the peritoneal cavity and liver before residing in the bile ducts the increase in mast cell numbers observed at these sites during infection would suggest that they have a significant role to play. Given mast cells role in wound healing and tissue remodelling [51], they are likely to be recruited in order to combat the extensive damage caused by flukes during their migratory phase [52]. Although there is currently no evidence to support this hypothesis.

The interaction of Fasciola antigens with mast cells could play an important role in shaping the adaptive immune response. However, mast cells activated with FhTeg fail to secrete key Th2 promoting cytokines and or induce the differentiation of Th2 subsets. Its interactions with mast cells was shown to be similar to that of DCs as it directly inhibits the ability of mast cells to promote Th1 immune responses [53]. The inhibition of Th1 immune responses is through the suppression of TNF-α, IL-6, IFN-γ, IL-10 cytokines and ICAM1, a cell surface molecule that has an important role in mast cell/T-cell communication [54]. Similar to DCs FhTeg suppresses LPS and microbial induced NF-κB and ERK activation in mast cells and enhances SOCS3 expression. Th1 immune responses are important in immune protection against *Fasciola* infection and mast cells were shown to promote Th1 immunity during microbial infections. It is plausible that these cells are recruited to promote Th1 immune responses in the early stages of infection and these responses are inhibited by the release of FhTeg into the micro-environment in order to suppress host immunity.

To support this hypothesis Th1 immune response were induced in mice following injecting with *B- pertussis* antigen. Co-infection with FhTeg caused suppression of *B. pertussis* induced TNF-α expression in mast cells. This would suggest that like dendritic cells and macrophages mast cells may be targeted by helminth antigens during bystander infections. This could explain the failure of *F. hepatica* co-infected mice to clear *B. pertussis* infection as mast cells are inhibited from secreting protective pro-inflammatory mediators like TNF-α and IFN-γ [24].

Similarly, mast cells promote the pathology associated with EAE in mice as mast cell knockout mice are protected from developing this disease [19]. This suppression of pro-inflammatory mast cells by FhTeg could also explain how *Fasciola* attenuates EAE in mice [19]. Further studies are required to examine mast cells-helminth interaction during these processes and these studies would shed further light on the impact of helminths on communicable and non-communicable diseases.

CONCLUSION

The suppression in Th1 type responses is necessary for the development of Th2 immune response during infection with *Fasciola* infection and is critical given that Th1 responses are important for immune protection with this parasite. Therefore, proteins secreted and released by the parasite co-operate immediately and effectively to modulate the host immune response to prevent expulsion and protect the host from excessive immune-mediated tissue pathology. While this chapter highlights the importance of innate immune cells, the focus upon DCs, macrophages and mast cells reflects current research in the field. However, further studies are required to examine to role of other innate immune cells such as basophils and nuocytes that are early sources of Th2 derived cytokines. *F. hepatica* is an excellent model to fully elucidate mechanisms of Th1-immune suppression and the induction of Th2/Treg immune responses. Furthermore, due its uncomplicated migration through the host and the immediate modulation of immune responses, this model affords an opportunity to characterise the role of individual parasite molecules and also the contribution of host-tissue molecules to the developing Th2/Treg immune responses.

ACKNOWLEDGEMENTS

All individuals listed as authors contributed equally to the manuscript. S.M. O'Neill is funded by Science Foundation Ireland (11/RFP.1/BIC/3109), the Wellcome Trust (WT094907) and the Programme for Research in Third Level Institutions (PRTLI) Cycle 4. The PRTLI is co-funded through the European Regional Development Fund (ERDF), part of the European Union Structural Funds Programme 2007-2013. We also would like to acknowledge support by the

COST Action BM1007 "Mast cells and basophils – Targets for innovative therapies". S. Donnelly was funded by the Australian National Health and Medical Research Council, project grant APP1010197.

CONFLICT OF INTEREST

The authors confirms that this chapter contents have no conflicts of interest.

REFERENCES

[1] Donnelly S, O'Neill SM, Sekiya M, *et al*. Thioredoxin peroxidase secreted by *Fasciola hepatica* induces the alternative activation of macrophages. Infect Immun 2005; 73: 166-73.
[2] Pearce EJ, MacDonald AS. The immunobiology of schistosomiasis. Nat Rev Immunol 2002; 7: 499-511.
[3] O'Neill SM, Mills KH, Dalton JP. *Fasciola hepatica* cathepsin L cysteine proteinase suppresses *Bordetella pertussis*-specific interferon-gamma production *in vivo*. Parasite Immunol 2001; 10: 541-7.
[4] Dowling DJ, Hamilton CM, Donnelly S, *et al*. Major secretory antigens of the helminth *Fasciola hepatica* activate a suppressive dendritic cell phenotype that attenuates Th17 cells but fails to activate Th2 immune responses. Infect Immun 2010; 78: 793-801.
[5] LaCourse EJ, Perally S, Morphew RM, *et al*. The Sigma class glutathione transferase from the liver fluke *Fasciola hepatica*. PLoS Negl Trop Dis 2012; 6: e1666.
[6] Robinson MW, Donnelly S, Hutchinson AT, *et al*. A family of helminth molecules that modulate innate cell responses *via* molecular mimicry of host antimicrobial peptides. PLoS Pathog 2011; 7: e1002042.
[7] Robinson MW, Dalton JP, Donnelly S. Helminth pathogen cathepsin proteases: it's a family affair. Trends Biochem Sci 2008; 33: 601-8.
[8] McManus DP, Dalton JP. Vaccines against the zoonotic trematodes *Schistosoma japonicum*, *Fasciola hepatica* and *Fasciola gigantica*. Parasitology 2006; 133 Suppl: S43-61.
[9] WHO. Fascioliasis: infection with the "neglected" neglected worms, 2009; Available from: http://www.who.int/neglected_diseases/integrated_media/integrated_media_fascioliasis/en/
[10] Mas-Coma S. Epidemiology of fascioliasis in human endemic areas. J Helminthol 2005; 79: 207-16.
[11] Parkinson M, O'Neill SM, Dalton JP. Endemic human fasciolosis in the Bolivian Altiplano. Epidemiol Infect 2007; 135: 669-74.
[12] Andrews SJ. "The life cycle of *Fasciola hepatica*" in *Fasciolosis*, ed. J.P. Dalton, CAB International, Oxon, Wallingford, UK, 1998; pp. 1-24.
[13] Moxon JV, LaCourse EJ, Wright HA, *et al*. Proteomic analysis of embryonic *Fasciola hepatica*: characterization and antigenic potential of a developmentally regulated heat shock protein. Vet Parasitol 2010; 169: 62-75.
[14] Flynn RJ, Mulcahy G, Welsh M, *et al*. Co-Infection of cattle with *Fasciola hepatica* and *Mycobacterium bovis*- immunological consequences. Transbound Emerg Dis 2009; 56: 269-74.

[15] Clery DG, Mulcahy G. Lymphocyte and cytokine responses of young cattle during primary infection with *Fasciola hepatica*. Res Vet Sci 1998; 65: 169-71.
[16] Mulcahy G, O'Connor F, McGonigle S, et al. Correlation of specific antibody titre and avidity with protection in cattle immunized against *Fasciola hepatica*. Vaccine 1998; 16: 932-9.
[17] Donnelly S, Stack CM, O'Neill SM, et al. Helminth 2-Cys peroxiredoxin drives Th2 responses through a mechanism involving alternatively activated macrophages. FASEB J 2008; 22: 4022-32.
[18] O'Neill SM, Brady MT, Callanan JJ, et al. *Fasciola hepatica* infection downregulates Th1 responses in mice. Parasite Immunol 2000; 22: 147-55.
[19] Walsh KP, Brady MT, Finlay CM, et al. Infection with a helminth parasite attenuates autoimmunity through TGF-beta-mediated suppression of Th17 and Th1 responses. J Immunol 2009; 183: 1577-86.
[20] Haçariz O, Sayers G, Flynn RJ, et al. IL-10 and TGF-beta1 are associated with variations in fluke burdens following experimental fasciolosis in sheep. Parasite Immunol 2009; 31: 613-22.
[21] Osman MM, Abo-El-Nazar SY. IL-10, IFN-gamma and TNF-alpha in acute and chronic human fascioliasis. J Egypt Soc Parasitol 1999; 29: 13-20.
[22] O'Neill SM, Parkinson M, Strauss W, et al. Immunodiagnosis of *Fasciola hepatica* infection (fascioliasis) in a human population in the Bolivian Altiplano using purified cathepsin L cysteine proteinase. Am J Trop Med Hyg 1998; 58: 417-23.
[23] el-Shabrawi M, el-Karaksy H, Okasha S, et al. Human fascioliasis: clinical eatures and diagnostic difficulties in Egyptian children. J Trop Pediatr 1997; 43: 162-6.
[24] Brady MT, O'Neill SM, Dalton JP, et al. *Fasciola hepatica* suppresses a protective Th1 response against *Bordetella pertussis*. Infect Immun 1999; 67: 5372-8.
[25] Hamilton CH, Dowling DJ, Loscher CE, et al. Suppression of LPS-induced dendritic cell maturation by *Fasciola hepatica* tegumental antigen. Infection and Immunity 2009; 77: 2488-98.
[26] Falcón C, Carranza F, Martínez FF, et al. Excretory-secretory products (ESP) from *Fasciola hepatica* induce tolerogenic properties in myeloid dendritic cells. Vet Immunol Immunopathol 2010; 137: 36-46.
[27] Falcón CR, Carranza FA, Aoki P, et al. Adoptive transfer of dendritic cells pulsed with *Fasciola hepatica* antigens and lipopolysaccharides confers protection against fasciolosis in mice. J Infect Dis 2012; 205: 506-14.
[28] Vukman KV, Adams PN, O'Neill SM. *Fasciola hepatica* tegumental coat antigen suppresses MAPK signalling in dendritic cells and up-regulates the expression of SOCS3. Parasite Immunol 2013; Mar 18. doi: 10.1111/pim.12033. [Epub ahead of print]
[29] Dalton JP, Mulcahy G. Parasite vaccines--a reality? Vet Parasitol 2001; 98: 149-67.
[30] Morphew RM, Hamilton CM, Wright HA, et al. Identification of the major proteins of an immune modulating fraction from adult Fasciola hepatica released by Nonidet P40. Vet Parasitol 2013; 191: 379-85.
[31] Wilson RA, Wright JM, de Castro-Borges W, et al. Exploring the *Fasciola hepatica* tegument proteome.Int J Parasitol 2011; 41: 1347-59.
[32] Marcilla A, Trelis M, Cortés A, et al. Extracellular vesicles from parasitic helminths contain specific excretory/secretory proteins and are internalized in intestinal host cells. PLoS One 2012; 7: e45974.

[33] Silverman JM, Clos J, Horakova E, et al. Leishmania exosomes modulate innate and adaptive immune responses through effects on monocytes and dendritic cells. J Immunol. 2010; 185: 5011-22.

[34] Kane CM, Cervi L, Sun J, et al. Helminth antigens modulate TLR-initiated dendritic cell activation. J Immunol 2004; 173: 7454-61.

[35] Everts B, Hussaarts L, Driessen NN, et al. Schistosome-derived omega-1 drives Th2 polarization by suppressing protein synthesis following internalization by the mannose receptor. J Exp Med 2012; 209: 1753-67.

[36] van Riet E, Everts B, Retra K, et al. Combined TLR2 and TLR4 ligation in the context of bacterial or helminth extracts in human monocyte derived dendritic cells: molecular correlates for Th1/Th2 polarization. BMC Immunol 2009; 10: 9.

[37] Yoshimura A, Suzuki M, Sakaguchi R, et al. SOCS, Inflammation, and Autoimmunity. Front Immunol 2012; 3: 20. doi: 10.3389/fimmu.2012.00020.

[38] Donnelly S, Dalton JP, Robinson MW. How pathogen-derived cysteine proteases modulate host immune responses. Adv Exp Med Biol 2011; 712: 192-207.

[39] Reyes JL, Terrazas LI. The divergent roles of alternatively activated macrophages in helminthic infections. Parasite Immunol 2007; 29: 609-19.

[40] Barron L, Wynn TA. Macrophage activation governs schistosomiasis-induced inflammation and fibrosis. Eur J Immunol 2011; 41: 2509-14.

[41] Jenkins SJ, Allen JE. Similarity and diversity in macrophage activation by nematodes, trematodes, and cestodes. J Biomed Biotechnol 2010; 2010: 262609.

[42] Donnelly S, O'Neill SM, Stack CM, et al. Helminth cysteine proteases inhibit TRIF-dependent activation of macrophages *via* degradation of TLR3. J Biol Chem 2010; 285: 3383-92.

[43] Robinson MW, Alvarado R, To J, et al. A helminth cathelicidin-like protein suppresses antigen processing and presentation in macrophages *via* inhibition of lysosomal vATPase. FASEB J 2012; 26: 4614-27.

[44] Rahko T. The pathology of natural *Fasciola hepatica* infection in cattle. Pathol Vet 1969; 6: 244-56.

[45] Ferreras MC, García-Iglesias MJ, Manga-González MY, et al. Histopathological and immunohistochemical study of lambs experimentally infected with *Fasciola hepatica* and *Schistosoma bovis*. J Vet Med B Infect Dis Vet Public Health 2000; 47: 763-73.

[46] Van Milligen FJ, Cornelissen JB, Bokhout BA. Location of induction and expression of protective immunity against *Fasciola hepatica* at the gut level: a study using an *ex vivo* infection model with ligated gut segments. J Parasitol 1998; 84: 771-7.

[47] Taub D, Dastych J, Inamura N, et al. Bone marrow-derived murine mast cells migrate, but do not degranulate, in response to chemokines. J Immunol 1995; 154, 2393-2402.

[48] Gilfillan AM, Austin SJ, Metcalfe DD. Mast cell biology: introduction and overview. Adv Exp Med Biol 2011; 716, 2-12.

[49] Kunii J, Takahashi K, Kasakura K, et al. Commensal bacteria promote migration of mast cells into the intestine. Immunobiology 2011; 216, 692-7.

[50] Hashimoto K, Uchikawa R, Tegoshi T, et al. Immunity-mediated regulation of fecundity in the nematode *Heligmosomoides polygyrus*--the potential role of mast cells. Parasitology 2009; 137: 881-7.

[51] Metcalfe DD, Peavy RD, Gilfillan AM. Mechanisms of mast cell signaling in anaphylaxis. J Allergy Clin Immunol 2009; 124, 639-46.

[52] Robinson MW, Hutchinson AT, Donnelly S, *et al*. Worm secretory molecules are causing alarm. Trends Parasitol 2010; 26, 371-2.

[53] Vukman KV, Adams PN, Metz M, *et al*. *Fasciola hepatica* tegumental coat impairs mast cells' ability to drive Th1 immune responses. J Immunol 2013; 190: 2873-9.

[54] Vukman KV, Adams PN, Dowling D, *et al*. The effects of *Fasciola hepatica* tegumental antigens on mast cell function. Int J Parasitol 2013; doi:pii: S0020-7519(13)00085-4.

Chapter 4: Parasite-Mediated Immune Modulation During the Development of Human Cystic Echinococcosis

CHAPTER 4

Parasite-Mediated Immune Modulation During the Development of Human Cystic Echinococcosis

Elisabetta Profumo[*], Alessandra Ludovisi[*], Brigitta Buttari, Maria Angeles Gomez Morales and Rachele Riganò

Department of Infectious, Parasitic and Immune-mediated Disease, Istituto Superiore di Sanità, Viale Regina Elena 299, 00161, Rome, Italy

Abstract: Cystic echinococcosis (CE) is a neglected zoonosis caused by the larval stage of the cestode *Echinococcus granulosus*. It represents one of the major health priorities in developing countries and its global prevalence is about three million. *E. granulous* modulates anti-parasite immunity and persists in infected humans despite the occurrence of detectable parasite-specific humoral and cellular responses. In particular, the up-regulation of the Th2-type response and of anti-inflammatory cytokines production is involved in the chronicity of the infection and in the inhibition of host protective mechanisms. In this chapter, we underline findings about the human immune response during the development of CE and new insights regarding to the ability of *E. granulosus* to directly modulate and even to exploit the host's immune system. New knowledge into the host immune response to the parasite will increase our understanding of this parasitic infection and will give the opportunity to design new preventive or therapeutic strategies.

Keywords: Cystic echinococcosis, host-parasite interaction, immune system, antigen, T helper response.

INTRODUCTION

Cystic echinococcosis (CE) is a zoonotic infection due to the larval stage (metacestode) of the cestode *Echinococcus granulosus* (family *Taeniidae*). Globally, the echinococcosis (hydatidosis) is one of the major parasitic diseases, with more than 95% of the worldwide estimated 3 million cases [1]. The parasite is present in the Mediterranean area, the Balkans, the Middle East, North and East

---

*Corresponding author Rachele Riganò: Department of Infectious, Parasitic and Immune-mediated Disease, Istituto Superiore di Sanità, Viale Regina Elena 299, 00161, Rome, Italy; Tel: +390649902760; Fax: +390649902886; E-mail: rachele.rigano@iss.it
*These authors contributed equally.

Emilio Jirillo, Thea Magrone and Giuseppe Miragliotta (Eds)
All rights reserved-© 2014 Bentham Science Publishers

Africa, part of South America, and in Central Asia, Mongolia, Sinkiang, Tibet and China [2]. The highest prevalence in humans and animals can be found in geographic areas with higher livestock production, where many livestock guard dogs (definitive host) can come into contact and ingest larval stages of the parasite from dead animal carcasses or illegal slaughter offal [3]. Herbivores (sheep, horse, cattle, pig, goat and camel) represent the intermediate hosts.

The small bowel of the definitive hosts houses the adult stage of *E. granulosus* of a 3 to 6 mm length (Fig. 1). Gravid proglottids release parasite eggs that are eliminated with the faeces (Fig. 2). The egg, once ingested by a suitable intermediate host, hatches in the small bowel. The penetration of released oncospheres into the bowel wall and their entrance into the bloodstream lead to their location in internal organs, in particular liver and lungs, where they develop into hydatid cysts. These cysts develop as unilocular fluid-filled bladder that slowly grows, giving origin to protosoleces and daughter cysts filling the interior of the cyst [4]. The cyst wall is constituted by an inner nucleated germinal layer and an outer acellular laminated layer which are two parasite-derived layers, surrounded by a fibrous capsule which is host-derived because it is the consequence of the host immune response. The infection of definitive hosts is due to ingestion of cyst-containing organs from parasitized intermediate hosts.

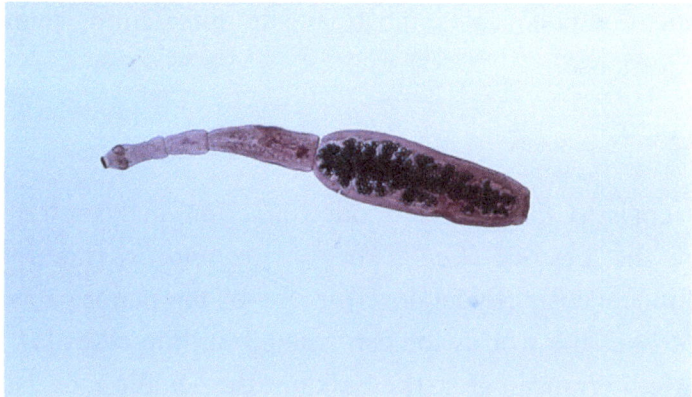

Figure 1: Morphology of the adult stage of *Echinococcus granulosus* from a dog. Adults range from 3mm to 6mm in length and usually consist of a scolex, and three proglottids. The third (terminal) proglottid is gravid, and is longer than wide, as shown in this picture. The scolex is constituted by four suckers and a rostellum with 25-50 hooks. The only definitive hosts for *Echinococcus* are dogs and other canids, consequently, adults are not expected to be found in the human host. Source: Center for Diseases Control and Prevention, Dr. Peter M. Schantz.

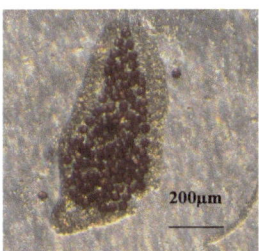

Figure 2: The terminal gravid proglottid of the adult cestode *Echinococcus granulosus*, from an infected dog. Source: European Union Reference Laboratory for Parasites, Dr. A. Casulli.

Ingested evaginated protoscoleces attach to the intestinal mucosa, and proceed to develop to the adult worm in 32 to 80 days (Fig. **3**). Humans are infected accidentally after ingestion of embryonated eggs present in food, drinks or other materials contaminated with feces from infected dogs. The small size of the proglottids or their disruption may facilitate the accidental contamination of the animal coat, making possible the transmission to the human hosts during playing; this is of particular importance in children.

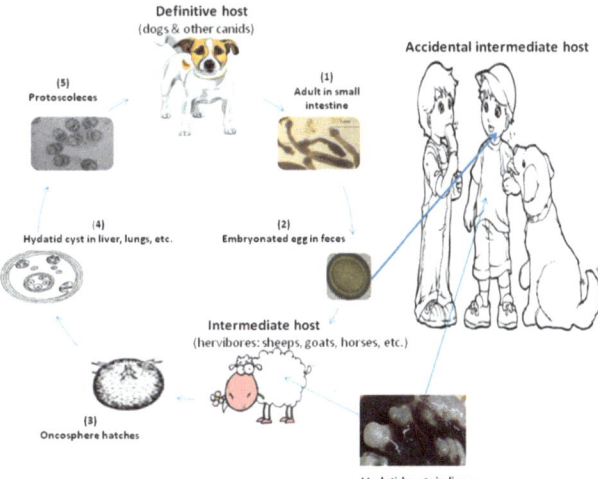

Figure 3: *Echinococcus granulosus* life cycle. The adult stage of *E. granulosus* (1) lives in the small bowel of dogs or other canids which represent the definitive hosts. Gravid proglottids in the feces release eggs (2) that when ingested by a suitable intermediate host, release the oncosphere (3) The oncosphere penetrates into the bowel wall and migrates through the bloodstream into internal organs, in particular liver and lungs. In these organs, the oncosphere develops into a hydatid cyst (4) that produces protoscoleces (5) and daughter cysts filling the cyst interior. The definitive host becomes infected after ingestion of cyst-containing organs from the parasitized intermediate host. In the definitive host evaginated protoscoleces, attached to the intestinal mucosa, develop into adult worm (1) in 32 to 80 days.

The peculiar aspects of *E. granulosus* infection are: (1) different mammalian species used by the parasite as intermediate hosts. New species, other than those classically recognised as intermediate hosts, in which fertile cysts may develop, can quickly adapt to become intermediate hosts. Examples are Australian marsupials that are now the main responsible for CE transmission in Australia, having become highly susceptible to CE after introduction of the parasite in this continent at the time of European settlement. (2) A long-term growth of the metacestode (hydatid) cysts in internal organs of the intermediate host (53 years) and (3) the consequent chronic disease in this host. The unilocular fluid-filled cysts can be detected in many internal organs, mostly in the liver (70%) and in the lung (20%). The remaining 10% is localized in different organs (kidney, spleen, brain, heart, and bone) [4].

There are ten genetic types (G1-10) within *E. granulosus*, with different geographical distributions, isolated from different intermediate hosts. These types have been identified by molecular studies based on mitochondrial DNA sequences [5,6], namely: two from sheep (G1 and G2), two from bovids (G3 and G5), one from the horse (G4), one from camelids (G6), two from pigs (G7 and the variant pig strain G9), one from American cervids (G8), and one from European cervids (G10).

Host–Parasite Interaction

After being ingested by the natural or accidental (humans) intermediate host, *E. granulosus* eggs release embryos (oncospheres) that penetrate the intestinal wall, migrate *via* the blood or lymph stream, and finally are trapped in the liver, lungs, and other sites where cysts begin to develop. This process leads up to transformation of the oncospheral stage to reach the metacestode stage, *i.e.* hydatid cyst [2] (Figs. **4-5**). The hydatid cyst enlarges concentrically within the organ parenchyma where can reach a diameter of 20 cm in some cases, with a fluid-filled bladder structure. It is linked by the hydatid cyst wall, formed by an inner cellular layer, (germinal layer, GL), and an outer protective acellular layer (laminated layer, LL). The other cyst component is the host's tissue surrounding the metacestode, called pericyst.

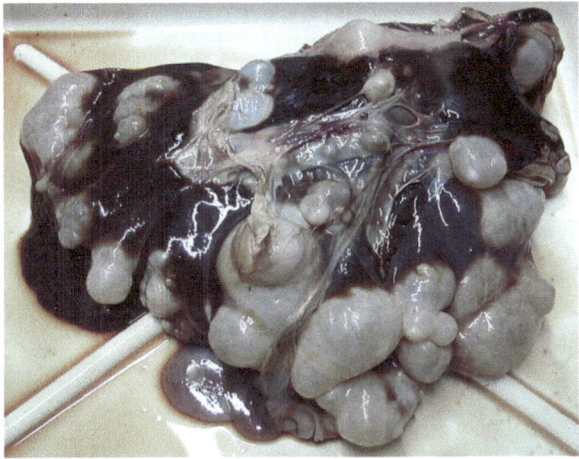

Figure 4: Sheep liver extracted during necropsy, showing numerous *Echinococcus granulosus* cysts. Source: European Union Reference Laboratory for Parasites, Dr. A. Casulli.

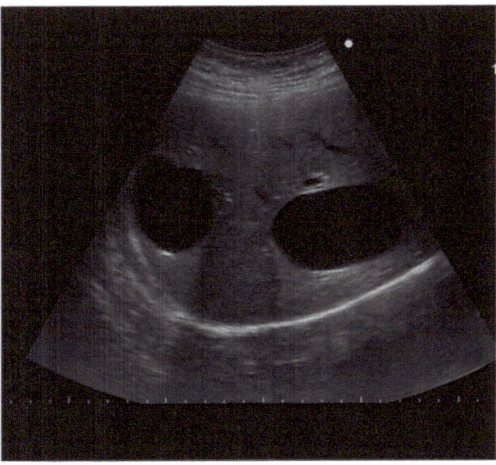

Figure 5: Two large hydatid cysts in the right lobe of human liver. Source: Università di Pavia, Dr. E. Brunetti.

The LL is a massive carbohydrate-rich structure secreted by the GL, containing abundant anti-carbohydrate antibodies from the host; it is usually encircled by an adventitial layer which is a host-derived collagen capsule, but can also be surronded by inflammatory cells from the host. The GL gives rise towards the cyst cavity to cellular buds that upon become brood capsules, turn towards their inside to generate protoscoleces. Daughter cysts, with their own complete cyst wall, occasionally are formed within larger cysts [7]. Thus the LL, found only in the genus *Echinococcus,* is related as a specialized extracellular matrix, specialized to maintain the metacestode physical integrity and to protect GL cells from the host immune response. Moreover, the LL, which is an essential element of the host–parasite interfaces in the intermediate host, seems to elicit non-inflammatory host immune responses, protecting the metacestode from antibodies. Hydatid cyst fluid (HCF) fills the cyst cavity and is responsible for the antigenic stimulation. In the early stages of the cyst, the HCF is clean and clear, including secretions of parasite and host origin, and all the components from the cyst "inner wall", called hydatid sand [8]. The HCF is identical to the host's serum regarding potassium, chlorine and CO_2 concentration. It has an alkaline pH, a density between 1.008 and 1.015; moreover, it contains specific proteins responsible for its antigenicity, such as antigen 5 (Ag5) and antigen B (AgB).

Immune Response to *E. Granulosus*

Since early stages of the echinococcal infection, there is a strong activation of host cellular immunity in both human and sheep infections. At these stages, pathological changes occur, including cellular inflammatory responses characterized by the infiltration of eosinophils, neutrophils, macrophages, and fibrocytes. However, in severe inflammatory response this infiltration generally does not result, and aged cysts become surrounded by a fibrous layer separating the LL from the host tissue [4]. The immune responses to *E. granulosus* have been largely studied in both patients with *E. granulosus* infection as well as in experimentally infected animals. Once established in the host, the parasite produces great quantities of antigens modulating the host immune responses. The immune responses are characterized by balanced Th2/Th1 responses. In most patients elevated levels of Th1 cytokines, especially interferon (IFN)-γ, and of Th2 cytokines including interleukin (IL)-4, IL-5, IL-6 and IL-10, coexist. Moreover, as the cyst develops and becomes established, IgG, especially IgG1 and IgG4, IgE and IgM are elevated. When the cyst dies, naturally or following chemotherapy, or it is surgically removed, Th2 responses decrease rapidly whereas Th1 responses increase. IgG antibody levels can persist in humans for several years after cyst removal. In patients with a relapse, the Th2 responses are rapidly regenerated [4]. Moreover, the degree of the antibody response depends on mature cyst location and condition. Indeed, hydatid cysts in human lung, spleen, or kidney are associated to a lower level of serum antibodies [4, 10].

Another important characteristic of the humoral response to CE, is that antibody detection, while indicating exposure to *Echinococcus*, may not necessarily correlate to the presence of an established and viable infection. In fact, antibodies can persist in the serum for up to 10 years after hydatid cyst removal [9]. Furthermore, in *Echinococcus*-endemic villages, it has been shown that more than 26% of the inhabitants may have antibodies to HCF antigens, but hydatid cysts were found only in 2% of the examined persons [11-13], showing that the true prevalence of CE infection may not necessarily be correlated to the antibody levels. For this reason, antigen detection may be considered a suitable alternative to confirm the presence of the parasite. The detection of antigens in serum may be less influenced by the hydatid cyst location and may provide a useful tool for the follow-up after the antiparasitic therapy [14]. Unfortunately, circulating CE antigen detection tests are not routinely available yet.

In mice and sheep orally challenged with *E. granulosus* eggs or oncospheres, the earliest anti-oncospheral IgG response can be detected after 11 weeks [2]. Since these antibodies play a major role in the parasite killing, they are considered to be central in the protective immune response against *E. granulosus*. Even if *E. granulosus* induces a strong humoral response, and numerous studies demonstrated the presence of high levels of *E. granulosus*-specific IgG, IgM, and IgE antibodies in patients' sera, none of these antibodies are associated with protection. Since IgG antibodies remain detectable for several years after radical surgery, they cannot be used as immunological markers to evaluate the therapy outcome. However, for a long time the analysis of IgG subclasses has been considered useful in patients follow-up, due to their variation according to the outcome of the disease. Indeed, in progressive human CE, a switch from predominant IgG1 is observed response to IgG4 as the infection proceeds. IgG4 subclass is associated to prolonged chronic infection and can reduce allergic pathology in the host by preventing IgE-mediated degranulation of effector cells. On the contrary, IgG1, IgG2, and IgG3 responses occur predominantly when cysts become infiltrated by inflammatory cells or are destroyed by the host (see above). In accordance with these studies, albendazole-treated patients with a good clinical outcome, showed levels of serum IgG4 antibodies significantly lower than patients poor or non-responders to therapy, whereas a reverse trend was observed for IgG1 antibody levels [2].

During CE infection, the levels of IgG4 and IgE isotypes and the frequent eosinophilia, indicated that the immune response to established *E. granulosus* infection is Th2 dominated. However, immunological studies have shown high *in vitro* production of parasite antigen-driven IL-4, IL-5, IL-6, IL-10, as well as IFN-γ by peripheral blood mononuclear cells (PBMC) from infected patients, suggesting that Th1 and Th2 responses coexist in this disease [15]. Published data support that in *E. granulosus* infection a strong Th2 response is associated with susceptibility to disease (active cyst), whereas a Th1 response is related to protective immunity (inactive cyst). Data obtained in *E. granulosus* experimental infection suggest the hypothesis that early production of IL-10, secreted by B cells in response to non-protein antigens, may favour parasite-survival and the establishment of a polarized type-2 cytokine response [16]. Other studies also suggest that IL-4/IL-10 impair the Th1 protective response and allow parasite survival in the human host [17]. Data underlining the important role of cytokines in the host-parasite relationship come from studies on parasite-driven cytokine production in albendazole-treated patients. PBMC from patients who responded to chemotherapy produced high amounts of IFN-γ whereas PBMC from patients who did not respond produced predominantly IL-4 and IL-10 [18]. Furthermore, T cell lines from *E. granulosus* infected people with an inactive cyst were reported to have a Th1 profile whereas those obtained from patients with active and transitional cysts showed mixed Th1/Th2 and Th0 profiles [19].

Since PBMC from seronegative infected patients were known to produce no parasite antigen-driven IL-5 and scarce IL-4 and IL-10, it has been suggested that during CE infection the seronegativity occurs because host or parasite factors or both avoid the Th2 cell activation, limiting or preventing production of IL-5, the cytokine that has a critical role in immunoglobulin expression [20].

Regulatory Mechanisms to Favour *E. Granulosus* Survival

Helminth parasites are capable to persist for long periods in the adverse environment of the host, determining a chronic infection. They have developed various mechanisms that allow them to perform their physiological functions, and to protect themselves from host immune aggressions by modulating the host immune response [21-23].

The life-span of an *E. granulosus* hydatid cyst can be up to 53 years in humans [24]. Of interest, this chronic infection runs in parallel with detectable immune responses to the parasite. *E. granulosus* uses two main strategies to defend itself from the host humoral and cellular responses, passive escape and immunomodulation. *E. granulosus*, by developing into larval stage, forms a physical barrier to protect the protoscoleces from cellular and molecular mediators of the host immune system. The external wall component LL is resistant to proteolysis and surrounded by a capsule or host-produced fibrous adventitious layer which helps to protect the parasite physically from host immune attacks [1,25,26].

However, an intact LL does not give complete protection to the parasite. The most effective strategy adopted by *E. granulosus* to survive in host tissues is modulation/suppression of the host immune response. To limit the impact of the host response, the helminth actively interacts with the host immune system [27]. Indeed, the metacestode of *E. granulosus* secretes several molecules with immunomodulatory properties, favoring the immune evasion and survival in the host [4,28]. Every parasite-derived molecule has to pass the metacestode LL to reach the host microenvironment [29]. These molecules can interfere with innate and adaptive immunity, stimulate regulatory responses and cause cell death, as summarized in Table **1**.

Table 1: Immunomodulant antigens from *Echinococcus granulosus*. An overview of selective *Echinococcus granulosus*-derived products with immunomodulatory activity

E. granulosus-Derived Products	Impact on Innate Immunity	Impact on Adaptive Immunity
Laminated layer	Poor activation of complement; anti-inflammatory and/or suppressive signal induction on innate immune cells.	Stimulation of T-independent antibody responses; induction of antigen-specific regulatory cells.
Hydatid Cyst Fluid	Chemotaxis inhibition and reduction of H_2O_2 production in neutrophils; impaired differentiation of monocytes in dendritic cells (DCs); polarization of immature DC differentiation towards Th0/Th1/Th2 priming.	Proliferation of mixed Th1/Th2 and Th0 cells; induction of lymphocyte apoptosis.
Antigen B	Chemotaxis inhibition and reduction of H_2O_2 production in neutrophils; impaired differentiation of monocytes in DCs; polarization of immature DC differentiation towards an anti-inflammatory phenotype.	Stimulation of a Th2 response; induction of IgG4 production by B lymphocytes.
Elongation factor 1β/δ	Unknown	Stimulation of a Th2 response; induction of IgG4 and IgE production by B lymphocytes.

Table 1: contd....

Cyclophilin	Unknown	Stimulation of a Th2 response; induction of IgG4 and IgE production by B lymphocytes.
Echinococcus granulosus heat shock protein 70	Unknown	Induction of IgE and IL-4 production; induction of regulatory T cells.
Echinococcus granulosus Tegumental antigen	Chemotaxis inhibition and reduction of H_2O_2 production in neutrophils.	Induction of IL-4 and IgG4 production.
Echinococcus granulosus Thioredoxin peroxidase	Unknown	Induction of IgG1 and IgG4 production by B lymphocytes.
Eg19	Unknown	Induction of IgG1 and IgG4 production by B lymphocytes.

Molecules Implicated in Immunomodulatory Mechanisms that Alter Normal Host-Immune System

Since the different developmental stages of the parasite express different antigens, the human host responses are independent from the invading oncosphere, the metacestode in transformation from the oncosphere, and the mature metacestode [28]. The immune response to CE infection is characterized by two phases: an "establishment" phase, in which the parasite is more susceptible to host effector mechanisms, and an "established metacestode (hydatid cyst)" phase in which the disease becomes chronic. *E. granulosus* surface molecules as well as excretory/secretory products are important key players. The LL undertakes innumerable interactions with the host immune system, and shapes the immune responses by down-regulating inflammation [30]. This parasite-derived structure has few T-cell epitopes and induces a non-inflammatory innate response and an adaptive response characterized by low-avidity antibodies specific for α-galactose [30]. The innate immune system considers the LL as a non-threatening material, that induces adaptive regulatory responses, and, in opposition to hydatid cyst fluid and protoscoleces, induces a weak activation of complement cascade, due to the absorbance of Complement inhibitor factor H on LL surface [31-34]. *E. granulosus* LL has adapted to prevent the entire activation of complement, while permitting diminished deposition of complement early components. This causes the opsonization of the LL by the C3 inactivation fragment iC3b, a situation that conditions dendritic cells (DCs) towards tolerogenic phenotypes [35]. Interestingly, the LL carbohydrates interact with the liver-specific Kupffer cell receptor and hepatocyte asialoglycoprotein receptor, able to recognize galactose-terminated glycans which are very abundant in the LL. Evidence exists that the LL does not contain agonists for Toll-like receptors (TLRs), thus being unable to promote DC maturation. Furthermore, *E. granulosus* LL extracts do not induce nitric oxide from macrophages [36], which is toxic for the parasite, and inhibit nitric oxide production by macrophages in response to lipopolysaccharide (LPS) or IFN-γ [36,37]. So the LL, with its peculiar structure, exerts a regulatory role on innate immune cells and can influence the adaptive immunity promoting regulatory, anti-inflammatory mechanisms. LL components may also influence T-cell responses by inducing innate cells to produce polarizing or suppressive signals. The liver, which represents the primary localization for *Echinococcus* larvae, is now considered as an immune organ able to induce regulatory T cell responses [38]. It has been reported that the galactose-specific receptors present in this organ induce tolerance towards allogeneic desialylated cells [39]. LL carbohydrates can be an adaptation of the parasite to interact with liver receptors able to present parasite antigens in a tolerogenic way. Even when metacestodes are lodged in other organs the tolerance induced in the liver by LL-derived mucin aggregates can impact on these infected sites [38].

Extensive studies on immune response and immune modulation in *E. granulosus* infection have focused on HCF that contains the main antigens for diagnostic assays [40]. HCF can have a direct influence on the main cellular effectors of host immune response, *i.e.* DCs and T lymphocytes. *E. granulosus* HCF is able to modulate the differentiation of DCs and their cytokine production [41]. We have demonstrated that it impairs the differentiation of immature DCs from monocyte precursors thus making DCs unable to mature in response to LPS [42]. HCF also impacts on adaptive immunity by promoting apoptosis of human lymphocytes [43].

The main parasitic antigens present in HCF are Ag5 and AgB [44,45]. These antigens were initially used for immunodiagnosis of CE, and only later evaluated for their function in the host-parasite relationship. Native Ag5, a 400 kDa thermolabile glycoprotein, generates two subunits at 55 and 65′ kDa in sodium-dodecyl-sulphate-polyacrylamide gel electrophoresis (SDS-PAGE) under non reducing conditions, and two subunits at 38/39 and 22/24 kDa under reducing conditions [46,47]. Although the biological function of Ag5 is unknown, its high concentration in HCF suggests an important role in the metacestode development. The 38/39 kDa component of Ag5, which contains phosphorylcholine epitopes, may be the cause of many non-specific reactions with sera from patients infected with nematodes, cestodes and trematodes [46,48]. Ag5 has been largely applied in the serodiagnosis of human CE, mostly in immunoelectrophoresis assays, where produced a precipitation line (arc 5) [40]. AgB, which represents as much as 10% of HCF content, is a 160 kDa thermostable lipoprotein that generates three subunits at 8/12, 16, and 20/24 kDa in SDS-PAGE under reducing and nonreducing conditions [48-50]. This antigen is localized in the protoscolex tegument and germinal membrane of the metacestode and secreted into the cyst fluid [51,52]. The oligomeric organization of AgB has been investigated in detail by González et al. [53], who reported at least two components in the 8 kDa subunit, which forms the building pieces of the higher molecular weight subunits. Evidence exists of an important role of this antigen in evasion mechanisms from the early innate host immune response [54]. AgB can modulate both innate and adaptive host immunity to the advantage of the parasite. The 12 kDa subunit of AgB actively modulates innate immune cell infiltration. This subunit is a serine protease inhibitor able to inhibit human neutrophil chemotaxis, leaving random migration and oxidative metabolism unaltered [49, 54]. Also, AgB is involved in switching the Th1/Th2 cytokine ratio towards a predominant Th2 polarization which is related to chronic CE disease [49,55,56]. PBMC of infected people stimulated with AgB raised high levels of IL-4 and IL-13, with low IFN-γ and no IL-12, indicating the presence of a Th2 polarization [49]. Our additional studies offered a rationale for this polarization with the demonstration that AgB suppresses IL-12p70 production by immature DCs and induces the immunoregulatory cytokine IL-10. Furthermore AgB impairs the increase of IL-12p70 but not of IL-6 by DCs in response to LPS, thus providing further evidence to the ability of AgB to actively modulate DC response towards a Th2 outcome [42]. In line with a Th2 polarization, a qualitative analysis of specific IgG isotype responses identified IgG4 as the predominant AgB-induced isotype [56].

Molecular and proteomic studies designed to identify new antigens and/or immunomodulatory molecules in CE, determined numerous other proteins which contribute, in a different way, to the final orientation of the host immune response.

Two *E. granulosus*-derived immunomodulatory molecules are *E. granulosus* elongation factor (EgEF)-1 β/δ and cyclophilin (EA21). Both are able to induce a polarization of T lymphocytes towards a Th2 response. It has been demonstrated that the IgE reactivity to EgEF-1 β/δ is significantly higher in infected people with allergic manifestations than in those without them [57]. Interestingly, EgEF-1 β/δ is a conserved constitutive protein located predominantly in the endoplasmic reticulum, that continues to be discharged into the HCF after protoscoleces degeneration. Accordingly, the percentage of antibodies specific for this protein was higher in *E. granulosus* infected people with inactive cysts than in those with active cysts [57,58]. EA21 is a protein expressed in protoscoleces and hydatid fluid. A study conducted in CE patients with and without allergic manifestations demonstrated the presence of IgE specific for *E. granulosus* cyclophilin in 80% of those with allergic manifestations [59]. Of note, 63% of CE patients without allergic symptoms showed IgG4 antibodies specific for this antigen [59]. These results indicate that in chronic disease a preferential Th2 IgE-mediated immune response is promoted by EA21, and suggest that IgG4 may prevent pathogenic allergic processes, in CE and in other parasitic diseases, decreasing severe clinical manifestations in the host.

E. granulosus Heat Shock Protein 70 (Eg2HSP70) is another antigenic molecule able to induce both B and T cell responses in the host. Total IgG, IgG4 and IgE specific for this protein were detected in an elevated percentage of patients' sera [60]. Furthermore, patients' PBMC stimulated with Eg2HSP70 produced high levels of Th1 (IFN-γ and TNF-α) and Th2 (IL-4 and IL-10) cytokines. In particular, this antigen stimulated high IL-4 levels only in PBMC from CE patients with allergic manifestations. Allergen-induced IgE synthesis depends on Th2 cells that interact with B cells promoting the production of this class of immunoglobulins. In CE, different antigens influence the Th1/Th2 balance by stimulating the production of IL-4, IL-10 and IL-13 and promoting a highly Th2-polarized microenvironment. Eg2HSP70 probably stimulates IgE production and elicits IL-4 secretion not directly, but by strengthening the already established Th2 polarization [60]. Also, recently HSP70 from other helminths was reported to increase IL-10 production and elicit regulatory T cells through the activation of TLR4 [61].

E. granulosus tegumental antigen (EgTeg) is a protein located in the protoscolex tegument and on the cyst wall germinal layer, and it is involved in immune escape. It inhibits polymorphonuclear cell chemotaxis and induces high percentages of T lymphocytes producing more IL-4 than IFN-γ [62]. The movement of neutrophils from the blood to tissue inflammatory sites is a peculiarity of the innate immunity and plays a crucial role in the defense against invading microorganisms and tissue damage. Thus, by modulating innate immune cell infiltration and, similarly to AgB, by promoting a preferential Th2 response, it contributes to build the anti-inflammatory environment which supports parasite survival [62].

An unclear role in immunomodulation is played by *E. granulosus* thioredoxin peroxidase (EgTPx) [63] and by Eg19 [64]. To elicit the host immune response, these molecules located in the protoscoleces are actively secreted in HCF. The humoral response to these antigen is characterized by the production of both IgG1 and IgG4 antibodies. The percentage of EgTPx-specific IgG4 serum positivity was significantly higher in patients with active than in those with inactive disease, and Eg19-specific antibodies were detected exclusively in sera from patients with active cysts, indicating these parasite-derived molecules as possible markers of disease status. It is well known that, upon *E. granulosus* infection, the host-parasite interaction can be influenced by cyst type [65]. Our data, showing that EgTPx- and Eg19-specific immune responses are not related to protection, question the role of anti-EgTPx and anti-Eg19 antibodies in *E. granulosus* infection, particularly in immune evasion mechanisms.

Immune Modulation: New Tools to Develop CE Control Programs

Despite large efforts put into its control, echinococcosis still represents a worldwide important disease. In some geographical areas, CE caused by *E. granulosus* is a re-emerging disorder. Although the leading role of ultrasound and benzoimidazole carbamates in the diagnosis and treatment of CE, a deeper understanding of the immunological events that occur during cyst development could be useful to set up new therapeutic strategies to achieve the complete healing of infection [44]. Considerable attempts have been made in Australia and New Zealand to develop protective vaccines for livestock against infections with the metacestode stage of taeniid cestodes [66], and to characterize protective immune responses in *E. granulosus* intermediate hosts. Many studies demonstrated that *E. granulosus* infection elicits an immune response that confers resistance to re-infection, and protection against an initial infection can be achieved in naive hosts by immunization with parasite extracts [1]. In particular, the immune response during metacestode infection causes destruction of incoming oncospheres through antibody-dependent, complement-mediated lysis. Antibodies are critical immune mediators against taeniid metacestodes, with IgG1, IgG2a, IgG2b, and IgE having an important major role in oncosphere killing, although the implication of other mechanisms cannot be excluded [1,67-73]. In particular, it has been *in vitro* demonstrated that sera from infected or actively immunized hosts are able to kill activated oncospheres [49,54,74-76]. Studies aimed to elucidate protective immune responses against *E. granulosus* identified some oncosphere antigens able to confer protection to vaccinated hosts [77-79]. *E. granulosus*-specific antibodies have provided a powerful tool to screen cDNA libraries and to identify genes encoding for specific antigens useful to develop effective recombinant vaccines [73]. Controlled studies performed in sheep have provided evidence that vaccination with EG95, a recombinant oncospheral *E. granulosus* antigen, leads to protection by a significant reduction of the cyst numbers in vaccinated animals [66,80-84]. A high level of immunity persists for 6 months in the absence of reinfection, and pregnant ewes vaccinated before lambing transfer high levels of protective antibodies to their offspring [85]. The mechanism of protection has been correlated with the presence of antibodies and with the complement-mediated lysis of the incoming oncospheres [70]. Another possible candidate antigen useful for *E. granulosus*-specific vaccine development is the recombinant preparation of 14-3-3 protein [86]. Mice vaccinated with this protein and challenged with protoscoleces showed significant protective immunity of about 80%, characterized by high serum levels of specific IgG1 and IgG2a.

The role played in host protection by cell-mediated responses against *E. granulosus* is unknown. However, indirect evidence exists that they should be important. *In vitro* experiments have demonstrated that neutrophils in combination with antibodies can kill *E. granulosus* oncospheres [87], indicating the involvement of antibody-dependent cell-mediated cytotoxicity responses. Furthermore, parasite-specific T cell lines obtained from patients at different clinical stages of disease may allow to identify Th1 protective epitopes on *Echinococcus* antigens, useful for vaccine development [19]. There is scarce information on cell-mediated immune response generated by *E. granulosus* recombinant vaccines. The secondary *E. granulosus* hydatid cyst mass in mice immunized with the recombinant *E. granulosus*-derived protein EG95 was reduced by nearly 93%, and this result was associated with elevated levels of IL-2, IFN-γ and TNF-α, and decreased levels of IL-4. Furthermore, splenocytes obtained from mice immunized with 14-3-3 protein secreted high levels of IFN-γ and IL-2. These data in vaccine models suggest that Th1 responses play a major protective role against challenge infection [86,88]. It is clear that host immunity plays a major role in the natural host-parasite relationship in CE, and it is associated to the presence of protective antibodies. However, although some protective immune responses against *E. granulosus* infection, such as antibodies responses, have been elucidated, the precise mechanisms involved in protection need to be better clarified. Understanding these mechanisms will benefit the research aimed to *E. granulosus* vaccine development [1].

CONCLUSION

Presently there is an increased request of alternatives to chemicals for managing parasitic diseases. The control of CE by vaccination holds great promises. Researches directed towards a better knowledge of the complex host-parasite relationship might one day contribute to make treatment more efficacious. A number of molecules of *E. granulosus* are able to modulate the host immune response and to favour its survival (Fig. **6**). New information can derive from the study of patients' immune status to unravel the underlying host protective responses [89]. Although the extensive studies on the immune responses during *E. granulosus* infection, the precise immunological mechanisms involved in protection need a better elucidation to improve research on vaccines and the control of CE.

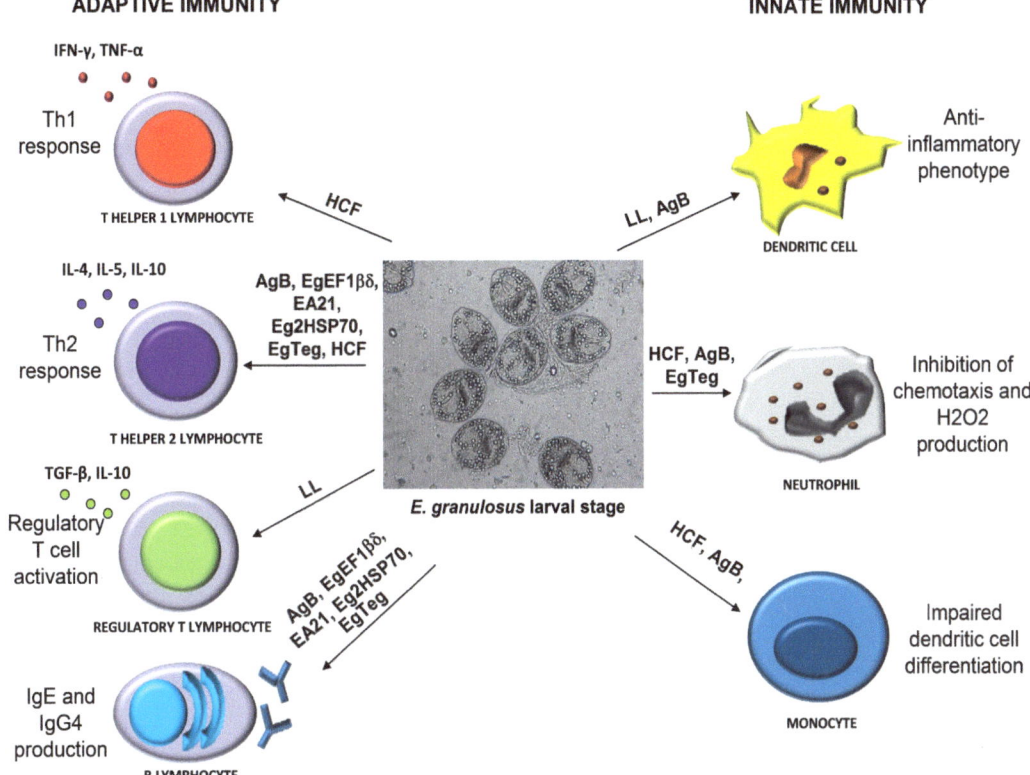

Figure 6: *Echinococcus granulosus* produces different molecules able to modulate the host immune response and favour parasite survival. In particular, the larval stage of the parasite (hydatid cyst), secretes proteins inhibiting neutrophil chemotaxis, promoting the development of an anti-inflammatory phenotype of dendritic cells, and activating a preferential Th2 response, thus inhibiting the Th1 pro-inflammatory mechanisms associated to the presence of inactive cyst in human intermediate host. HCF: hydatid cyst fluid; AgB: antigen B; EgEF-1β/δ: *E. granulosus* elongation factor 1 β/δ; EA21: cyclophilin; Eg2HSP70: *E. granulosus* Heat Shock Protein 70; EgTeg: *E. granulosus* tegumental antigen; LL: laminated layer.

ACKNOWLEDGEMENT

We thank Dr. Adriano Casulli who provided Figs. **2** and **4**, and Dr. E. Brunetti who provided Fig. **5**.

CONFLICT OF INTEREST

The author(s) confirm that this chapter contents have no conflict of interest.

REFERENCES

[1] Zhang W, Ross AG and McManus DP. Mechanisms of immunity in hydatid disease: implications for vaccine development. J Immunol 2008; 181: 6679-85.

[2] Siracusano A, Delunardo F, Teggi A, Ortona E. Host-parasite relationship in cystic echinococcosis: an evolving story. Clin Dev Immunol 2012; 2012: 1-12.

[3] Mastrandrea S, Stegel G, Piseddu T, Ledda S, Masala G. A retrospective study on burden of human echinococcosis based on Hospital Discharge Records from 2001 to 2009 in Sardinia. Acta Trop 2012; 123: 184-9.

[4] Zhang W, Wen H, Li J, Lin R, McManus DP. Immunology and immunodiagnosis of cystic echinococcosis: an update. Clin Dev Immunol 2012; 2012: 101895.

[5] McManus DP, Thompson RC. Molecular epidemiology of cystic echinococcosis. Parasitology 2003; 127 Suppl: S37-51.

[6] Thompson RC, McManus DP. Towards a taxonomic revision of the genus *Echinococcus*. Trends Parasitol 2002; 18: 452-7.

[7] Díaz A, Casaravilla C, Irigoín F, Lin G, Previato JO, Ferreira F. Understanding the laminated layer of larval *Echinococcus* I: structure. Trends Parasitol 2011; 27: 204-13.

[8] Pawlowski ZS, Eckert J, Vuitton DA. A public health problem of global concern. In: Eckert J, Gemmel MA, Meslin FX, Pawlowski ZS, Eds. WHO/OIE Manual on Echinococcosis in Humans and Animals. 2001; pp. 20–71.

[9] Li J, Zhang WB, McManus DP. Recombinant antigens for immunodiagnosis of cystic echinococcosis. Biol Proced Online 2004; 6: 67-77.

[10] Zhang W, McManus DP. Recent advances in the immunology and diagnosis of echinococcosis. FEMS Immunol Med Microbiol 2006; 47: 24–41.

[11] Gavidia, CM, Gonzalez AE, Zhang W, McManus DP, Lopera L, Ninaquispe B, Garcia HH, Rodríguez S, Verastegui M, Calderon C, Pan WK, Gilman RH. Diagnosis of cystic echinococcosis, central Peruvian Highlands. Emerg Infect Dis 2008; 14: 260-6.

[12] Craig PS, Zeyhle E, Romig T. Hydatid disease: research and control in Turkana. II. The role of immunological techniques for the diagnosis of hydatid disease. Trans R Soc Trop Med Hyg 1986; 80: 183-92.

[13] Chai J, Sultan Y, Wei M. An investigation on the epidemiologic baseline of hydatid disease in Xinjiang, China. I. A sero-epidemiological survey of human hydatidosis. End Dis Bull 1989; 4: 1–8.

[14] Craig PS, Nelson GS. The detection of circulating antigen in human hydatid disease. Ann Trop Med Parasitol 1984; 78: 219-27.

[15] Riganò R, Profumo E, Di Felice G, Ortona E, Teggi A, Siracusano A. *In vitro* production of cytokines by peripheral blood mononuclear cells from hydatic patients. Clin Exp Immunol 1995; 99: 433-9.

[16] Baz A, Ettlin GM, Dematteis S. Complexity and function of cytokine responses in experimental infection by *Echinococcus granulosus*. Immunobiology 2006; 211: 3-9.

[17] Amri M, Mezioug D, Touil-Boukoffa C. Involvement of IL-10 and IL-4 in evasion strategies of *Echinococcus granulosus* to host immune response. Eur Cytokine Netw 2009; 20: 63-8.

[18] Riganò R, Profumo E, Ioppolo S, Notargiacomo S, Ortona E, Teggi A, Siracusano A. Immunological markers indicating the effectiveness of pharmacological treatment in human hydatid disease. Clin Exp Immunol 1995; 102: 281-5.

[19] Riganò R, Buttari B, De Falco E, Profumo E, Ortona E, Margutti P, Scottà C, Teggi A, Siracusano A. *Echinococcus granulosus*-specific T-cell lines derived from patients at various clinical stages of cystic echinococcosis. Parasite Immunol 2004; 26: 45-52.

[20] Riganò R, Profumo E, Ioppolo S, Notargiacomo S, Teggi A, Siracusano A. Cytokine patterns in seropositive and seronegative patients with *Echinococcus granulosus* infection. Immunol Lett 1998; 64: 5-8.

[21] Maizels RM, Yazdanbakhsh M. Immune regulation by helminth parasites: cellular and molecular mechanisms. Nat Rev Immunol 2003; 3: 733–44.

[22] Rosenzvit MC, Camicia F, Kamenetzky L, Muzulin PM, Gutierrez AM. Identification and intra-specific variability analysis of secreted and membrane-bound proteins from *Echinococcus granulosus*. Parasitol Int 2006; 55: S63–7.

[23] Siracusano A, Margutti P, Delunardo F, Profumo E, Riganò R, Buttari B, Teggi A, Ortona E. Molecular cross-talk in host-parasite relationships: the intriguing immunomodulatory role of *Echinococcus* antigen B in cystic echinococcosis. Int J Parasitol 2008; 38: 1371-6.

[24] Spruance SL. Latent period of 53 years in a case of hydatid cyst disease. Arch Intern Med 1974; 134: 741-2.

[25] Slais J, and Vanek M. Tissue reaction to spherical and lobular hydatid cysts of *Echinococcus granulosus* (Batsch, 1786). Folia Parasitol 1980; 27: 135–43.

[26] Richards KS, Arme C, and Bridges JF. *Echinococcus granulosus* equinus: an ultrastructural study of murine tissue response to hydatid cysts. Parasitology 1983; 86: 407–17.

[27] Zhang W, Li J, McManus DP. Concepts in immunology and diagnosis of hydatid disease. Clin Microbiol Rev 2003; 16: 18–36.

[28] Siracusano A, Delunardo F, Teggi A, Ortona E. Cystic echinococcosis: aspects of immune response, immunopathogenesis and immune evasion from the human host. Endocr Metab Immune Disord Drug Targets 2012; 12: 16-23.

[29] Vuitton DA, Gottstein B. *Echinococcus* multilocularis and its intermediate host: a model of parasite-host interplay. J Biomed Biotechnol 2010; 2010: 923193.

[30] Diaz A, Casaravilla C, Allen JE, Sim RB and Ferreira AM. Understanding the laminated layer of larval *Echinococcus* II: immunology. Trends Parasitol 2011; 27: 263-72.

[31] Diaz A and Allen JE. Mapping immune response profiles: the emerging scenario from helminth immunology. Eur J Immunol 2007; 37: 3319–26.

[32] Ferreira AM, Irigoín F, Breijo M, Sim RB, Diáz A. How *Echinococcus granulosus* deals with complement. Parasitol Today 2000; 16: 168–72.

[33] Irigoín F, Würzner R, Sim RB, Ferreira AM. Comparison of complement activation *in vitro* by different *Echinococcus granulosus* extracts. Parasite Immunol 1996; 18: 371–5.

[34] Díaz A, Ferreira A, Sim RB. Complement evasion by *Echinococcus granulosus*: sequestration of host factor H in the hydatid cyst wall. J Immunol 1997; 158: 3779–86.

[35] Verbovetski I, Bychkov H, Trahtemberg U, Shapira I, Hareuveni M, Ben-Tal O, Kutikov I, Gill O, Mevorach D. Opsonization of apoptotic cells by autologous iC3b facilitates clearance by immature dendritic cells, down-regulates DR and CD86, and up-regulates CC chemokine receptor 7. J Exp Med 2002; 196: 1553–61.

[36] Andrade MA, Siles-Lucas M, Espinoza E, Pérez Arellano JL, Gottstein B, Muro A. *Echinococcus multilocularis* laminated layer components and the E14t 14-3-3 recombinant

protein decrease NO production by activated rat macrophages *in vitro*. Nitric Oxide 2004; 10: 150–5.

[37] Steers NJ, Rogan MT, Heath S. In-vitro susceptibility of hydatid cysts of *Echinococcus granulosus* to nitric oxide and the effect of the laminated layer on nitric oxide production. Parasite Immunol 2001; 23: 411–7.

[38] Carambia A and Herkel J. CD4 T cells in hepatic immune tolerance. J Autoimmun 2010; 34: 23–8.

[39] Suda T, Sano S, Hori S, Azuma T, Tateishi N, Hamaoka T, Fujiwara H. Prevention of suppression of alloreactive capacity following intravenous injection of neuraminidase-treated allogeneic cells by co-injection of agents competing for asialoglycoprotein receptor. Reg Immunol 1988; 1: 24–31.

[40] Carmena D, Benito A, Eraso E. Antigens for the immunodiagnosis of *Echinococcus granulosus* infection: an update. Acta Trop 2006; 98: 74–86.

[41] Kanan JH, Chain BM. Modulation of dendritic cell differentiation and cytokine secretion by the hydatid cyst fluid of *Echinococcus granulosus*. Immunology 2006; 118: 271–8.

[42] Riganò R, Buttari B, Profumo E, Ortona E, Delunardo F, Margutti P, Mattei V, Teggi A, Sorice M, Siracusano A. *Echinococcus granulosus* antigen B impairs human dendritic cell differentiation and polarizes immature dendritic cell maturation towards a Th2 cell response. Infect Immun 2007; 75: 1667–78.

[43] Mokhtari Amirmajdi M, Sankian M, Eftekharzadeh Mashhadi I, Varasteh A, Vahedi F, Sadrizadeh A, Spotin A. Apoptosis of human lymphocytes after exposure to hydatid fluid. Iran J Parasitol 2011; 6: 9-16.

[44] Siracusano A, Teggi A, Ortona E. Human cystic echinococcosis: old problems and new perspectives. Interdiscip Perspect Infect Dis 2009; 2009: 474368.

[45] Lightowlers MW, Liu DY, Haralambous A, Rickard MD. Subunit composition and specificity of the major cyst fluid antigens of *Echinococcus granulosus*. Mol Biochem Parasitol 1989; 37: 171-82.

[46] Capron A, Vernes A, and Biguet J. Le diagnostic immune-electrophoretique de l'hydatidose. In: SIMEP, Eds. Le Kyste Hydatique du Foie. Lyon, France, 1967; pp. 20–7.

[47] Yarzabal LA, Dupas H, Bout D. *Echinococcus granulosus*: the distribution of hydatid fluid antigens in the tissues of the larval stage. II. Localization of the thermostable lipoprotein of parasitic origin (antigen B). Exp Parasitol 1977; 42: 115–20.

[48] Shepherd JC, McManus DP. Specific and cross-reactive antigens of *Echinococcus granulosus* hydatid cyst fluid. Mol Biochem Parasitol 1987; 25: 143-54.

[49] Riganò R, Profumo E, Bruschi F, Carulli G, Azzarà A, Ioppolo S, Buttari B, Ortona E, Margutti P, Teggi A, Siracusano A. Modulation of human immune response by *Echinococcus granulosus* antigen B and its possible role in evading host defenses. Infect Immun 2001; 69: 288–96.

[50] Maddison SE, Slemenda SB, Schantz PM, Fried JA, Wilson M, Tsang VC. A specific diagnostic antigen of *Echinococcus granulosus* with an apparent molecular weight of 8kDa. Am J Trop Med Hyg 1989; 40: 377-83.

[51] Rickard M D, Davies C, Bout DT, and Smith JD. Immunohistological localization of two hydatid antigens (antigen 5 and antigen B) in the cyst wall, brood capsules and protoscoleces of *Echinococcus granulosus* (ovine and equine) and E. multilocularis using immunoperoxidase methods. J Helminthol 1977; 51: 359–64.

[52] Sanchez F, March F, Mercader M, Coll P, Munoz C, and Prats G. Immunochemical localization of major hydatid fluid antigens in protoscoleces and cysts of *Echinococcus granulosus* from human origin. Parasite Immunol 1991; 13: 583–92.

[53] González G, Nieto A, Fernández C, Orn A, Wernstedt C, Hellman U. Two different 8 kDa monomers are involved in the oligomeric organization of the native *Echinococcus granulosus* antigen B. Parasite Immunol 1996; 18: 587–96.

[54] Shepherd JC, Aitken A, McManus DP. A protein secreted *in vivo* by *Echinococcus granulosus* inhibits elastase activity and neutrophil chemotaxis. Mol Biochem Parasitol 1991; 44: 81-90.

[55] Virginio VG, Taroco L, Ramos AL, Ferreira AM, Zaha A, Ferreira HB, Hernández A. Effects of protoscoleces and AgB from *Echinococcus granulosus* on human neutrophils: possible implications on the parasite's immune evasion mechanisms. Parasitol Res 2007; 100: 935-42.

[56] Ioppolo S, Notargiacomo S, Profumo E, Franchi C, Ortona E, Rigano R, Siracusano A. Immunological responses to antigen B from *Echinococcus granulosus* cyst fluid in hydatid patients. Parasite Immunol 1996; 18: 571-8.

[57] Ortona E, Margutti P, Vaccari S, Riganò R, Profumo E, Buttari B, Chersi A, Teggi A, Siracusano A. Elongation factor 1 â/ä of *Echinococcus granulosus* and allergic manifestations in human cystic echinococcosis. Clin Exp Immunol 2001; 125: 110-6.

[58] Margutti P, Ortona E, Vaccari S, Barca S, Riganò R, Teggi A, Muhschlegel F, Frosch M, Siracusano A. Cloning and expression of a cDNA encoding an elongation factor 1β/δ protein from *Echinococcus granulosus* with immunogenic activity. Parasite Immunol 1999; 21: 485-92.

[59] Ortona E, Vaccari S, Margutti P, Delunardo F, Rigano R, Profumo E, Buttari B, Rasool O, Teggi A, Siracusano A. Immunological characterization of *Echinococcus granulosus* cyclophilin, an allergen reactive with IgE and IgG4 from patients with cystic echinococcosis. Clin Exp Immunol 2002; 128: 124-30.

[60] Ortona E, Margutti P, Delunardo F, Vaccari S, Riganò R, Profumo E, Buttari B, Teggi A, Siracusano A. Molecular and immunological characterization of the C-terminal region of a new *Echinococcus granulosus* Heat Shock Protein 70. Parasite Immunol 2003; 25: 119-26.

[61] Ludwig-Portugall I, Layland LE. TLRs, Treg, and B cells, an interplay of regulation during helminth infection. Front Immunol 2012; 3: 8.

[62] Ortona E, Margutti P, Delunardo F, Nobili V, Profumo E, Riganò R, Buttari B, Carulli G, Azzarà A, Teggi A, Bruschi F, Siracusano A. Screening of an *Echinococcus granulosus* cDNA library with IgG4 from patients with cystic echinococcosis identifies a new tegumental protein involved in the immune escape. Clin Exp Immunol 2005; 142: 528-38.

[63] Margutti P, Ortona E, Delunardo F, Tagliani A, Profumo E, Riganò R, Buttari B, Teggi A, Siracusano A. Thioredoxin peroxidase from *Echinococcus granulosus*: a candidate to extend the antigenic panel for the immunodiagnosis of human cystic echinococcosis. Diagn Microbiol Infect Dis 2008; 60: 279-85.

[64] Delunardo F, Ortona E, Margutti P, Perdicchio M, Vacirca D, Teggi A, Sorice M, Siracusano A. Identification of a novel 19 kDa *Echinococcus granulosus* antigen. Acta Trop 2010; 113: 42-7.

[65] Rogan MT, Hai WY, Richardson R, Zeyhle E, Craig PS. Hydatid cysts: does every picture tell a story? Trends Parasitol 2006; 22: 431–8.

[66] Eckert J, Deplazes P. Biological, epidemiological, and clinical aspects of Echinococcosis, a zoonosis of increasing concern. Clin Microbiol Rev 2004; 17: 107-35.

[67] Lightowlers MW, Colebrook AL, Gauci CG, Gauci SM, Kyngdon CT, Monkhouse JL, Vallejo Rodriquez C, Read AJ, Rolfe RA, Sato C. Vaccination against cestode parasites: anti-helminth vaccines that work and why. Vet Parasitol 2003; 115: 83–123.

[68] Dempster RP, Harrison GB. Maternal transfer of protection from *Echinococcus granulosus* infection in sheep. Res Vet Sci 1995; 58: 197–202.

[69] Dempster RP, Harrison GB, Berridge MV, Heath DD. *Echinococcus granulosus*: use of an intermediate host mouse model to evaluate sources of protective antigens and a role for antibody in the immune response. Int J Parasitol 1992; 22: 435–41.

[70] Heath DD, Holcman B, Shaw RJ. *Echinococcus granulosus*: the mechanism of oncosphere lysis by sheep complement and antibody. Int J Parasitol 1994; 24: 929–35.

[71] Heath DD, Parmeter SN, Osborn PJ, Lawrence SB. Resistance to *Echinococcus granulosus* infection in lambs. J Parasitol 1981; 67: 797–9.

[72] Herd RP. The cestocidal effect of complement in normal and immune sera *in vitro*. Parasitology 1976; 72: 325–34.

[73] Lightowlers MW. Cestode vaccines: origins, current status and future prospects. Parasitology 2006; 133 (Suppl.): S27–42.

[74] Alkarmi T, Behbehani K. *Echinococcus* multilocularis: inhibition of murine neutrophil and macrophage chemotaxis. Exp Parasitol 1989; 69: 16–22.

[75] Kizaki T, Ishige M, Bingyan W, Day NK, Good RA, and Onoe K. Generation of CD8+ suppressor T cells by protoscoleces of *Echinococcus* multilocularis *in vitro*. Immunology 1993; 79: 412–7.

[76] Kizaki T, Kobayashi S, Ogasawara K, Day N K, Good RA, and Onoe K. Immune suppression induced by protoscoleces of *Echinococcus* multilocularis in mice. Evidence for the presence of CD8dull suppressor cells in spleens of mice intraperitoneally infected with E. multilocularis. J Immunol 1991; 147: 1659–66.

[77] Heath DD, Lawrence SB. Antigenic polypeptides of *Echinococcus granulosus* oncospheres and definition of protective molecules. Parasite Immunol 1996; 18: 347–57.

[78] Woollard DJ, Heath DD, Lightowlers MW. Assessment of protective immune responses against hydatid disease in sheep by immunization with synthetic peptide antigens. Parasitology 2000; 121: 145–53.

[79] Woollard DJ, Gauci CG, Heath DD, Lightowlers MW. Protection against hydatid disease induced with the EG95 vaccine is associated with conformational epitopes. Vaccine 2000; 19: 498–507.

[80] Heath DD, Jensen O, Lightowlers MW. Progress in control of hydatidosis using vaccination—a review of formulation and delivery of the vaccine and recommendations for practical use in control programmes. Acta Trop 2003; 85: 133-43.

[81] Heath DD, Pusheng Q, Zhuangzhi Z, Jincheng W, Jinglan F, Lightowlers MW. Role of immunization of the intermediate host in hydatid disease control. Arch Int Hidatid 1999; 33: 14–6.

[82] Jensen O. Immunizacion ovina: factibilidad te´cnica en Argentina. Arch Int Hidatid 1999; 33: 17–9.

[83] Lightowlers MW. Vaccines for control of cysticercosis and hydatidosis, In Craig P and Pawlowski Z Eds. Cestode zoononoses: echinococcosis and cysticercosis, an emergent and global problem. IOS Press, 2002; pp. 381–91.

[84] Lightowlers MW, Heath DD, Jensen O, Fernandez E, Iriarte JA. Intermediate host vaccination and prospects for a human vaccine. Arch Int Hidatid 1999; 33: 13–4.

[85] Heath DD, Lightowlers MW. Vaccination on hydatidology—state of the art. Arch Int Hidatid 1997; 33: 14–6.

[86] Li ZJ, Wang YN, Wang Q, Zhao W. *Echinococcus granulosus* 14-3-3 protein: a potential vaccine candidate against challenge with *Echinococcus granulosus* in mice. Biomed Environ Sci 2012; 25: 352-8.

[87] Rogan MT, Craig PS, Zehyle E, Masinde G, Wen H, Zhou P. *In vitro* killing of taeniid oncospheres, mediated by human sera from hydatid endemic areas. Acta Trop 1992; 51: 291–6.

[88] Li WG, Wang H, Zhu YM. Change of splenocyte lymphokines in mice induced by recombinant BCG-Eg95 vaccine against *Echinococcus granulosus* (in Chinese). Zhongguo Ji Sheng Chong Xue Yu Ji Sheng Chong Bing Za Zhi (Chin J Parasitol Parasitic Dis) 2007; 25: 109–13.

[89] Siracusano A, Margutti P, Delunardo F, Profumo E, Riganò R, Buttari B, Teggi A, Ortona E. Molecular cross-talk in host-parasite relationships: the intriguing immunomodulatory role of *Echinococcus* antigen B in cystic echinococcosis. Int J Parasitol 2008; 38: 1371-6.

Chapter 5: The Immunobiology of Urogenital Schistosomiasis

CHAPTER 5

The Immunobiology of Urogenital Schistosomiasis

Luke F. Pennington[1,*] and Michael H. Hsieh[1,2]

[1]Stanford Immunology, Stanford University, Stanford, California, USA and [2]Department of Urology, Stanford University, Stanford, California, USA

Abstract: *Schistosoma haematobium*, the infectious agent responsible for urogenital schistosomiasis, infects over 112 million people annually in Sub-Saharan Africa alone. Despite a complicated life-cycle within the human host, the vast majority of clinical manifestations occur in response to eggs deposited into the bladder and ureter walls by adult worms. Egg-associated inflammatory lesions feature markedly dysregulated fibrosis responsible for obstructive disease, and urothelial alterations linked to human bladder cancers. Epidemiologic evidence suggests that S. haematobium is responsible for 32 million cases of dysuria, 10 million cases of hydronephrosis, and 150,000 deaths from renal failure annually, making *S. haematobium* the world's deadliest schistosome. Despite the fundamental role of urogenital pathology in human disease, few animal models have been able to recreate natural infection. This review gathers the existing body of knowledge regarding the immunological events during S. haematobium infection, and surveys novel *S. haematobium* infection models to reflect on how we can move forward towards understanding both the pathologic and protective immune responses to the world's deadliest schistosome.

Keywords: Bladder, cancer, co-infection, eosinophils, fibrosis, granuloma, haematobium, immunity, Immunoglobulin-E, Immunoglobulin-G4, immune-modulatory, immunopathology, injection, innate, Interleukin-10, Interleukin-5, Schistosoma, schistosomiasis, urogenital, urothelial.

INTRODUCTION

Epidemiological studies continue to expose the damage caused by schistosomiasis throughout the developing world [1-3]. In 1993 the World Health Organization estimated that 200 million people were infected with at least one of the *Schistosoma* species, and it has become increasingly clear that the morbidity of schistosomiasis reaches far beyond those acutely infected [4,5]. Taking into

---

*Corresponding author Luke Pennington: Stanford University, Grant Building Rm S229, 300 Pasteur Drive, Stanford, CA 94305, 650-498-6350, USA; E-mail: lukepenn@stanford.edu

Emilio Jirillo, Thea Magrone and Giuseppe Miragliotta (Eds)
All rights reserved-© 2014 Bentham Science Publishers

account the lifelong sequelae of chronic infection and the insidious role of schistosomiasis in the acquisition or development of other diseases, new research suggests that between 586-659 million individuals are affected globally [5]. It is now well-established that various forms of schistosomiasis precipitate chronic fibrotic organ damage, promote the transmission of sexually transmitted infections (including HIV), and act as a carcinogen [5-7].

Human schistosomiasis arises primarily from infection by three species of trematode worms of the *Schistosomatidae* family: *Schistosoma haematobium, Schistosoma mansoni,* and *Schistosoma japonica* [3]. *Schistosoma* infection begins when cercariae emerge from their intermediate snail host, penetrate a human host's skin and pass into the circulation. Within the host vasculature the cercariae mature into adult worms and form mating pairs capable of laying eggs for many years [8]. These adult worm mating pairs reside in different venous plexi and their eggs are deposited in adjacent tissues. Eggs are eventually secreted through urine or stool back to fresh water sources, where they hatch into miracidia, infect snail hosts, and complete the *Schistosoma* life cycle [9]. All of the stages of the parasite life cycle within the human host are capable of eliciting immune responses, yet the majority of ensuing morbidity and mortality results from the pronounced immune response to eggs within host tissues. Human infections with *S. mansoni* and *S. japonicum* are primarily responsible for schistosomiasis of the liver, intestines, and spleen, while infection with *S. haematobium* is chiefly responsible for urogenital schistosomiasis [10,11]. The anatomic preference for egg deposition across species is dependent on the venous plexus that adult worm mating pairs ultimately inhabit, as is evident from rodent models of *S. haematobium* infection, in which adult mating pairs cannot be found in the bladder plexus, as in human infection, but instead in the portal system where they predispose to liver, intestinal, and splenic disease [12,13]. The hepatic and enteric egg deposition seen in most rodent *S. haematobium* infection models has limited their human relevance, thus precluding the use of rodent species with established experimental reagents. Non-human primates appear to be the best animal models capable of recapitulating the full course of urogenital schistosomiasis, but are unwieldy, expensive, and ethically contentious to employ [14-16]. Recently, our laboratory has published a new model of *S. haematobium-*

induced bladder pathology employing microinjections of parasite eggs into the mouse bladder wall, providing a promising new approach to understand the immunopathology of *S. haematobium* infection [9, 17].

Historically, the characterization of *S. haematobium* egg-induced pathology has been driven by extrapolations from mouse studies of *S. mansoni* infection, case studies of biopsies and organ samples, and clinical studies of serum surrogates of bladder pathology, such as cytokine or antibody responses [18-21]. These studies have provided an invaluable basis for our understanding of egg-induced inflammation and systemic immune modulation, and yet have not characterized species-specific and organ-specific *S. haematobium*-associated pathology. Regardless, the wealth of mouse reagents and transgenic mouse strains have allowed *S. mansoni* researchers to uncover the essential role of Th2-polarized immune responses and alternative macrophage activation in both the progression and resolution of liver fibrosis, and in the prevention of uncontrolled systemic inflammation during infection [22,23]. This work has constructed a model of egg-associated granuloma formation driven by an admixture of T-cells, B-cells, alternatively activated macrophages, myofibroblasts, eosinophils, basophils, and neutrophils [10,11,24]. Many, but not all, of the same cell populations and cytokine networks have also been implicated in our new model of *S. haematobium* egg-induced pathology, providing a promising opportunity to identify conserved immunopathological pathways between species, and the features of organ pathology which diverge between schistosome species.

Prior rodent models of *S. haematobium* infection generally fail to recapitulate natural oviposition in pelvic organs. In golden hamsters infected with *S. haematobium* or *S. mansoni*, *S. haematobium* infection-induced liver granulomata were smaller and featured fewer eosinophils, a higher percentage of polymorphonuclear cells and histiocytes, and similar numbers of lymphocytes relative to *S. mansoni* infection-induced liver granulomata [25]. Histopathologic analyses of hamster infection models have also noted that *S. haematobium*-induced liver granulomas often resolve without scarring, and many associated eggs are degraded, fragmented, or calcified [26]. In these early papers the relatively smaller granulomata were attributed to the attenuated virulence of *S. haematobium* relative to other human *Schistosoma* infections. Newer clinical and epidemiologic data have reinforced that *S. haematobium* infection is not only the most prevalent *Schistosoma* infection among humans, but also has a unique constellation of pathological sequelae that cause significant morbidity, and cannot be thought of simply as a less virulent species [3,7]. Ultimately *S. haematobium* is primarily a pathogen of the urogenital tract, and conclusions drawn from models of hepatic and enteric infection may fail to recapitulate essential immunological features of human urogenital pathology.

Efficient egg expulsion is an essential portion of the *Schistosoma* life cycle, and it is reasonable to assume that there would be significant evolutionary pressure for *Schistosoma* species to feature specialized egg expulsion strategies for their anatomic niches within their definitive hosts. The primary organs within which *Schistosoma* eggs must be deposited and subsequently expulsed to continue each species' life cycle are the intestine (*S. mansoni* and *S. japonicum*) and the bladder (*S. haematobium*). Although both the intestines and the bladder store and excrete human waste, they are fundamentally different organ systems. The intestines are lined with an absorptive and secretory epithelium, while the bladder is lined with the barrier function-oriented urothelium. The bladder is exposed to the mostly sterile filtrate of the kidney and the occasional bladder infection, while the intestines are constantly bombarded by ingested food particles and gut microbiota. Disturbances of tolerogenic mechanisms in the gut lead to pathologic inflammation, and the interplay between gut IL-10-producing macrophages and regulatory T-cells is essential for local tolerance [27]. In the liver, where *S. mansoni* and *S. japonicum* also reside, Kupffer cells have emerged as central regulators of organ fibrosis [28,29]. This is in stark contrast to the bladder where relatively little is known about resident immune cells, and no functionally distinct resident macrophages or dendritic cells have been identified. Only recently, populations of bladder-resident mast cells have been implicated in bladder disease [30]. Given the heterogeneity of tissues affected across different species of *Schistosoma*, it is likely that tissue-specific inflammatory processes also exist, and that *Schistosoma* species-specific parasite products may shape the immunologic response.

Identifying potentially diverse parasite products is now possible with the advent of high throughput molecular techniques, and the publication of the genomes of *S. japonicum, S. mansoni,* and *S. haematobium*. A significant degree of homology exists between the three species, but *S. haematobium* also produces 73 unique predicted protein products with no known conserved domains or homologs [31]. Combining new models of *S. haematobium* pathology with tools based on observations regarding key mediators of *Schistosoma-induced* inflammation should provide unique insights into future therapeutic approaches. This review aims to collate what is currently known about the immunologic events during *S. haematobium* infection. Numerous parallels exist between *Schistosoma* species, and many of the studies discussed here were inspired from findings first made in the field of *S. mansoni* and *S. japonicum* research. However, in the interest of establishing species-specific observations and areas for future study, these studies will not be emphasized.

HUMAN *S. HAEMATOBIUM* INFECTION

The majority of overt *S. haematobium*-induced pathology is associated with egg deposition and inflammation within host tissues, and can only be directly sampled through invasive procedures, such as tissue biopsy, which are not routinely practical in human research. Instead, human blood samples have been used to dissect out systemic immunologic events and immune response gene alleles relevant to *S. haematobium* infection. These studies have provided invaluable insights into many features of human immune responses to *S. haematobium* infection, but face several challenging obstacles. The first of these challenges is the ubiquitous nature of *S. haematobium* infection in endemic regions, and the subsequent difficulty of characterizing the exposure history of any given study participant. Some research groups even suggest that individuals may be first exposed to maternal infection-associated antigens before birth, and have identified fetal-derived IgE specific for *S. haematobium* egg antigens and expanded populations of $CD5^-CD19^+$ circulating mature fetal B-cells in the cord blood of children born to *S. haematobium*-infected mothers [32] The second challenge to conducting *S. haematobium* immunoepidemiologic studies lies in the marked differences in infection intensity as a function of age, which makes comparisons across studies with differently aged cohorts difficult. Finally, geographic differences in infection intensity provide challenges to identifying control populations and comparing studies across regions. The following sections of this review aim to highlight features of these studies. It is important to acknowledge that not all published observations have proved reproducible, and in some instances, groups have reported outright contradictory results. The immunological mediators and events described in these studies are summarized in Fig. (1), and references related to these findings are provided.

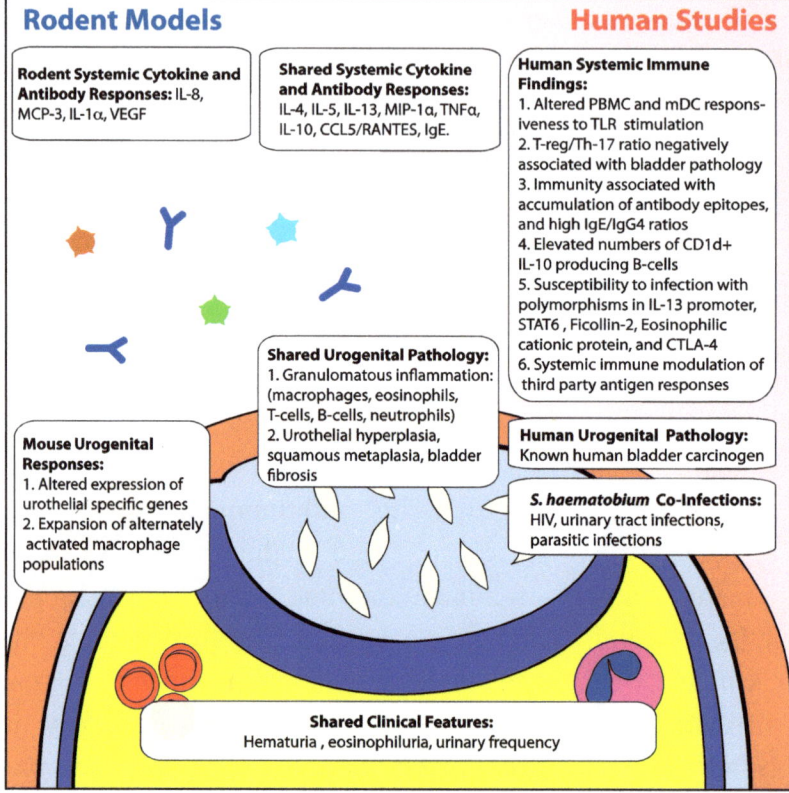

Figure 1. Summary of immunologic, pathologic, and clinical findings during *S. haematobium* infection from human and rodent studies. This table provides a summary of the features of *S. haematobium* infection shared by humans and rodents, as well as those found only in human studies or only in rodent studies to date. The PubMed or PubMed Central ID is provided below for each reference related to these findings.

Rodent cytokine and antibody responses: IL-8, MCP-3, IL-1a, VEGF (PMC3315496). **Human systemic immune findings:** Altered PBMC and mDC responsiveness to TLR stimulation (PMC2857749, PMC3459871, PMC2291570,14999608, PMC3169609). T-reg/Th-17 ratio negatively associated with bladder pathology (PMC3571236). Systemic immune modulation of third party antigen responses (11095260, PMC3398828, PMC3089602, 15679634, PMC2939900, PMC1594876). Immunity associated with accumulation of antibody epitopes, and high IgE/IgG4 ratios (PMC3033519,1898985, 18549316, PMC3084999, PMC1523344) Elevated numbers of CD1d+ IL-10 producing B-cells (PMC3275567). Susceptibility to infection with polymorphisms in IL-13 promoter (20861864), STAT6 (18273035), Ficollin-2 (22693230), and CTLA-4 (PMC3405286). **Shared Cytokine and Antibody Responses:** IL-4 (PMC3315496,PMC3033519). IL-5 (PMC3315496, PMC3033519, 9593042, 12404164, 11095260). IL-13 (PMC3315496,19392635, 11095260) MIP-1α (PMC3315496,19392635, PMC2770052). TNFα (PMC3315496, 23045617, 15529268). IL-10 (2PMC3315496, PMC3033519, 11095260, PMC3089602, 12706745,15529268, PMC3275567). CCL5/RANTES (PMC3510078, 19392635). IgE (PMC3315496, 1898985, PMC3084999). **S. haematobium co-infections:** HIV (22327410, 16406034, PMC3232194, 15838790, 15776378, 11101053). UTI (18338685, 869608, 6926771). Parasitic Infections: (15679634, PMC2939900, PMC1594876, PMC3279404). **Shared Urogenital Pathology:** Granulomatous inflammation (PMC3315496, 16083060, PMC1903998,19082376). Urothelial Hyperplasia, Squamous Metaplasia, Bladder Fibrosis (PMC3315496, PMC3510078, 8673838, 22786992, 19143123, 11388504). **Mouse Urogenital Responses:** Altered expression of urothelial specific genes (PMC3510078). Expansion of alternately activated macrophage populations (PMC3510078). **Human Urogenital Pathology:** Known human bladder carcinogen (9880476, 19143123). **Shared Clinical Features:** Hematuria (PMC3315496, 16997665). Eosinophiluria (PMC3315496, 2505608). Urinary Frequency (PMC3315496, 20427427).

S. Haematobium Infection and Innate Immunity

Danger signals propagated by innate immune receptors are essential for the coordination and potency of subsequent immunologic events. Diverse arrays of innate receptors are capable of recognizing foreign pathogen associated molecular motifs or PAMPs. These receptors include the toll like receptors (TLRs), C-type lectin receptors, cytoplasmic pattern recognition receptors, and secreted receptors such as mannose binding lectin. A wide variety of cells in the peripheral blood mononuclear cell (PBMC) pool express some of these receptors and are capable of responding to stimuli by secreting pro-inflammatory cytokines and increasing expression of molecules associated with the activation of the adaptive immune system. Early inflammatory stimuli from PAMPs, as well as host systems capable of secreting inflammatory mediators after tissue damage, are important for guiding subsequent immunologic activity. Emerging evidence suggests that innate immune mediators are important for defense against *S. haematobium* infection, and that this schistosome is able to alter innate immune responsiveness of PBMC.

For example, ficolin-2, a secreted innate immune receptor similar to mannose binding lectin (MBL), has recently been associated with *S. haematobium* infection. Ficolin-2 initiates inflammatory events by recognizing multiple PAMPs [glycosylation motifs, bacterial cell wall lipoteichoic acids, and fungal cell wall 1, 3-β-D-glucan] and activating the lectin complement cascade [33]. Some of the glycosylation motifs recognized by ficolin-2, including N-acetylglucosamine, have been found on *Schistosoma* antigens, and are reported to decorate potent immunomodulatory *S. mansoni* proteins, including Interleukin-4-inducing principle from *Schistosoma mansoni* eggs (IPSE/Alpha-1) and Kappa-5 [34,35]. Polymorphisms in the ficolin-2 promoter region, which lead to reduced serum ficolin-2 levels, have been associated with susceptibility to *S. haematobium* infection, and provide evidence that innate recognition of parasite-associated glycoproteins plays a role in human infection [33].

Others studies which emphasize the role of early innate inflammatory events in *S. haematobium* infection have described alterations in PBMC responsiveness to stimulation *via* a wide variety of innate inflammatory receptors. One study performed in an *S. haematobium*-endemic region found diminished populations of myeloid dendritic cells (mDCs) in *S. haematobium*-infected *versus* uninfected subjects, and showed that mDCs from infected patients expressed lower levels of HLA-DR than those from uninfected controls [36]. These same mDCs from infected subjects were less responsive to stimulation by TLR4 and TLR7/8 agonists, and showed a decreased ability to drive T-cell proliferation and activation *in vitro* [36]. Subsequent studies have also observed lower HLA-DR expression levels on circulating mDCs in cohorts of young infected individuals (5-9 years old), but offer contrasting data about HLA-DR expression levels in various age groups, underscoring the variability of the findings in different patient populations [37]. It is not apparent why *S. haematobium* would benefit from suppressing TLR4 signaling, a receptor primarily known for its reactivity to components of the bacterial cell wall, or TLR7 and 8 signaling, two receptors which recognize viral-associated single stranded RNA. However, all three of these TLRs signal through a MyD88-dependent pathway, which is activated downstream of many inflammatory receptors, including TLR2, and it is possible that suppression of this pathway could blunt many *S. haematobium*-directed inflammatory events. For example, TLR2 has been shown to interact with schistosomal lyso-phosphatidylserine (lyso-PS), and PBMCs from *S. haematobium*-infected children show a diminished capacity to produce IL-8 and TNF-α in response to lyso-PS [38,39]. The mechanism by which *S. haematobium* suppresses multiple TLR signaling cascades is not known, but this finding appears to be TLR-specific. Other innate stimuli, including *S. haematobium* worm glycolipids, which drive cytokine production in PBMC through a TLR-independent pathway, drive elevated IL-8 and IL-6 production in schistosome-infected children relative to uninfected controls [39]. Taken collectively, it is tempting to conclude that *S. haematobium* infection suppresses multiple TLR signaling cascades sharing the MyD88-dependent activation pathway, but numerous studies contradict each other and suggest that differences in the reported data may arise from variations in control arms across studies [40]. Therefore, further investigation is warranted before definitive conclusions regarding these findings can be made.

S. Haematobium Infection and Systemic Cytokine Responses

Systemic cytokine levels have been measured in both case-control studies and in cohorts before and after praziquantel treatment. These two approaches have revealed numerous distinct features of the systemic immune response to

S. haematobium infection and several cytokines associated with disease pathology. A third body of literature has also identified susceptibility loci in several Th2 cytokine genes and their promoters in endemic populations, which suggests there is heterogeneity in the magnitude of cytokine responses across individuals. Taking all of these factors into account, it is difficult to dissect which trends in cytokine responses correlate with increasing infection intensity because they are conserved features of the human immune response, and which cytokine responses are altered in infected subjects simply because of an individual's intrinsic ability to secrete *S. haematobium*-triggered cytokines.

Cytokine Susceptibility Loci

Epidemiologic studies of *S. haematobium* infection intensity have revealed that in many endemic areas, virtually all members of a population have been exposed to infection, as evident from IgM titers directed towards worm, egg, or cercarial antigens [41]. However, not all individuals are currently or chronically infected, and not all individuals with active infection have urogenital morbidity. Early studies documented that high levels of worm-specific IgE and low levels of worm- and egg-specific IgG4 were associated with immunity, and these two isotypes were associated with high levels of IL-4 and IL-13 in humans [42]. Many other clinical features of disease, including eosinophiluria, eosinophilia, and elevated serum IgE levels are also characteristic of Th2-polarized responses, leading to the notion that individual differences in Th2 immunity may determine infection susceptibility. Several studies have stratified populations in endemic areas by infection intensity, measured by egg counts in urine samples, and identified associated risk alleles for *S. haematobium* infection. The major risk loci identified in these studies were mapped to the 5q31-q33 region, which contains many prototypical Th2 genes (*IL4, IL5, IL13*) [43]. Specifically, several polymorphisms within the IL-13 gene promoter and the STAT6 gene, a transcription factor that is phosphorylated downstream of both IL-4 and IL-13 signaling, were positively associated with infection intensity and showed additive effects when inherited together [44]. Conversely, IL-13 promoter polymorphisms associated with resistance to infection were linked to increased IL-13 gene expression, underscoring this cytokine's role in protective immunity [45]. The same study populations were also evaluated for bladder and kidney pathology by ultrasound, circulating anodic antigen (CAA) levels, and eosinophilic cationic protein (ECP) levels in prior studies. These measures demonstrated that kidney pathology was associated with increased CAA levels, and severe bladder pathology was associated with either increased egg counts or elevated ECP levels [43]. These additional clinical measures suggest that within *S. haematobium*-infected populations, increased infection intensity as measured by egg count correlates with bladder pathology. Thus, polymorphisms in alleles of the IL-13 promoter region and the STAT6 gene may also be important in resulting urogenital pathology.

Praziquantel Treatment and Systemic Cytokine Levels

Numerous studies have suggested that treatment with praziquantel releases otherwise "cryptic" antigens from dying worms and eggs which alter host immune responses during subsequent infections [46-48]. Nevertheless, it is likely that circulating cytokine levels before and after treatment also reflect both the clearance of pro-inflammatory, parasite-derived antigens which drive cytokine production, as well as contracting populations of cytokine-secreting effector cells that expanded during active infection. Interpreting studies from these two perspectives reveals both cytokines associated with active infection, and systemic immune changes altered in the wake of praziquantel treatment, and helps draw comparisons to findings seen in case control studies.

In one study which measured cytokine responses to adult worm antigen (AWA) re-challenge in individuals with poly- and mono- parasitic infections, the PBMC of individuals mono-infected with *S. haematobium* and poly-infected with *S. haematobium, S. mansoni,* and *E. hystolitica/dispar* produced more IL-13 and CCL-17 and less MIP-1α, MIP-1β, and RANTES post-praziquantel treatment [49]. A similar drop in MIP-1α production has also been observed after praziquantel treatment in HIV and *S. haematobium* co-infected individuals [46]. The finding that AWA-driven IL-13 and CCL-17 production increased after praziquantel treatment is consistent with the notion that otherwise cryptic adult worm antigens were released following treatment and worm death and subsequently fueled a stronger recall response to antigen stimulation *in vitro*. However, the findings that MIP-1α (CCL3), MIP-1β (CCL4), and RANTES

(CCL5) production decreased with antigen re-challenge after treatment would suggest that cell populations expanded or activated only during ongoing infection produce these cytokines. These findings are consistent with PBMC cell populations associated with *Schistosoma* infection and the functions of MIP-1α and MIP-1β, chemokines which recruit monocytes/macrophages, and RANTES, a chemokine which can recruit multiple cell populations, including T-cells and eosinophils [50,51].

Eosinophilia and eosinophiluria are well-described features of *S. haematobium* infection [10,19]. Likewise, eosinophil-associated cytokines, including IL-5 and RANTES, have also been tied to anti-parasite responses in human infection. Grogan *et al.* investigated PBMC responses to AWA or soluble egg antigen (SEA) in individuals who cleared infection two years prior, and were subsequently tested for reinfection. These studies indicated that individuals who were not re-infected produced higher levels of IL-5 after AWA or SEA challenge than those who had succumbed to a second infection, while IL-4 and IL-13 production was similar between groups [52]. IL-5 has also been demonstrated to rise with age in long-term egg-negative individuals in endemic areas, along with IL-4 and IL-10 levels, and decrease in those with persistent infections [41]. The notion that IL-5 production is associated with resistance to infection is not surprising, given that IL-5 is a classic Th2-associated cytokine with a known role in driving antibody production and activating eosinophils. Interestingly, IL-5 has also been associated with microhematuria in infected individuals, suggesting that although IL-5 may drive events which play a central role in combating infection, these same events may be associated with end organ (bladder) pathology [48]. However, in studies conducted by Van den Biggelaar *et al.*, in which children were followed for resolution of infection and PBMC cytokine production after praziquantel treatment, somewhat contradictory findings were observed. Newly infected children and children re-infected after a single dose of praziquantel produced markedly more IL-5 upon AWA challenge as compared to uninfected counterparts [48]. Yet, this finding does not necessarily challenge the role of strong IL-5 recall responses in protective immunity. When the control groups across related studies are compared, the age range of subjects within Van den

Biggelaar's study are only within the age range of highest infection intensity, while the aforementioned studies also included individuals who are past this window and likely have developed true resistance to infection. It is therefore reasonable to conclude the relatively elevated levels of IL-5 in Van den Biggelaar's young cohort are associated with populations of IL-5 producing cells expanded during active infection, and that these cells are being compared to those from uninfected controls who are not truly infection-resistant, but instead are not currently infected. Given the reproducible eosinophil expansion seen clinically during infection, it is likely that IL-5 and other eosinophil-associated cytokines play a central role in combating infection.

Many of the aforementioned studies evaluating the effect of praziquantel treatment on host immunity have focused on recall responses to adult worm antigens (AWA) before and after treatment, as these responses are suspected to be associated with host immunity to reinfection. Recently, an analysis of Th1, Th2, and Th17 cytokines expressed in response to antigens from all human stages of the parasite life cycle has provided a new perspective on the immune polarizing effects of praziquantel treatment [53]. In this study, egg antigen stimulation of peripheral blood after praziquantel treatment drove increased levels of the pro-inflammatory cytokines TNFα, IL-6, IL-8, IFN-γ, IL-12p70, and IL-23 as compared to pretreatment PBMC pools. Cercarial *versus* AWA antigen stimulation of post-treatment PBMC resulted in increased levels of IL-8 *versus* lower amounts of IL-6, respectively, than pretreatment PBMC pools. Although this study did not recapitulate all findings noted in the aforementioned studies, the significance of the observations are twofold. First, this work has provided a comprehensive analysis of the effect of praziquantel treatment on host immune responses to parasite re-challenge, and suggests that treated and subsequently re-infected individuals may experience more pronounced inflammatory responses to eggs recently deposited in tissues. Second, this study demonstrated that responses to egg antigens, and not cercariae or adult worm antigens, changed most drastically after treatment. No mechanism can be easily inferred from this observation, but it is possible that, prior to elimination by drug therapy, live eggs or adult worms are capable of actively suppressing host immune responses towards egg antigens, or that eggs are uniquely suited to conceal their own antigens in the schistosome antigen-naïve host.

IL-10 and the S. haematobium Immune Response

Numerous case-control studies in *S. haematobium*-endemic regions have attempted to correlate systemic pro-inflammatory and anti-inflammatory markers with disease susceptibility or infection-associated pathology. In a landmark study investigating the effect of *S. haematobium* infection on allergic responses, stimulation of PBMC from *S. haematobium*-infected children with AWA resulted in significantly more production of IL-5, IL-13, and IL-10 than in uninfected counterparts [54]. These elevated IL-10 levels were negatively associated with skin test reactivity to house mite allergens. The inverse correlation between infection intensity and dust mite reactivity has since been confirmed in subsequent studies [55], and both serum IL-10 levels and positive infection status have also been correlated with lower auto-reactive antibody titers in *S. haematobium*-infected individuals [56]. This schistosome-driven IL-10 response may begin in the earliest stages of infection. Groups using a human foreskin culture model of cercarial infection have documented IL-10 production in tissues harvested from individuals naïve to *S. haematobium* infection [57]. Recently, a human field study has also demonstrated that the excretory/secretory material of cercariae drives elevated IL-10 production in the PBMC of infected individuals as compared to uninfected controls [58]. Collectively, these findings suggest that elevated IL-10 levels are present throughout schistosome infection and may globally suppress inflammation, which is consistent with IL-10's known anti-inflammatory activity [59]. In agreement with these observations, individuals with greater bladder morbidity (as detected by ultrasound) have 8-fold greater levels of SEA-driven TNF-α production and 99-fold greater TNF-α/IL-10 ratios compared to subjects without observed pathology [60]. Intriguingly, a recent publication demonstrated that *S. mansoni* infection of mice induced $CD1d^+$ B-cells capable of suppressing allergic inflammation in an IL-10-dependent fashion [61]. This same group identified an expanded population of $CD1d^+$ B-cells producing IL-10 in *S. haematobium*-infected children, suggesting that these cells could be a potential source of the cytokine observed during infection. Furthermore, *S. mansoni* infection models have identified similar populations of B-cells capable of producing IL-10 in response to oligosaccharides found in *S. mansoni* egg isolates [62]. CD1d is an MHC Class I-like molecule capable of presenting lipid molecules to NKT cells, and could conceivably present schistosome-derived glycolipid antigens [39]. However, these CD1d/schistosome-based studies cannot conclusively identify the source of IL-10, a cytokine produced by a wide variety of cell types, and IL-10 could have many tissue-specific or systemic sources during inflammation [59]. Nonetheless, numerous publications have demonstrated elevated IL-10 levels in *S. haematobium* infection capable of altering responses to third party antigens, including host immune responses to *P. falciparum* co-infection, underscoring the potential role of this cytokine in the course of *S. haematobium* infection [56,63-65]. Consistent with the aforementioned immunosuppressive effects of IL-10, *S. mansoni* infection models have even suggested that systemic IL-10 is partially responsible for slow acquisition of immunity to *Schistosoma* infection [66]. Given the biologically plausible role of IL-10 in the global suppression of host immune responses, and evidence from experimental models in *S. mansoni* literature, further investigation into the role of IL-10 in the development of host immunity is warranted.

S. haematobium Infection and T-Cells

T-cells are believed to be important for preventing *S. haematobium* infection, and polymorphisms in cytotoxic T-lymphocyte antigen 4 (CTLA-4), an inhibitory co-receptor expressed on T-cells, have been positively linked with *S. haematobium* infection [67]. These polymorphisms confer a gain of signaling function, and may lead to mild global immune suppression by inhibiting activation and proliferation of T-cells. However, T-cell responses may not be strictly protective against *S. haematobium* infection. One group has demonstrated that the fecundity and maturation of adult worms is deficient in Rag-1 (-/-) mice lacking mature B and T lymphocytes, and that T-cell-mediated events may promote parasite maturation [68]. The notion that portions of the human inflammatory response may improve *S. haematobium*'s reproductive success is also supported by the finding that egg expulsion is reduced in HIV co-infected individuals [68]. To date, it is not well understood how T-cells drive this phenomenon, but studies have begun to characterize how certain T-cell subsets are involved in the immunopathology of *S. haematobium* infection.

Building on work that identified alterations in regulatory T-cell (T-reg) populations during *S. mansoni* infection, several human studies have investigated T-regs in *S. haematobium* infection. One study found that T-reg populations were positively correlated with increasing infection intensity in young individuals, and negatively correlated with infection intensity in older individuals [69]. This divergence in patterns across age groups has been previously documented and is attributed to the gradual transformation of immune responses as individuals in endemic areas acquire immunity, and may also be a product of age-related immune senescence. In a second study of children co-infected with *P. falciparum*, reduced numbers of regulatory T-cells were seen in those concurrently infected with *S. haematobium*, and this effect diminished months later during periods of lower malaria transmission [70]. Although these studies do not provide a clear consensus on the function of regulatory T-cells during infection, the ratio of regulatory T-cells to pro-inflammatory Th-17 cells does seem to correlate with bladder pathology. *S. haematobium*-infected children with bladder pathology were demonstrated to have higher circulating levels of Th-17 cells and higher Th17/Treg ratios than infected children without pathology and uninfected children [71]. This finding is one of the first to implicate Th-17 activity in *S. haematobium* infection, and provides another example of how infections with and without overt pathology may represent distinct inflammatory states.

S. haematobium Antibody Responses and Immunity

Epidemiologic studies have documented that virtually all individuals living in endemic areas have been exposed to *S. haematobium* antigens as indicated by positive anti-parasite IgM titers [41]. In these regions the development of immunity is a gradual process that correlates with the accumulation of a diverse anti-parasite antibody repertoire [72]. It is also evident that a high ratio of IgE/IgG4 is important for the development of immunity [42]. Subsequent analyses which employed proteomic techniques to examine individual epitope responses have documented a similar pattern of IgE /IgG4 ratios, including an inverse relationship with infection intensity [73]. It is suspected that IgG4 modulates IgE activity by competitively binding shared epitopes and preventing IgE-mediated effector functions, and that the differential expression of IgE and IgG4 can be regulated by IL-10, a cytokine clearly associated with *S. haematobium* infection

[74]. The suppressive impact of IgG4 on IgE function are exemplified by the finding that IgG4 antibodies only recognize several dominant epitopes, and that these epitopes are shared with IgE antibodies [73]. Although IgE/IgG4 ratios appear to play a central role in immunity, other antibody isotypes have also been correlated with immunity, including anti-AWA IgG1 antibodies, and IgG3 directed to the adult worm tegument associated antigen 13 (Sh13) [73,75].

Amidst ongoing research into the essential features of naturally acquired immunity to *S. haematobium* infection, a phase I clinical trial of the recombinant *S. haematobium* 28kda glutathione S-transferase (rShGST) vaccine was recently completed [76]. The results of the study showed that the vaccine was capable of increasing titers of IgG1a, IgG2, IgG3, and IgG4 antibodies which all inhibited ShGST enzymatic function *in vitro*. The vaccine, along with several other proposed vaccine targets [77], offers a promising start towards a *S. haematobium* vaccine, yet induction of one of the isotypes most strongly correlated with immunity, IgE, was not observed in this study.

S. haematobium Co-Infection

Co-infection is one of the best "natural experiments" to demonstrate the systemic immune effects of one pathogen on another. Concurrent *S. haematobium* infection has been shown to alter transmission rates and immune responses to a variety of pathogens, including *P. falciparum,* HIV, and bacterial urinary tract infections [6,78,79]. As discussed elsewhere in this review *P. falciparum* studies have demonstrated reduced numbers of regulatory T-cells, altered systemic cytokine responses, and changes in anti-*P. falciparum* antibody responses in individuals co-infected with *S. haematobium* [63-65,70].

Schistosoma infection is also thought to promote HIV/AIDS susceptibility, progression, and transmission [6]. During *S. haematobium* infection eggs are primarily deposited in the urinary bladder plexus, and to a lesser extent throughout the pelvic vascular network, seeding inflammatory lesions in multiple genital organs [80]. In girls and women with female genital schistosomiasis, egg-associated lesions increase cervical and vaginal vascularity, contact bleeding, and numbers of HIV-susceptible $CD4^+$ T-cells near the genital mucosa both before and months after treatment with praziquantel [80,81]. These lesions are thought to facilitate viral transmission. In males, *S. haematobium* infection has also been proposed to increase transmission of HIV by both increasing the viral load and $CD4^+$ lymphocyte counts in semen [6,82].

Beyond modulating transmission of HIV, *S. haematobium* and *S. mansoni* co-infection have also been shown to affect HIV disease progression. Early praziquantel treatment of *S. haematobium* or *S. mansoni* infected HIV-positive individuals improved their $CD4^+$ T-cell counts and lowered viral loads, as compared to those who were initially untreated with praziquantel [83], though earlier studies conducted on other co-infected populations have not observed this trend [84]. The mechanisms behind the enhanced viral progression in *S. haematobium* infected HIV^+ patients has been ascribed to increased rates of viral replication within $CD4^+$ central memory cells, as observed in SHIV-C-*Schistosoma* co-infection models, and increased surface expression of the HIV co-receptors CCR5 and CXCR4 on T-cells and monocytes [85,86].

S. haematobium co-infection has also been demonstrated to alter host susceptibility to bacterial urinary tract infections, and *S. haematobium* infected individuals feature higher rates of bacteriuria [79,87,88]. Several groups have also demonstrated that there is not only a higher rate of co-infection, but also increased rate of infection with bacteria capable of reducing nitrates to N-nitrosamine precursors, a potential bladder carcinogen [79,88]. Relatively few studies have investigated the mechanism or clinical impact of these associations, and this field represents an important overlooked source of morbidity associated with *S. haematobium* infection. Taken together, *S. haematobium* co-infection plays an insidious role in the course of bacterial, viral, and parasitic disease, and likely alters many facets of host immune responses.

EXPERIMENTAL MODELS OF *S. HAEMATOBIUM*

Much of the research to date on the features of *S. haematobium* infection has been gathered from field studies of populations in endemic areas. These studies, by nature, tend to be limited to questions surrounding systemic immune responses that correlate with infection intensity and pathology. However, the logistical design of these studies cannot directly investigate the mechanisms of egg-induced pathology and immune modulation within tissues. Previous attempts to develop a higher fidelity experimental model of urogenital schistosomiasis are nothing short of heroic. In a series of studies in the 1950s, Robert Kuntz and George Malakatis investigated the susceptibility of hundreds of mammalian species to *S. haematobium* infection [89-91]. They found that the overwhelming majority of rodents investigated failed to either carry *S. haematobium* infection or recapitulate the urogenital pathology seen in human disease. Notably, several rodents in their study [the African Grass Rat (*Arvicanthis niloticus*), the Greater Egyptian Gerbil (*Gerbillus pyramidum*), Shaw's Jird (*Meriones shawi*), and the Short-tailed Bandicoot Rat (*Nesokia indica suilla*)] displayed occasional urogenital egg deposition. Other groups have also identified bladder lesions in additional species [the Common African Rat (*Mastomys natalensis*), the Highveld Gerbil (*Tatera brantsii*), and the South African Pouched Mouse (*Saccostomus campestris*)] but urogenital pathology was only noted in a minority of these animals as well [13]. Many of these studies suggested that the natural course of human *S. haematobium* infection (*i.e.*, urogenital pathology) could not be recreated in rodents because the small size of the rodent vesical plexus would not accommodate adult worm mating pairs. In contrast to this body of work, one study suggested that rodent models may be possible, and was able to identify urogenital pathology reliably in the Brazilian Marsh Rat (*Holochilus brasiliensis*), the Shaw's Jird (*Meriones shawi*), and the Mongolian jird (*Meriones unguiculatus*) [92]. Given the small size of these successfully infected rodents, the study authors suggested that theories concerning failed urogenital oviposition due to the minute caliber of the rodent pelvic venous plexus may be erroneous. In theory, the permissive species identified in this study, namely the Shaw's Jird, could provide alternate models to study the natural course of *S. haematobium* infection, including urogenital organ oviposition. However, virtually no experimental reagents are available for any of these species. Moreover, these exotic species are not widely available for research use. Although reliable rodent models of natural *S. haematobium* infection and urogenital pathology remain out of reach, *S. haematobium* infection of the golden hamster (*Mesocricetus auratus*) is frequently used to maintain *S. haematobium* strains in the laboratory. Nevertheless, infected hamsters feature adult worms which preferentially migrate to the portal venous system and predispose to hepatoenteric rather than urogenital disease [12,26]. Finally, it is also noteworthy that several species of baboon, chimpanzees, and other non-human primates have been able to recreate features of natural infection [16,93-95]. Unfortunately, the logistical difficulties associated with these models and the paucity of species-specific reagents still present significant obstacles to their widespread adoption for urogenital schistosomiasis research.

Recently, our group published a novel mouse model of *S. haematobium* egg-induced pathology. In this model, *S. haematobium* eggs are microinjected into the mouse bladder wall [9,17]. Although this protocol is not a surrogate for the full course of natural infection in humans, it offers several unique advantages. The most important advantage lies in the host species. The diversity of mouse-specific reagents and transgenic strains of mice greatly exceeds the repertoire of experimental tools available for any other species. The second advantage lies in the fact that the synchronous deposition of eggs allows for reliable, precise, temporally-based experiments. In contrast, natural infection studies inevitably feature uncertainty regarding whether and when oviposition has commenced. This may allow for the application of new techniques to genetically manipulate the parasite at specific time points in the egg life stage, including the use of dsRNA to temporarily silence gene expression in *Schistosoma* eggs [96].

Although our model focuses on a single stage in the *S. haematobium* lifecycle, it induces many cytokines in the mouse host that have also been documented in human studies. These include bladder tissue increases in TNFα, MIP-1α, and IL-10, which is also seen in systemic human immune responses. Moreover, systemic features seen in human infection are also noted in the sera of egg-injected mice, including elevated IL-5 and high serum IgE levels [9]. Finally, microarray analysis of egg-injected bladders has revealed increased expression of CCL5/RANTES, a cytokine produced by PBMC during *S. haematobium* infection [49]. However, the most striking similarities between this model and the clinical course of human infection lie in associated bladder pathology. Egg instillation into the bladder wall produces characteristic granulomatous inflammation also seen in human infection. These lesions are characterized by CD68$^+$ macrophages encapsulating *S. haematobium* eggs, with populations of infiltrating eosinophils, B-cells, T-cells, and neutrophils. The prototypical Th2-associated cytokines IL-4 and IL-13 are also elevated in bladder tissue, along with known clinical features of infection including eosinophiluria, hematuria, urinary frequency, and bladder fibrosis [9]. The synchronous nature of our model has also allowed us to demonstrate that following egg deposition, many of the cytokines produced and cells recruited precede the window of adaptive immune responses. This provides compelling evidence that innate immunological events may play a prominent role in early urogenital immune responses. Finally, our urogenital schistosomiasis model induces egg-dependent hyperplasia and squamous metaplasia of the urothelium, and therefore may provide a valuable model for *S. haematobium*-associated bladder cancer. More broadly, our model will allow us to glean general principles regarding the links between chronic inflammation and neoplastic transformation.

Major Immunomodulatory Molecules Produced by *S. haematobium*

In mouse models of *S. mansoni* infection, significant headway has been made into uncovering a number of the egg-derived molecular mediators of host pathology. Some pathogen-associated molecular motifs, such as schistosomal lyso-PS and parasite glycolipids, have been isolated from both *S. mansoni* and *S. haematobium*, and may drive conserved inflammatory events across *Schistosoma* species [39]. Evidence from the *S. mansoni* literature also suggests that carbohydrate moieties and parasite dsRNA can provide innate inflammatory signals [97,98]. Despite the important role that these glycosylated inflammatory triggers play in schistosomal pathogenesis, perhaps one of the most interesting classes of immunomodulatory parasite products is a class of secreted proteins which can mediate potent immunomodulatory effects regardless of glycosylation status [99-102]. The publication of the *S. haematobium* genome has facilitated comparisons of homology between these proteins across species, and the homologs identified provide evidence for divergent evolution of inflammatory mediators [103]. This divergence may reflect the evolutionary specialization of each species for its anatomical niche and serve as the basis for future research avenues. (Table 1) contains a list of some of the immunomodulatory proteins identified in *S. mansoni* studies that are shared with *S. haematobium*.

CONCLUSION

With the advent of new models of *S. haematobium* infection, the recently published *S. haematobium* genome, and the advancing field of human immunologic research, *S. haematobium* research is now more feasible than ever. As we begin to push the frontiers of our knowledge about *Schistosoma* infection, these tools will allow us to identify conserved and divergent features of each *Schistosoma* species, and develop appropriate interventions and vaccines. Much as *S. mansoni* research has provided a valuable tool for understanding the molecular mediators of liver fibrosis and pathology, *S. haematobium* studies may provide unique insight into bladder biology, and the immunological events that mediate neoplastic transformation in the setting of chronic inflammation.

Table 1: Proposed Immunomodulatory Proteins of *Schistosoma haematobium*

Immunomodulatory Proteins[1]	Homolog Identified:	*S. mansoni*	*S. japonicum*
Cathepsin-B Cysteine Protease		yes	yes
Cercarial Serine Protease		yes	?
Estradiol 17 β dehydrogenase		yes	yes
IPSE/Alpha-1		yes	?
Omega-1		yes	yes
Peroxiredoxin		yes	yes
Sjc23 Tetraspanin		yes	yes
Sm16/SPO-1/Sj16		yes	yes
Venom Allergen-like Proteins		yes	yes

All predicted *S. haematobium* homologs from Young *et al. 2012 [32] and* unpublished data (M. Hsieh)

ACKNOWLEDGEMENT

Declared none.

CONFLICT OF INTEREST

The author(s) confirm that this chapter contents have no conflict of interest.

ABBREVIATIONS

(AWA)	=	Adult Worm Antigen
(CAA)	=	Circulating Anodic Antigen
(CTLA-4)	=	Cytotoxic T-Lymphocyte Antigen 4
(GST)	=	Glutathione S-Transferase
(IPSE/alpha-1)	=	Interleukin-4-inducing Principle from Schistosome Eggs
(lyso PS)	=	Lyso-phosphatidylserine
(MBL)	=	Mannose-Binding Lectin
(mDC)	=	Myeloid Dendritic Cell
(PAMPs)	=	Pathogen Associated Molecular Patterns
(PBMC)	=	Peripheral Blood Mononuclear Cell
(pDC)	=	Plasmacytoid Cendritic Cell
(SEA)	=	Soluble Egg Antigens
(TLRs)	=	Toll-Like Receptors
(VEGF)	=	Vascular Endothelial Growth Factor

REFERENCES

[1] Mathers CD, Ezzati M, Lopez AD. Measuring the burden of neglected tropical diseases: the global burden of disease framework. PLoS Negl. Trop. Dis. [Internet]. 2007 Jan [cited 2012 Oct 5];1(2):e114. Available from: http://www.pubmedcentral.nih.gov/articlerender.fcgi?artid=2100367&tool=pmcentrez&rendertype=abstract

[2] King CH, Dickman K, Tisch DJ. Reassessment of the cost of chronic helmintic infection: a meta-analysis of disability-related outcomes in endemic schistosomiasis. Lancet [Internet]. 2005 Jan 30 [cited 2012 Oct 17];365(9470):1561-9. Available from: http://www.thelancet.com/journals/a/article/PIIS0140-6736(05)66457-4/fulltext

[3] Rollinson D. A wake up call for urinary schistosomiasis: reconciling research effort with public health importance. Parasitology [Internet]. 2009/07/25 ed. 2009;136(12):1593-610. Available from: http://www.ncbi.nlm.nih.gov/pubmed/19627633

[4] Van der Werf MJ, de Vlas SJ, Brooker S, et al. Quantification of clinical morbidity associated with schistosome infection in sub-Saharan Africa. Acta Trop [Internet]. 2003/05/15 ed. 2003 May [cited 2012 Apr 23];86(2-3):125-39. Available from: http://www.ncbi.nlm.nih.gov/pubmed/12745133

[5] King CH. Parasites and poverty: the case of schistosomiasis. Acta Trop [Internet]. 2009/12/08 ed. 2010 Feb [cited 2012 Apr 8];113(2):95-104. Available from: http://www.ncbi.nlm.nih.gov/pubmed/19962954

[6] Secor WE. The effects of schistosomiasis on HIV/AIDS infection, progression and transmission. Curr. Opin. HIV AIDS [Internet]. 2012 May [cited 2012 Jul 20];7(3):254-9. Available from: http://www.ncbi.nlm.nih.gov/pubmed/22327410

[7] Mostafa MH, Sheweita SA, O'Connor PJ. Relationship between schistosomiasis and bladder cancer. Clin. Microbiol. Rev. [Internet]. 1999/01/09 ed. 1999;12(1):97-111. Available from: http://www.ncbi.nlm.nih.gov/pubmed/9880476

[8] Smith P, Fallon RE, Mangan NE, et al. Schistosoma mansoni secretes a chemokine binding protein with antiinflammatory activity. J Exp Med [Internet]. 2005/11/23 ed. 2005;202(10):1319-25. Available from: http://www.ncbi.nlm.nih.gov/pubmed/16301741

[9] Fu C-L, Odegaard JI, De'Broski RH, et al. A novel mouse model of Schistosoma haematobium egg-induced immunopathology. PLoS Pathog. [Internet]. 2012 Jan [cited 2012 Sep 21];8(3):e1002605. Available from: http://www.pubmedcentral.nih.gov/articlerender.fcgi?artid=3315496&tool=pmcentrez&rendertype=abstract

[10] Wynn TA, Thompson RW, Cheever AW, et al. Immunopathogenesis of schistosomiasis. Immunol Rev [Internet]. 2004/09/14 ed. 2004;201:156-67. Available from: http://www.ncbi.nlm.nih.gov/pubmed/15361239

[11] Pearce EJ, MacDonald AS. The immunobiology of schistosomiasis. Nat Rev Immunol [Internet]. 2002/07/03 ed. 2002;2(7):499-511. Available from: http://www.ncbi.nlm.nih.gov/pubmed/12094224

[12] Ghandour AM. The development of Schistosoma haematobium in the hamster. Ann. Trop. Med. Parasitol. [Internet]. 1978 Jun [cited 2012 Dec 27];72(3):219-25. Available from: http://www.ncbi.nlm.nih.gov/pubmed/666393

[13] Gear JH, Davis DH, Pitchford RJ. The susceptibility of rodents to schistosome infection, with special reference to Schistosoma haematobium. Bull. World Health Organ. [Internet]. 1966 Jan [cited 2012 Dec 30];35(2):213-21. Available from: http://www.pubmedcentral.nih.gov/articlerender.fcgi?artid=2476116&tool=pmcentrez&rendertype=abstract

[14] Farah IO, Kariuki TM, King CL, et al. An overview of animal models in experimental schistosomiasis and refinements in the use of non-human primates. Lab. Anim. [Internet]. 2001 Jul;35(3):205-12. Available from: http://www.ncbi.nlm.nih.gov/pubmed/11463066

[15] Ordan P, Goatly KD. Experimental schistosomiasis in primates in Tanzania. I. A preliminary note on the susceptibility of Cercopithecus aethiops centralis to infection with Schistosoma haematobium and Schistosoma mansoni. Ann. Trop. Med. Parasitol. [Internet]. 1966 Mar [cited 2012 Dec 27];60(1):3-9. Available from: http://www.ncbi.nlm.nih.gov/pubmed/4960090

[16] Jordan P, Von Lichtenberg F, Goatly KD. Experimental schistosomiasis in primates in Tanzania. Preliminary observations on the susceptibility of the baboon Papio anubis to

[17] Ray D, Nelson TA, Fu C-L, et al. Transcriptional Profiling of the Bladder in Urogenital Schistosomiasis Reveals Pathways of Inflammatory Fibrosis and Urothelial Compromise. Davies SJ, editor. PLoS Negl. Trop. Dis. [Internet]. Public Library of Science; 2012 Nov 29 [cited 2012 Nov 30];6(11):e1912. Available from: http://dx.plos.org/10.1371/journal.pntd.0001912

[18] Silva IM da, Pereira Filho E, Thiengo R, et al. Schistosomiasis haematobia: histopathological course determined by cystoscopy in a patient in whom praziquantel treatment failed. Rev. Inst. Med. Trop. Sao Paulo [Internet]. [cited 2012 Jul 20];50(6):343-6. Available from: http://www.ncbi.nlm.nih.gov/pubmed/19082376

[19] Eltoum IA, Ghalib HW, Sualaiman S, et al. Significance of eosinophiluria in urinary schistosomiasis. A study using Hansel's stain and electron microscopy. Am. J. Clin. Pathol. [Internet]. 1989 Sep [cited 2013 Feb 18];92(3):329-38. Available from: http://www.ncbi.nlm.nih.gov/pubmed/2505608

[20] Mutapi F. Helminth parasite proteomics: from experimental models to human infections. Parasitology [Internet]. Cambridge University Press; 2012 Aug 1 [cited 2012 Dec 22];139(9):1195-204. Available from: /pmc/articles/PMC3417537/?report=abstract

[21] Bourke CD, Nausch N, Rujeni N, et al. Integrated Analysis of Innate, Th1, Th2, Th17, and Regulatory Cytokines Identifies Changes in Immune Polarisation Following Treatment of Human Schistosomiasis. J. Infect. Dis. [Internet]. Oxford University Press; 2012 Oct 8 [cited 2012 Dec 23]; Available from: http://jid.oxfordjournals.org/content/early/2012/09/25/infdis.jis524.full

[22] Herbert DR, Holscher C, Mohrs M, et al. Alternative macrophage activation is essential for survival during schistosomiasis and downmodulates T helper 1 responses and immunopathology. Immunity [Internet]. 2004/05/15 ed. 2004;20(5):623-35. Available from: http://www.ncbi.nlm.nih.gov/pubmed/15142530

[23] Pesce JT, Ramalingam TR, Mentink-Kane MM, et al. Arginase-1-expressing macrophages suppress Th2 cytokine-driven inflammation and fibrosis. PLoS Pathog [Internet]. 2009/04/11 ed. 2009;5(4):e1000371. Available from: http://www.ncbi.nlm.nih.gov/pubmed/19360123

[24] Burke ML, Jones MK, Gobert GN, et al. Immunopathogenesis of human schistosomiasis. Parasite Immunol [Internet]. 2009/03/19 ed. 2009;31(4):163-76. Available from: http://www.ncbi.nlm.nih.gov/pubmed/19292768

[25] Hussein MR, Abu-Dief EE, El-Hady HA, et al. Quantitative comparison of infected Schistosomiasis mansoni and Haematobium: animal model analysis of the granuloma cell population. J. Egypt. Soc. Parasitol. [Internet]. 2005 Aug [cited 2012 Dec 27];35(2):467-76. Available from: http://www.ncbi.nlm.nih.gov/pubmed/16083060

[26] Von Lichtenberg F, Erickson DG, Sadun EH. Comparative histopathology of schistosome granulomas in the hamster. Am. J. Pathol. [Internet]. 1973 Aug [cited 2012 Dec 27];72(2):149-78. Available from: http://www.pubmedcentral.nih.gov/articlerender.fcgi?artid=1903998&tool=pmcentrez&rendertype=abstract

[27] Hadis U, Wahl B, Schulz O, et al. Intestinal tolerance requires gut homing and expansion of FoxP3+ regulatory T cells in the lamina propria. Immunity [Internet]. 2011 Feb 25 [cited

2012 Nov 22];34(2):237-46. Available from: http://www.ncbi.nlm.nih.gov/pubmed/21333554

[28] Ten Hagen TL, van Vianen W, Bakker-Woudenberg IA. Isolation and characterization of murine Kupffer cells and splenic macrophages. J Immunol Methods [Internet]. 1996/06/14 ed. 1996;193(1):81-91. Available from: http://www.ncbi.nlm.nih.gov/pubmed/8690933

[29] Hayashi N, Matsui K, Tsutsui H, et al. Kupffer Cells from Schistosoma mansoni-Infected Mice Participate in the Prompt Type 2 Differentiation of Hepatic T Cells in Response to Worm Antigens. J. Immunol. [Internet]. 1999 Dec 15 [cited 2012 Dec 31];163(12):6702-11. Available from: http://www.jimmunol.org/content/163/12/6702.full

[30] Chan CY, St. John AL, Abraham SN. Mast Cell Interleukin-10 Drives Localized Tolerance in Chronic Bladder Infection. Immunity [Internet]. 2013 Feb 14 [cited 2013 Feb 15]; Available from: http://www.ncbi.nlm.nih.gov/pubmed/23415912

[31] Young ND, Jex AR, Li B, et al. Whole-genome sequence of Schistosoma haematobium. Nat. Genet. [Internet]. 2012 Feb [cited 2012 Mar 17];44(2):221-5. Available from: http://www.ncbi.nlm.nih.gov/pubmed/22246508

[32] Seydel LS, Petelski A, van Dam GJ, et al. Association of in utero sensitization to Schistosoma haematobium with enhanced cord blood IgE and increased frequencies of CD5- B cells in African newborns. Am. J. Trop. Med. Hyg. [Internet]. 2012 Apr [cited 2012 Jul 20];86(4):613-9. Available from: http://www.ncbi.nlm.nih.gov/pubmed/22492145

[33] Ouf EA, Ojurongbe O, Akindele AA, et al. Ficolin-2 levels and FCN2 genetic polymorphisms as a susceptibility factor in schistosomiasis. J. Infect. Dis. [Internet]. 2012 Aug 15 [cited 2012 Dec 23];206(4):562-70. Available from: http://www.ncbi.nlm.nih.gov/pubmed/22693230

[34] Wuhrer M, Balog CI, Catalina MI, et al. IPSE/alpha-1, a major secretory glycoprotein antigen from schistosome eggs, expresses the Lewis X motif on core-difucosylated N-glycans. FEBS J. [Internet]. 2006/05/03 ed. 2006;273(10):2276-92. Available from: http://www.ncbi.nlm.nih.gov/pubmed/16650003

[35] Meevissen MHJ, Driessen NN, Smits HH, et al. Specific glycan elements determine differential binding of individual egg glycoproteins of the human parasite Schistosoma mansoni by host C-type lectin receptors. Int. J. Parasitol. [Internet]. 2012 Feb 16 [cited 2012 Jun 14]; Available from: http://www.ncbi.nlm.nih.gov/pubmed/22673410

[36] Everts B, Adegnika AA, Kruize YCM, et al. Functional impairment of human myeloid dendritic cells during Schistosoma haematobium infection. PLoS Negl. Trop. Dis. [Internet]. 2010 Jan [cited 2012 Jul 29];4(4):e667. Available from: http://www.pubmedcentral.nih.gov/articlerender.fcgi?artid=2857749&tool=pmcentrez&rendertype=abstract

[37] Nausch N, Louis D, Lantz O, et al. Age-related patterns in human myeloid dendritic cell populations in people exposed to Schistosoma haematobium infection. PLoS Negl. Trop. Dis. [Internet]. 2012 Sep [cited 2012 Dec 23];6(9):e1824. Available from: http://www.pubmedcentral.nih.gov/articlerender.fcgi?artid=3459871&tool=pmcentrez&rendertype=abstract

[38] Hartgers FC, Obeng BB, Kruize YCM, et al. Lower expression of TLR2 and SOCS-3 is associated with Schistosoma haematobium infection and with lower risk for allergic reactivity in children living in a rural area in Ghana. PLoS Negl. Trop. Dis. [Internet]. 2008 Jan [cited 2012 Jul 20];2(4):e227. Available from: http://www.pubmedcentral.nih.gov/articlerender.fcgi?artid=2291570&tool=pmcentrez&rendertype=abstract

[39] Van der Kleij D, van den Biggelaar AHJ, Kruize YCM, et al. Responses to Toll-like receptor ligands in children living in areas where schistosome infections are endemic. J.

Infect. Dis. [Internet]. 2004 Mar 15 [cited 2012 Jul 30];189(6):1044-51. Available from: http://www.ncbi.nlm.nih.gov/pubmed/14999608

[40] Meurs L, Labuda L, Amoah AS, et al. Enhanced pro-inflammatory cytokine responses following Toll-like-receptor ligation in Schistosoma haematobium-infected schoolchildren from rural Gabon. PLoS One [Internet]. 2011 Jan [cited 2012 Jul 18];6(9):e24393. Available from: http://www.pubmedcentral.nih.gov/articlerender.fcgi?artid=3169609&tool=pmcentrez&rendertype=abstract

[41] Milner T, Reilly L, Nausch N, et al. Circulating cytokine levels and antibody responses to human Schistosoma haematobium: IL-5 and IL-10 levels depend upon age and infection status. Parasite Immunol. [Internet]. [cited 2012 Jul 20];32(11-12):710-21. Available from: http://www.pubmedcentral.nih.gov/articlerender.fcgi?artid=3033519&tool=pmcentrez&rendertype=abstract

[42] Hagan P, Blumenthal UJ, Dunn D, et al. Human IgE, IgG4 and resistance to reinfection with Schistosoma haematobium. Nature [Internet]. 1991 Jan 17 [cited 2012 Dec 31];349(6306):243-5. Available from: http://www.ncbi.nlm.nih.gov/pubmed/1898985

[43] Kouriba B, Traore HA, Dabo A, et al. Urinary disease in 2 Dogon populations with different exposure to Schistosoma haematobium infection: progression of bladder and kidney diseases in children and adults. J. Infect. Dis. [Internet]. 2005 Dec 15 [cited 2012 Sep 1];192(12):2152-9. Available from: http://www.ncbi.nlm.nih.gov/pubmed/16288382

[44] He H, Isnard A, Kouriba B, et al. A STAT6 gene polymorphism is associated with high infection levels in urinary schistosomiasis. Genes Immun. [Internet]. 2008 Apr [cited 2012 Jul 20];9(3):195-206. Available from: http://www.ncbi.nlm.nih.gov/pubmed/18273035

[45] Isnard A, Kouriba B, Doumbo O, et al. Association of rs7719175, located in the IL13 gene promoter, with Schistosoma haematobium infection levels and identification of a susceptibility haplotype. Genes Immun. [Internet]. 2011 Jan [cited 2012 Jul 20];12(1):31-9. Available from: http://www.ncbi.nlm.nih.gov/pubmed/20861864

[46] Zinyama-Gutsire R, Gomo E, Kallestrup P, et al. Downregulation of MIP-1alpha/CCL3 with praziquantel treatment in Schistosoma haematobium and HIV-1 co-infected individuals in a rural community in Zimbabwe. BMC Infect. Dis. [Internet]. 2009 Jan [cited 2012 Jul 20];9:174. Available from: http://www.pubmedcentral.nih.gov/articlerender.fcgi?artid=2770052&tool=pmcentrez&rendertype=abstract

[47] Rujeni N, Nausch N, Midzi N, et al. Schistosoma haematobium infection levels determine the effect of praziquantel treatment on anti-schistosome and anti-mite antibodies. Parasite Immunol. [Internet]. 2012 Jun [cited 2012 Jul 20];34(6):330-40. Available from: http://www.ncbi.nlm.nih.gov/pubmed/22429049

[48] Van den Biggelaar AHJ, Borrmann S, Kremsner P, et al. Immune responses induced by repeated treatment do not result in protective immunity to Schistosoma haematobium: interleukin (IL)-5 and IL-10 responses. J. Infect. Dis. [Internet]. 2002 Nov 15 [cited 2012 Jul 30];186(10):1474-82. Available from: http://www.ncbi.nlm.nih.gov/pubmed/12404164

[49] Hamm DM, Agossou A, Gantin RG, et al. Coinfections with Schistosoma haematobium, Necator americanus, and Entamoeba histolytica/Entamoeba dispar in children: chemokine and cytokine responses and changes after antiparasite treatment. J. Infect. Dis. [Internet]. 2009 Jun 1 [cited 2012 Jul 20];199(11):1583-91. Available from: http://www.ncbi.nlm.nih.gov/pubmed/19392635

[50] De Souza RDP, Cardoso LS, Lopes GTV, et al. Cytokine and Chemokine Profile in Individuals with Different Degrees of Periportal Fibrosis due to Schistosoma mansoni

Infection. J. Parasitol. Res. [Internet]. 2012 Jan [cited 2013 Feb 19];2012:394981. Available from: http://www.pubmedcentral.nih.gov/articlerender.fcgi?artid=3540765&tool=pmcentrez&rendertype=abstract

[51] Souza ALS, Souza PRS, Pereira CA, et al. Experimental infection with Schistosoma mansoni in CCR5-deficient mice is associated with increased disease severity, as CCR5 plays a role in controlling granulomatous inflammation. Infect. Immun. [Internet]. 2011 Apr [cited 2013 Feb 26];79(4):1741-9. Available from: http://www.pubmedcentral.nih.gov/articlerender.fcgi?artid=3067544&tool=pmcentrez&rendertype=abstract

[52] Grogan JL, Kremsner PG, Deelder AM, et al. Antigen-specific proliferation and interferon-gamma and interleukin-5 production are down-regulated during Schistosoma haematobium infection. J. Infect. Dis. [Internet]. 1998 May [cited 2012 Dec 26];177(5):1433-7. Available from: http://www.ncbi.nlm.nih.gov/pubmed/9593042

[53] Bourke CD, Nausch N, Rujeni N, et al. Integrated Analysis of Innate, Th1, Th2, Th17, and Regulatory Cytokines Identifies Changes in Immune Polarisation Following Treatment of Human Schistosomiasis. J. Infect. Dis. [Internet]. 2012 Oct 8 [cited 2012 Dec 23]; Available from: http://www.ncbi.nlm.nih.gov/pubmed/23045617

[54] Van den Biggelaar AH, van Ree R, Rodrigues LC, et al. Decreased atopy in children infected with Schistosoma haematobium: a role for parasite-induced interleukin-10. Lancet [Internet]. 2000 Nov 18 [cited 2013 Jan 3];356(9243):1723-7. Available from: http://www.ncbi.nlm.nih.gov/pubmed/11095260

[55] Rujeni N, Nausch N, Bourke CD, et al. Atopy Is Inversely Related to Schistosome Infection Intensity: A Comparative Study in Zimbabwean Villages with Distinct Levels of Schistosoma haematobium Infection. Int. Arch. Allergy Immunol. [Internet]. 2012 Jan [cited 2012 Jul 20];158(3):288-98. Available from: http://www.ncbi.nlm.nih.gov/pubmed/22398631

[56] Mutapi F, Imai N, Nausch N, et al. Schistosome infection intensity is inversely related to auto-reactive antibody levels. PLoS One [Internet]. 2011 Jan [cited 2012 Jul 20];6(5):e19149. Available from: http://www.pubmedcentral.nih.gov/articlerender.fcgi?artid=3089602&tool=pmcentrez&rendertype=abstract

[57] He Y-X, Chen L, Ramaswamy K. Schistosoma mansoni, S. haematobium, and S. japonicum: early events associated with penetration and migration of schistosomula through human skin. Exp. Parasitol. [Internet]. 2002 Oct [cited 2013 Jan 2];102(2):99-108. Available from: http://www.ncbi.nlm.nih.gov/pubmed/12706745

[58] Turner JD, Meurs L, Dool P, et al. Schistosome infection is associated with enhanced whole blood IL-10 secretion in response to cercarial excretory/secretory products. Parasite Immunol. [Internet]. 2013 Feb 12 [cited 2013 Feb 18]; Available from: http://www.ncbi.nlm.nih.gov/pubmed/23398537

[59] Saraiva M, O'Garra A. The regulation of IL-10 production by immune cells. Nat. Rev. Immunol. [Internet]. 2010 Mar [cited 2012 Oct 29];10(3):170-81. Available from: http://www.ncbi.nlm.nih.gov/pubmed/20154735

[60] Wamachi AN, Mayadev JS, Mungai PL, et al. Increased ratio of tumor necrosis factor-alpha to interleukin-10 production is associated with Schistosoma haematobium-induced urinary-tract morbidity. J. Infect. Dis. [Internet]. 2004 Dec 1 [cited 2012 Jul 30];190(11):2020-30. Available from: http://www.ncbi.nlm.nih.gov/pubmed/15529268

[61] Van der Vlugt LEPM, Labuda LA, Ozir-Fazalalikhan A, et al. Schistosomes induce regulatory features in human and mouse CD1d(hi) B cells: inhibition of allergic

inflammation by IL-10 and regulatory T cells. PLoS One [Internet]. 2012 Jan [cited 2012 Jul 20];7(2):e30883. Available from: http://www.pubmedcentral.nih.gov/articlerender.fcgi?artid=3275567&tool=pmcentrez&rendertype=abstract

[62] Velupillai P, Harn DA. Oligosaccharide-specific induction of interleukin 10 production by B220+ cells from schistosome-infected mice: a mechanism for regulation of CD4+ T-cell subsets. Proc. Natl. Acad. Sci. U. S. A. [Internet]. 1994 Jan 4 [cited 2013 Jan 4];91(1):18-22. Available from: http://www.pubmedcentral.nih.gov/articlerender.fcgi?artid=42877&tool=pmcentrez&rendertype=abstract

[63] Diallo TO, Remoue F, Schacht AM, et al. Schistosomiasis co-infection in humans influences inflammatory markers in uncomplicated Plasmodium falciparum malaria. Parasite Immunol. [Internet]. [cited 2012 Jul 30];26(8-9):365-9. Available from: http://www.ncbi.nlm.nih.gov/pubmed/15679634

[64] Diallo TO, Remoue F, Gaayeb L, et al. Schistosomiasis coinfection in children influences acquired immune response against Plasmodium falciparum malaria antigens. PLoS One [Internet]. 2010 Jan [cited 2012 Jul 20];5(9):e12764. Available from: http://www.pubmedcentral.nih.gov/articlerender.fcgi?artid=2939900&tool=pmcentrez&rendertype=abstract

[65] Lyke KE, Dabo A, Sangare L, et al. Effects of concomitant Schistosoma haematobium infection on the serum cytokine levels elicited by acute Plasmodium falciparum malaria infection in Malian children. Infect. Immun. [Internet]. 2006 Oct [cited 2012 Jul 18];74(10):5718-24. Available from: http://www.pubmedcentral.nih.gov/articlerender.fcgi?artid=1594876&tool=pmcentrez&rendertype=abstract

[66] Wilson MS, Cheever AW, White SD, et al. IL-10 blocks the development of resistance to re-infection with Schistosoma mansoni. Pearce EJ, editor. PLoS Pathog. [Internet]. Public Library of Science; 2011 Aug [cited 2013 Jan 2];7(8):e1002171. Available from: http://dx.plos.org/10.1371/journal.ppat.1002171

[67] Idris ZM, Yazdanbakhsh M, Adegnika AA, et al. A pilot study on cytotoxic T lymphocyte-4 gene polymorphisms in urinary schistosomiasis. Genet. Test. Mol. Biomarkers [Internet]. 2012 Jun [cited 2012 Jul 20];16(6):488-92. Available from: http://www.ncbi.nlm.nih.gov/pubmed/22288822

[68] Lamb EW, Crow ET, Lim KC, et al. Conservation of CD4+ T cell-dependent developmental mechanisms in the blood fluke pathogens of humans. Int. J. Parasitol. [Internet]. 2007 Mar [cited 2012 Jul 29];37(3-4):405-15. Available from: http://www.pubmedcentral.nih.gov/articlerender.fcgi?artid=1858658&tool=pmcentrez&rendertype=abstract

[69] Nausch N, Midzi N, Mduluza T, et al. Regulatory and activated T cells in human Schistosoma haematobium infections. PLoS One [Internet]. 2011 Jan [cited 2012 Jul 20];6(2):e16860. Available from: http://www.pubmedcentral.nih.gov/articlerender.fcgi?artid=3037381&tool=pmcentrez&rendertype=abstract

[70] Lyke KE, Dabo A, Arama C, et al. Reduced T regulatory cell response during acute Plasmodium falciparum infection in Malian children co-infected with Schistosoma haematobium. PLoS One [Internet]. 2012 Jan [cited 2012 Jul 20];7(2):e31647. Available from: http://www.pubmedcentral.nih.gov/articlerender.fcgi?artid=3279404&tool=pmcentrez&rendertype=abstract

[71]   Mbow M, Larkin BM, Meurs L, *et al.* T-helper 17 cells are associated with pathology in human schistosomiasis. J. Infect. Dis. [Internet]. 2013 Jan [cited 2012 Dec 23];207(1):186-95. Available from: http://www.ncbi.nlm.nih.gov/pubmed/23087431

[72]   Mutapi F, Burchmore R, Mduluza T, *et al.* Age-related and infection intensity-related shifts in antibody recognition of defined protein antigens in a schistosome-exposed population. J. Infect. Dis. [Internet]. 2008 Jul 15 [cited 2012 Jul 20];198(2):167-75. Available from: http://www.ncbi.nlm.nih.gov/pubmed/18549316

[73]   Mutapi F, Bourke C, Harcus Y, *et al.* Differential recognition patterns of Schistosoma haematobium adult worm antigens by the human antibodies IgA, IgE, IgG1 and IgG4. Parasite Immunol. [Internet]. 2011 Mar [cited 2012 Jul 20];33(3):181-92. Available from: http://www.pubmedcentral.nih.gov/articlerender.fcgi?artid=3084999&tool=pmcentrez&rendertype=abstract

[74]   Jeannin P, Lecoanet S, Delneste Y, *et al.* IgE *versus* IgG4 production can be differentially regulated by IL-10. J. Immunol. [Internet]. 1998 Apr 1 [cited 2013 Jan 3];160(7):3555-61. Available from: http://www.ncbi.nlm.nih.gov/pubmed/9531318

[75]   Mutapi F, Mduluza T, Gomez-Escobar N, *et al.* Immuno-epidemiology of human Schistosoma haematobium infection: preferential IgG3 antibody responsiveness to a recombinant antigen dependent on age and parasite burden. BMC Infect. Dis. [Internet]. 2006 Jan [cited 2012 Jul 30];6:96. Available from: http://www.pubmedcentral.nih.gov/articlerender.fcgi?artid=1523344&tool=pmcentrez&rendertype=abstract

[76]   Riveau G, Deplanque D, Remoué F, *et al.* Safety and immunogenicity of rSh28GST antigen in humans: phase 1 randomized clinical study of a vaccine candidate against urinary schistosomiasis. PLoS Negl. Trop. Dis. [Internet]. 2012 Jan [cited 2012 Dec 23];6(7):e1704. Available from: http://www.pubmedcentral.nih.gov/articlerender.fcgi?artid=3389022&tool=pmcentrez&rendertype=abstract

[77]   McManus DP, Loukas A. Current status of vaccines for schistosomiasis. Clin. Microbiol. Rev. [Internet]. 2008 Jan [cited 2012 Jul 20];21(1):225-42. Available from: http://www.pubmedcentral.nih.gov/articlerender.fcgi?artid=2223839&tool=pmcentrez&rendertype=abstract

[78]   Lyke KE, Wang A, Dabo A, *et al.* Antigen-specific B memory cell responses to Plasmodium falciparum malaria antigens and Schistosoma haematobium antigens in co-infected Malian children. PLoS One [Internet]. 2012 Jan [cited 2012 Nov 16];7(6):e37868. Available from: http://www.pubmedcentral.nih.gov/articlerender.fcgi?artid=3367916&tool=pmcentrez&rendertype=abstract

[79]   Nmorsi OPG, Kwandu UNCD, Ebiaguanye LM. Schistosoma haematobium and urinary tract pathogens co-infections in a rural community of Edo State, Nigeria. J. Commun. Dis. [Internet]. 2007 Jun [cited 2013 Jan 27];39(2):85-90. Available from: http://www.ncbi.nlm.nih.gov/pubmed/18338685

[80]   Kjetland EF, Mduluza T, Ndhlovu PD, *et al.* Genital schistosomiasis in women: a clinical 12-month *in vivo* study following treatment with praziquantel. Trans R Soc Trop Med Hyg [Internet]. 2006/01/13 ed. 2006;100(8):740-52. Available from: http://www.ncbi.nlm.nih.gov/pubmed/16406034

[81]   Mbabazi PS, Andan O, Fitzgerald DW, *et al.* Examining the relationship between urogenital schistosomiasis and HIV infection. PLoS Negl. Trop. Dis. [Internet]. 2011 Dec

[cited 2012 Jul 20];5(12):e1396. Available from: http://www.pubmedcentral.nih.gov/article render.fcgi?artid=3232194&tool=pmcentrez&rendertype=abstract

[82] Leutscher PDC, Pedersen M, Raharisolo C, et al. Increased prevalence of leukocytes and elevated cytokine levels in semen from Schistosoma haematobium-infected individuals. J. Infect. Dis. [Internet]. 2005 May 15 [cited 2012 Jul 30];191(10):1639-47. Available from: http://www.ncbi.nlm.nih.gov/pubmed/15838790

[83] Kallestrup P, Zinyama R, Gomo E, et al. Schistosomiasis and HIV-1 infection in rural Zimbabwe: implications of coinfection for excretion of eggs. J. Infect. Dis. [Internet]. 2005 Apr 15 [cited 2012 Jul 30];191(8):1311-20. Available from: http://www.ncbi.nlm.nih.gov/pubmed/15776378

[84] Lawn SD, Karanja DM, Mwinzia P, et al. The effect of treatment of schistosomiasis on blood plasma HIV-1 RNA concentration in coinfected individuals. AIDS [Internet]. 2000 Nov 10 [cited 2013 Feb 19];14(16):2437-43. Available from: http://www.ncbi.nlm.nih.gov/pubmed/11101053

[85] Chenine A-L, Shai-Kobiler E, Steele LN, et al. Acute Schistosoma mansoni infection increases susceptibility to systemic SHIV clade C infection in rhesus macaques after mucosal virus exposure. Bethony J, editor. PLoS Negl. Trop. Dis. [Internet]. Public Library of Science; 2008 Jan [cited 2012 Nov 1];2(7):e265. Available from: http://dx.plos.org/10.1371/journal.pntd.0000265

[86] Secor WE, Shah A, Mwinzi PMN, et al. Increased density of human immunodeficiency virus type 1 coreceptors CCR5 and CXCR4 on the surfaces of CD4(+) T cells and monocytes of patients with Schistosoma mansoni infection. Infect. Immun. [Internet]. 2003 Nov [cited 2013 Jan 2];71(11):6668-71. Available from: http://www.pubmedcentral.nih.gov/articlerender.fcgi?artid=219584&tool=pmcentrez&rendertype=abstract

[87] Wilkins HA. Schistosoma haematobium in a Gambian community. III. The prevalence of bacteriuria and of hypertension. Ann. Trop. Med. Parasitol. [Internet]. 1977 Jun [cited 2013 Jan 27];71(2):179-86. Available from: http://www.ncbi.nlm.nih.gov/pubmed/869608

[88] Hicks RM, Ismail MM, Walters CL, et al. Association of bacteriuria and urinary nitrosamine formation with Schistosoma haematobium infection in the Qalyub area of Egypt. Trans. R. Soc. Trop. Med. Hyg. [Internet]. 1982 Jan [cited 2013 Jan 27];76(4):519-27. Available from: http://www.ncbi.nlm.nih.gov/pubmed/6926771

[89] KUNTZ RE, MALAKATIS GM. Susceptibility studies in schistosomiasis. II. Susceptibility of wild mammals to infection by Schistosoma mansoni in Egypt, with emphasis on rodents. Am. J. Trop. Med. Hyg. [Internet]. 1955 Jan [cited 2013 Feb 4];4(1):75-89. Available from: http://www.ncbi.nlm.nih.gov/pubmed/13228851

[90] KUNTZ RE, MALAKATIS GM. Susceptibility studies in schistosomiasis. III. Infection of various experimental hosts with Schistosoma haematobium in Egypt. Exp. Parasitol. [Internet]. 1955 Jan [cited 2013 Feb 4];4(1):1-20. Available from: http://www.ncbi.nlm.nih.gov/pubmed/13231838

[91] KUNTZ RE, MALAKATIS GM. Susceptibility studies in schistosomiasis. IV. Susceptibility of wild mammals to infection by Schistosoma haematobium in Egypt, with emphasis on rodents. J. Parasitol. [Internet]. 1955 Oct [cited 2013 Feb 4];41(5):467-75. Available from: http://www.ncbi.nlm.nih.gov/pubmed/13264019

[92] Vuong PN, Bayssade-Dufour C, Albaret JL, et al. Histopathological observations in new and classic models of experimental Schistosoma haematobium infections. Trop. Med. Int. Health [Internet]. 1996/06/01 ed. 1996;1(3):348-58. Available from: http://www.ncbi.nlm.nih.gov/pubmed/8673838

[93] Webbe G, Nelson GS, James C, et al. Urogenital lesions in 2 baboons (Papio anubis) infected with Schistosoma haematobium. Trans. R. Soc. Trop. Med. Hyg. [Internet]. 1970 Jan [cited 2012 Dec 29];64(1):22. Available from: http://www.ncbi.nlm.nih.gov/pubmed/4986061

[94] Sadun EH, Von Lichtenberg F, Cheever AW, et al. Experimental infection with Schistosoma haematobium in chimpanzees. Am. J. Trop. Med. Hyg. [Internet]. 1970 May [cited 2013 Jan 28];19(3):427-58. Available from: http://www.ncbi.nlm.nih.gov/pubmed/4911014

[95] Soliman LA, Cheever AW, Kuntz RE, et al. Lesions of bladder muscle in baboons and monkeys infected with schistosoma haematobium. Tropenmed. Parasitol. [Internet]. 1974 Sep [cited 2013 Jan 28];25(3):327-33. Available from: http://www.ncbi.nlm.nih.gov/pubmed/4215179

[96] Rinaldi G, Okatcha TI, Popratiloff A, et al. Genetic manipulation of Schistosoma haematobium, the neglected schistosome. PLoS Negl Trop Dis [Internet]. 2011/10/25 ed. 2011;5(10):e1348. Available from: http://www.ncbi.nlm.nih.gov/pubmed/22022628

[97] Aksoy E, Zouain CS, Vanhoutte F, et al. Double-stranded RNAs from the helminth parasite Schistosoma activate TLR3 in dendritic cells. J. Biol. Chem. [Internet]. 2005 Jan 7 [cited 2013 Jan 3];280(1):277-83. Available from: http://www.ncbi.nlm.nih.gov/pubmed/15519998.

[98] Okano M, Satoskar AR, Nishizaki K, et al. Induction of Th2 Responses and IgE Is Largely Due to Carbohydrates Functioning as Adjuvants on Schistosoma mansoni Egg Antigens. J. Immunol. [Internet]. 1999 Dec 15 [cited 2013 Jan 3];163(12):6712-7. Available from: http://www.jimmunol.org/content/163/12/6712.abstract?ijkey=0193433ae27535f4a2098e540dcb2af5bd36bcf2&keytype2=tf_ipsecsha

[99] Schramm G, Mohrs K, Wodrich M, et al. Cutting edge: IPSE/alpha-1, a glycoprotein from Schistosoma mansoni eggs, induces IgE-dependent, antigen-independent IL-4 production by murine basophils in vivo. J. Immunol. [Internet]. 2007/05/04 ed. 2007;178(10):6023-7. Available from: http://www.ncbi.nlm.nih.gov/pubmed/17475824

[100] Schramm G, Hamilton J V, Balog CIA, et al. Molecular characterisation of kappa-5, a major antigenic glycoprotein from Schistosoma mansoni eggs. Mol. Biochem. Parasitol. [Internet]. 2009 Jul [cited 2012 Mar 15];166(1):4-14. Available from: http://www.ncbi.nlm.nih.gov/pubmed/19428667

[101] Everts B, Perona-Wright G, Smits HH, et al. Omega-1, a glycoprotein secreted by Schistosoma mansoni eggs, drives Th2 responses. J. Exp. Med. [Internet]. 2009 Aug 3 [cited 2012 Aug 15];206(8):1673-80. Available from: http://www.pubmedcentral.nih.gov/articlerender.fcgi?artid=2722183&tool=pmcentrez&rendertype=abstract

[102] Donnelly S, Stack CM, O'Neill SM, et al. Helminth 2-Cys peroxiredoxin drives Th2 responses through a mechanism involving alternatively activated macrophages. FASEB J. [Internet]. 2008 Nov [cited 2012 Apr 5];22(11):4022-32. Available from: http://www.ncbi.nlm.nih.gov/pubmed/18708590

[103] Young ND, Jex AR, Li B, *et al.* Whole-genome sequence of Schistosoma haematobium. Nat. Genet. [Internet]. 2012/01/17 ed. 2012;44(2):221-5. Available from: http://www.ncbi.nlm.nih.gov/pubmed/22246508

CHAPTER 6

The Translational Immunology of Trichinellosis: From Rodents to Humans

Fabrizio Bruschi[1,*] and Maria Angeles Gómez-Morales[2]

[1]*Department of Translational Research, N.T.M.S., University of Pisa, Medical School, Via Roma, 55 56126 Pisa, Italy and* [2] *Department of Infectious, Parasitic and Immunomediated Diseases, Istituto Superiore di Sanità, viale Regina Elena 299, 00161 Rome, Italy*

Abstract: Trichinellosis is a worldwide zoonosis caused by the parasitic nematodes belonging to the *Trichinella* genus.

In this review we describe some aspects of the host immunity to the different species of *Trichinella* in humans, as well as in rodents which are one of the most studied experimental models. The role of humoral (antibodies) and cellular (T cells, mast cells, eosinophils and neutrophils), immune responses to this nematode will be considered in experimental as well as in human infections. Particular attention will be paid on the possibility to exploit such knowledge to improve the diagnostic possibilities of infection. Immunopathological aspects of infection will also be considered.

Finally, the evasion mechanisms of host immune responses exploited by *Trichinella* and the vaccination perspectives for control will be elucidated.

Keywords: Basophils, cytokines, dendritic cells, diagnosis, eosinophils, human trichinellosis, IgE, IgG, immunology, immunopathology, infection in rodents, macrophages, mast cells, myositis, neutrophils, nurse cell, *Trichinella spiralis*, *Trichinella britovi*, *Trichinella pseudospiralis*, vaccines

INTRODUCTION

Trichinellosis is a meat-borne infection/disease caused by *Trichinella*. This nematode has a wide host range as well as geographical distribution [1, 2]. In Fig. (**1**) the global distribution of different *Trichinella* species is shown.

---

*Corresponding author **Fabrizio Bruschi:** Department of Translational Research, N.T.M.S., University of Pisa, Medical School, *Via Roma*, 55 56126 Pisa, Italy; Tel: +39 050 2218547; Fax: +39 050 2218547557; E-mail: fabrizio.bruschi@med.unipi.it

Emilio Jirillo, Thea Magrone and Giuseppe Miragliotta (Eds)
All rights reserved-© 2014 Bentham Science Publishers

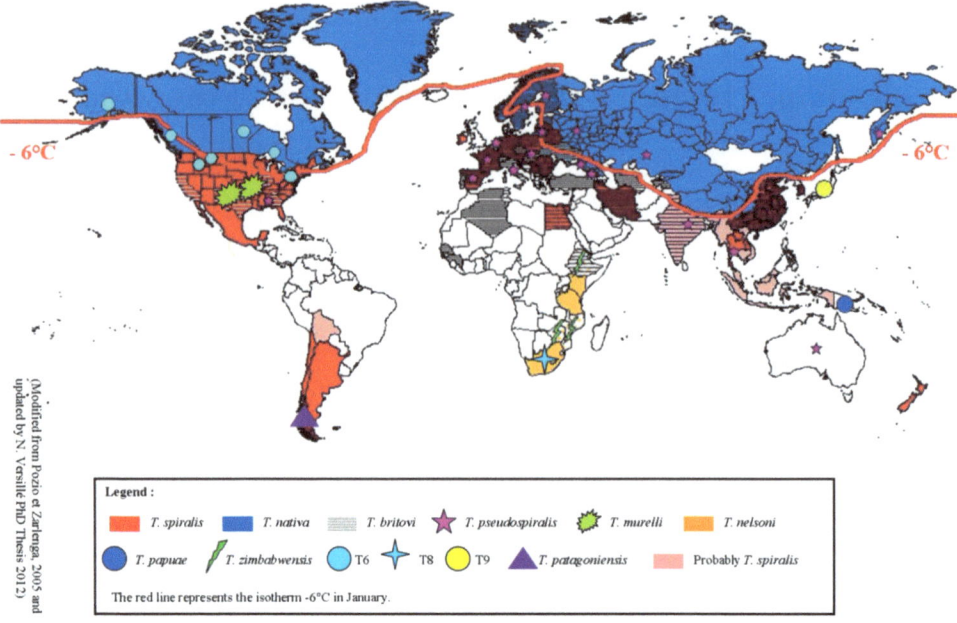

Figure 1: The global distribution of different *Trichinella* species. From (Ref. [2]) with permission.

Nowadays, nine different species have been described, the so-called encapsulating species such as *Trichinella spiralis*, *Trichinella nativa*, *Trichinella nelsoni*, *Trichinella britovi*, *Trichinella murrelli*, and the recently described *Trichinella patagoniensis* [3] and *Trichinella pseudospiralis*, *Trichinella papuae* and *Trichinella zimbabwensis* (which, viceversa are not able to induce the capsule formation) plus different genotypes. Trichinellosis is controlled in Europe and U.S.A., but it is now emerging in either high or low income countries [1].

In the U.S.A., Canada and European Union, human infections caused by the consumption of meat from domestic pigs have nearly or completely disappeared. The reasons are different: i) the improvement of pig-production facilities and practices; ii) the amelioration of detection technologies employed in the slaughterhouses. However, occasional infections with *T. spiralis* still occur in these countries, being mainly related to the consumption of pork from the so-called backyard pigs or pigs reared on organic farms [4]. The situation is completely different in countries, either developed or developing of Central and South America (Argentina), Eastern Europe and Asia, particularly China [5, 6].

Life Cycle of *Trichinella* (shown in Fig. 2)

Among helminths, *Trichinella* is unique as regards the life cycle since it has an intracellular localization, initially in enterocytes, then in skeletal muscle cells [1].

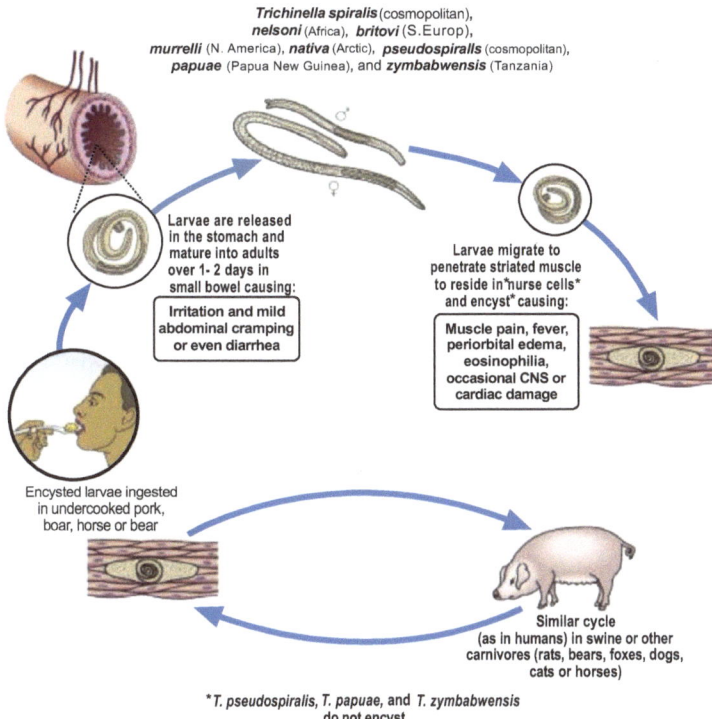

Figure 2: The life cycle of *Trichinella* spp. *Trichinella spiralis* (cosmopolitan), *T. nelsoni* (distributed in Africa), *T. britovi* (in South Europe), *T. murrelli* (in North America), *T. nativa* (in the Arctic), *T. pseudospiralis* (with a cosmopolitan distribution), *T. papuae* (in Papua New Guinea), *T. zymbabwensis* (in Tanzania), and *T. patagoniensis* (in South America), not yet described at that time. From (Ref. [162]) with permission.

All stages of the parasite (larval and adult) occur in the same host. Mammals are prone to be infected, along with birds and reptiles. Humans, swines and horses are the most relevant hosts from both medical and veterinary perspecives [1]. When a host ingests infected meat, the muscle larva, which corresponds to the first larval stage (L1), by the action of pepsin is released and migrates to the small intestine. The external part of the cuticle (epicuticle) is modified by the alkaline pH and the pancreatic enzymes [7, 8]. This process allows the free parasites to perceive environmental signals and to achieve their cellular localization in the host intestinal cell cytoplasm. Then, young adults are stimulated by yet unknown factors to pass through the villi basement [9]. There, the larvae invade the columnar epithelium, and after moulting four times, mature sexually (in about 10-30 hours after ingestion).

Adult female measures 2.5-3.5 mm in length with a diameter of 50 µm whereas males are shorter (between 1.0 and 1.5 mm) by 30 µm in width [10].

The mating occurs within three days after infection and the first newborn larvae (NBL) are released already one day after copulation.

This process occurs for the remaining life of the female. The number of NBL produced depends on the host immune status and the *Trichinella* species involved [11]. It is estimated that between 500 and 1,500 NBL are shed over the life span of an adult female worm before host immune response induces their expulsion from the small intestine [12]. According to the common opinion, the adult worms remain in the intestine for only few weeks, but they actually may maintain their viability longer, mainly in immunocompromised hosts, like nude mice, in experimental conditions in rodents [13]. The timing of worm expulsion is extremely variable, depending on host and *Trichinella* species, but the infection dose is a crucial factor [5]. The NBL measure 80-120 µm in length and 7 µm in diameter. NBL and are characterised by the presence of a stylet localised close to cephalic extremity. It allows to this stage to penetrate the *lamina propria*, then the mesenteric capillary walls or those of lymphatic vessels and finally the plasma membrane of skeletal muscle cell. After the NBL have penetrated into the submucosa, they enter the circulatory system and diffuse to the different organs, where they may cause mechanical tissue damage, but only the larvae which invade the skeletal muscle fibers can survive and grow. As expected, there is a relation between the blood supply to the muscle and the number of NBL which arrive to infect the tissue [2]. NBL penetrate the skeletal muscle cells after having grown and maturating of about 20- 30%. This step involves enzymes which are not yet identified [14]. The tropism of NBL for the skeletal muscle cell is very high and most of them arrive to this site in not immunised hosts [5]. Apparently, in intravenously administered infections, larval penetration of muscle can occur at anytime up to three days after the time of injection [14, 15].

In most parasite species such as those which are encapsulating (*i.e.* they induce the collagen capsule) they slowly encyst, developing into the infective stage about 3 to 4 weeks after infection.

In species which are not-encapsulated, the larvae are not surrounded by a collagen capsule. However, in any case the transformation of the skeletal muscle fiber in the "nurse cell" (NC). This new cell completely lacks the characteristics of contractile cell but it is mainly devoted to the survival and growth of the parasite [5]. This phenotypic change lasts about twenty days to be accomplished [14, 15]. Larval infectivity is kept for several years, being this period different from host to host. The parasite is non-pathogenic for the natural hosts (excluding humans) unless very large numbers of larvae are installed in the muscles.

THE HOST RESPONSES TO THE PARASITE

Trichinella spp. completes its natural life cycle in only one host, consequently, antigens from all of three life stages - adult (AD), NBL and muscle larvae (ML) play a crucial role in the development and maintenance of the host immunity. The host, which presents a genetically determined great variability [16], can activate different effector mechanisms able to eliminate the parasite or limit the parasite's ability to induce injury (see Table **1**, [17]).

The Intestinal Phase

During the intestinal phase the larval and adult worms of *Trichinella* are found in the jejunal intestinal epithelium, often at the crypt-villous junction, and do not to cross the basement membrane. Despite its relatively large size, the worm establishes an intracellular niche and appears to occupy several cells simultaneously, inducing an inflammatory response, sustained mainly by eosinophils. Other relevant changes in the epithelium occur, namely: infiltration by mucosal mast cells (MC), villus atrophy, crypt hyperplasia, goblet and Paneth cell hyperplasia and increased contractility of intestinal smooth muscle cells, by which worm expulsion is facilitated. Among all of them, the increased levels of eosinophils, the pronounced mastocytosis and the activation of mucosal MC are considered to be the hallmarks of *Trichinella* infection in both, experimental models [18, 19] and human infections [20]. However, the mechanisms which regulate the response to the parasite in humans are not completely clear at intestinal level.

Table 1: Scheme of the stages involved in the life cycle of *Trichinella spiralis* and the immune and inflammatory responses initiated in the infected mouse host (modified from Wakelin, [17])

Parasite life cycle	Host response
Entry of infective muscle larvae Invasion of enterocytes Release of stichosomal antigen Exposure of surface antigen	Uptake, processing and recognition of antigens, initial Th1 response
Maturation of adults Release of new born larvae (NBL) Exposure of adult and NBL antigens	**Antibody response** **Mast cell response** **Gut inflammation begins**
Expulsion of adult worms Migration of NBL	**Antibody response** **Mast cell response** Acute inflammation **Shift to Th2 response**
Invasion of muscles Nurse cell formation Release of stichocyte antigen Formation of capsule, when present	**Antibody response** **Eosinophilia** Gut inflammation subsides **Inflammation in muscle** **Consolidated Th2 response**

Processes described also in humans are written in red

Many experimental studies have been carried out in rodent models to demonstrate to which extent MC are crucial in the host response to the parasite. In both mice and rats, mast cell degranulation can be detected at the time of adult worm expulsion [21, 22]. The temporal alignment of intestinal mastocytosis and mast cell degranulation with the expulsion of adult worms provided evidence that MC play a fundamental role in intestinal defense against the parasite. Support for this notion has been provided by reports in which rejection of both primary and secondary intestinal infections with *T. spiralis* is delayed in mast cell-deficient W/Wv mice [23, 24] and in which the capacity to reject AD worms can be reconstituted with bone marrow cells [25]. Furthermore, mice unable to produce mast cell protease-1 (mMCP-1) show delayed rejection of *T. spiralis* [19]. It has been hypothesized that mMCP-1 increases intestinal permeability, providing antibodies access to parasite antigens [26]. In fact, previous studies had indicated that mMCP-1, which is a β-chymase (chymotrypsin-like-serine protease), can degrade proteins necessary for the formation of tight junctions between epithelial cells [26]. Consequently, mMCP-1 may disrupt tight junction structure, facilitating paracellular permeability [27].

In rats, primary intestinal infection with *T. spiralis* induces an accumulation of mast cells which degranulate at the same time of rapid expulsion in challenged rats, as shown by the increase of rat mast cell protease II (RMCPII) serum levels; however, there is no direct evidence that MC contribute to expulsion. Immunization of adult rats by infecting animals directly in the muscles (skipping the intestinal phase) did not cause intestinal mast cell accumulation, however such rats are able to mount a rapid expulsion when challenged orally. Despite the absence of mastocytosis, the RMCPII was present in sera during expulsion. Further, the evaluation of mast cell activity in neonatal rats that display rapid expulsion showed that pups born from infected dams underwent rapid expulsion, with RMCPII in their sera. By feeding pups with parasite-specific monoclonal antibodies (Abs) or polyclonal Abs specific for *Trichinella* prior to a secondary infection, the authors dissociated mast cell degranulation from worm expulsion, indicating that this phenomenon can occur in the absence of either intestinal mast cell accumulation or RMCPII release [28].

It has been documented in Inhuit populations living in the Canadian Arctic, especially in elderly patients a diarrheic syndrome, lasting even 100 days with abdominal pain, short muscle symptomatology and without fever. These individuals are regularly exposed to *T. nativa*, and their intestinal syndrome could be related with the worm expulsion phenomenon similar to that observed in rodents [29].

It has been shown that antigens derived from AD and ML, that, during the intestinal phase of the infection, interact with the host, can activate a rat MC line (HRMC) with mucosal characteristics through an immunoglobulin (Ig)-independent pathway. In fact the direct binding of *T. spiralis* muscle larva (TSL) group1 antigens to unsensitized MC, brought to their activation and to the release of histamine, increasing interleukin (IL)-4 and tumor necrosis factor (TNF) at the mRNA and protein levels [30, 31]. Moreover, AD total extract caused the release of histamine from unsensitized MC, the same effect is not observed with NBL crude extract or NBL purified antigens [32].

On the other hand, it has been demonstrated that secreted proteins from *T. spiralis* infective larvae inhibit nucleotide-induced MC activation, in particular the process is specifically blocked by parasite secretory 5'-nucleotidase when it is stimulated by adenosine diphosphate (ADP) or uridine diphosphate (UDP). Either parasite secreted products or the 5'-nucleotidase inhibit ADP-induced release of MC protease, whereas that stimulated by adenosine triphosphate (ATP) is partially inhibited by secreted products alone [33].

Eosinophilia is considered to be a hallmark of nematode infection. It was demonstrated that IL-5 deficient mice not only were unable to mount an intestinal eosinophilia, as expected, but also underwent a lower intestinal hyper-contractility with a transient delay of worm expulsion. The effect of IL-5 on intestinal smooth muscles is not direct, but rather due to the increase of eosinophil inflammation which might lead to hyper-contractility, through the release of products of arachidonic acid metabolism like for example, leukotrienes [34]. When eosinophil-ablated mice were infected with *Trichuris muris,* or *T. spiralis* no key role for eosinophils in the intestinal phase was observed [35, 36].

In most rodent models, after the first 2-4 days of *T. spiralis* infection parasite-specific T cells are produced in the intestinal mucosa [37], then these cells migrate progressively to the Peyer's patches and to the mesenteric lymph nodes to be distributed further to the tissues [16].

It has been investigated in monolayers of epithelial cells from the human colon the initial invasion of *T. spiralis*, showing that a high cell impairment and a transcriptional activation of pro-inflammatory cytokines, follows the invasion of intestinal epithelial cells by the parasite. These cytokines promote the inflammatory response inducing the recruitment and activation of cells in the *lamina propria*. With the loss of membrane integrity, the damaged cells undergo swelling of the whole volume, organelle increase, finally necrosis and crashing [38].

At intestinal level, the immune response triggered by *T. spiralis* in mice depends on T CD4+ cells [39, 40] with a pattern of cytokine response type 0 or type 1 [41, 42] which switch to a Th2 which produce cytokines such as IL-4, IL-5, IL-9 and IL-13 [27]. These factors are produced additionally by non-T cells like B cells, eosinophils, MC and basophils. Also by these cytokines, Th2-type responses are driven, but it is well established that worm expulsion is essentially CD4+ T cell-dependent and IL-4 and IL-13 are needed for such process. In fact, only these cytokines activate the signal transducer and activator of transcription 6 (Stat 6) through the binding to IL-4 receptor α. Stat 6 signaling promotes the immune response to *T. spiralis* both through effects on bone marrow- and non-bone marrow derived cells [43]. Instead, IL-9 does not influence *T. spiralis* expulsion, although it can promote protective immunity, increasing the jejunum muscle hyper-contractility, and consequently accelerating the worm expulsion [44].

IL-5 seems to be not essential in expulsion mechanisms during a primary infection with the parasite, but it is important during the secondary *T. spiralis* infection [45]. Intestinal eosinophils from infected rats unless activated by IL-5 are not able to kill NBL in an antibody dependent cellular cytotoxicity (ADCC) *in vitro*, contrary to peritoneal eosinophils [46].

In the intestinal phase of the *Trichinella* infection other cytokines may be involved, as for example IL-10, which plays a crucial role in as results from studies in mice in which the gene coding for this cytokine is disrupted. Also normal mice treated with an antibody neutralizing IL-10 receptor (by this treatment they become highly susceptible to a primary *T. spiralis* infection) delayed adult worm expulsion and showed an increased worm burden at muscular level [47]. IL-12 down-regulates the effects of Th2 activation, delaying worm expulsion and leading to an increased worm muscle burden in an interferon-γ (IFNγ)-independent way [48]. An increase in worm burden was also observed in mice treated with the Th1 adjuvant *Helicobacter pylori* neutrophil activating protein, a Toll like receptor 2 ligand [49]. Intestinal levels of IL-17 and IL-23 increase during infection with the parasite in mice, furthermore IL-17 can stimulate *in vitro* smooth muscle contractility [50]. IL-18 regulates either Th1 or Th2 responses, depending on the cytokine environment. Exogenous IL-18 in mice inhibits also the development of mast cell accumulation which follows the infection with *T. spiralis* and mice knock out (KO) for this cytokine expel *T. spiralis* faster than wild-type do [51].

The participation of Abs in rapid expulsion of *T. spiralis* AD has been documented in passively immunized rat pups: immune serum or parasite-specific monoclonal immunoglobulin (Ig)G1 or IgG2c confer an immunity on pups that is indistinguishable from that of the previously infected adult rats which lead to the rapid expulsion. Abs are protective when delivered to pups orally or by *i.p.* injection, or when passively transferred in milk from the mother. The two rat isotypes known to activate MC, IgE and IgG2a, do not protect neonates. In contrast to rat pups, passive immunization of adult rats is effective only after intestinal priming [52, 53]. Protective Abs are specific for β tyvelose-bearing glycans that are unique to L1 [54]. In the presence of tyvelose-specific Abs, L1 are excluded from the epithelium, entrapped in mucus, or encumbered in epithelial cells [55, 56].

Other possible effectors to *Trichinella* at intestinal level are mucins and intelectins secreted by the goblet cells. Mucins (Muc) are glycoproteins with several ramifications, forming the mucus layer which covers the epithelium, and contributes to the host protection during the lumen-dwelling stages of *T. spiralis*. Mice infected with *T. spiralis* show increased expression of Muc2 and Muc3, at a higher extent however, when animals deficient in T cells or cytokine signaling necessary to clear the parasite are infected they continue to express these proteins at high level. Intelectins, which belong to a family of galactofuranose-binding lectins were found primarily in goblet cells and Paneth cells of the intestine. BALB/c mice, a resistant strain, but not susceptible C57BL/10 mice, show increased expression of intelectin-2 early during *T. spiralis* infection, suggesting a role for this protein in parasite recognition or expulsion [57].

The Muscle Phase

Experimental studies have shown that larvae initiate the muscle phase of infection when they enter individual, myotubes which are completely-differentiated. Over a period of 3 weeks the infected myotube reenters the cell cycle, remodelling the cytoplasmic matrix, produces a collagen capsule - if the infective parasite is an encapsulating species-, and induces the formation of a capillary rete around the nurse cell-parasite complex. These changes correlate with a strong inflammatory response causing myositis and with dramatic modifications in host gene expression. Transcription of muscle-specific genes is down-regulated, whereas synthesis of syndecan-1 is induced, as well as vascular endothelial growth factor (VEGF) genes are activated and collagen transcripts are increased [58-62]. These modifications correlate with the formation of the NC. *Trichinella* species induce various grades of myositis around the NC-parasite complex, and differences between encapsulating and non-encapsulating species, probably due to their distinctive biological features are relevant [63]. Early histological studies of infected muscle revealed an accumulation of inflammatory cells surrounding individual infected muscle cells [13]. Similar to a granuloma, the focal infiltrate which surrounds individual NCs contains macrophages [59, 64], eosinophils, lymphocytes and MC. Macrophages can also be observed in the cytoplasm of the NC [65]. Once the larva completes development in the muscle, it continues to be infective for months to years. In mice, NBL arrive to the muscle at the same time when the intestinal Th2 driven immune response expels adult worms and stimulates blood and tissue eosinophilia [36]. Despite the intense local inflammation, intracellular muscle larvae mature and become infectious. Over the ensuing years, the clearance of the larvae can occur, in that case histopathology is characterized by patchy necrotic lesions with infiltration of eosinophils, lymphocytes, and macrophages, which later turn into calcified deposits, after parasite death [66]. Skeletal muscle is populated exclusively with a MC subpopulation, the connective tissue-type MC population that produces both the chymases (chymotryptic-like serine proteases) and the tryptases (tryptic-like serine proteases). *In vivo* analyses, using a strain of mMCP-6-deficient mice, have demonstrated that initially the adaptive immune response produces specific IgE that binds to *T. spiralis* larvae in skeletal muscle; these complex activates the connective tissue-type MC expressing mMCP-6, causing release of tryptase, responsible of the eosinophil recruitment [67].

Although eosinophil-ablated mice expel normally *T. spiralis* from the intestine, immunity to the larva is even enhanced in these animals; in fact, muscle larvae have a high mortality (50-75%) at the same time increased IFN-γ and diminished

IL-4 production is detected in draining lymph nodes [36, 68]. Without eosinophils, leukocytes, mainly macrophages, produce inducible NO synthase (iNOS) at sites of infection whereas parasites improve their viability when specific iNOS inhibitors are given to mice. There is an increase of the NO production and parasite killing up to 90% when IL-10 deficiency is introduced into the eosinophil-deficient mice. These studies suggest that eosinophils promote accumulation of Th2 cells and prevent induction of iNOS in macrophages and neutrophils, supporting parasite growth and survival [69].

Since inflammatory infiltrates are absent around NCs in T lymphocyte deficient mice, it can be deduced that the inflammatory response during the muscle phase is regulated by T cells [13]. IL-4 is produced by activated popliteal lymph node cells once activated by direct injection of NBL into thigh muscles of BALB/c [70]. Furthermore, cells recovered from cervical lymph nodes of C57BL/10 or C57BL/6 infected mice produce IL-5, IL-10, IL-13 and IFN-γ after stimulation with somatic larval antigens [68, 71]. To study the immune response induced and maintained by muscle infection, Fabre *et al.* [36] infected mice by intravenous inoculation of NBL, this procedure allows to establish a synchronous infection that is not influenced by the immune response induced at the intestinal phase. In this model, the infiltrated cells observed on the sites of infection were predominantly macrophages, numerous CD4+ T cells, fewer CD8+ T cells, and rare B lymphocytes. In these experiments the effect of the anti-inflammatory cytokine IL-10 was evident 20 days after muscle infection, since the numbers of cells in IL-10 deficient mice was higher than in the C57BL/6 wild-type mice; however the involved cells of muscle infiltrates was unvariated. Mice that were orally infected such that they experience intestinal infection prior to muscle infection develop stronger Th2 responses in cervical lymph nodes than did those mice directly injected with NBL into thigh muscles. Nevertheless, the influence of IL-10 on myositis is similar in infections initiated by either oral and muscular route [36]. Enhanced myositis in IL-10 deficient mice did not alter parasite establishment or survival [59]. Thus, in the context of a primary muscle infection, IL-10 functions largely protect the host against injury caused by inflammation [36]. Instead, chronic inflammation is independent of IL-10 because in the period of 20 to 50 days post-infection the inflammatory response ameliorates in both wild type and IL-10 deficient mice. Muscle infection induces an antibody response of mixed isotypes directed to somatic larval antigens that changes to an IgG1 dominated response directed to β tyvelose-bearing excretory-secretory antigens (ESA) [59]. The increase of IgG1 coexists with the IL-10 independent phase of the cellular response. Thus, IL-10 limits the local inflammatory response during the early stages of muscle infection while control of chronic inflammation is IL-10-independent and is coincident with a strong Th2 response. CD4+ CD25- T cells rather than CD4+ CD25+ T regulatory cells are central to IL-10 modulation of acute inflammation as resulted from cell depletion and adoptive transfer experiments [68]. In addition to IL-10, transforming growth factor (TGF)-β is known to mediate T cell suppression [72]. Treatment of wild-type mice with antibodies to TGF-β induces myositis; however, the combined deficiency in TGF-β and IL-10 leads to a much more severe inflammatory response in muscles. The abrogation of TGF-β alone did not affect parasite survival but the combined depletion of TGF-β and IL-10 was associated with parasite death in muscle [68]. Consequently, TGF-β helps with IL-10 in the control of local inflammation. In the absence of IL-10, TGF-β promotes parasite survival in muscles [36].

The cell-mediated immunity was studied during the muscle phase in infections caused by *T. spiralis* and *T. britovi* in humans [73]. The results have shown that during the infection period studied (up to 14 months p. i.) peripheral blood mononuclear cells are able to respond to parasite antigens and express and produce a type 2 cytokine pattern (IL-4, IL-5, IL-6, IL-10), irrespective of *Trichinella* species. The great amount of eosinophils surrounding the encysted parasites, which may be responsible for the muscle damage, may be explained by the type 2 cytokine pattern [63].

The circulating antibody responses to *T. spiralis* infection have been deeply studied in experimentally-infected mice. Parasite-specific IgG1, IgG2 [74] and IgE [75] increase significantly during last stages of the muscular phase of infection. Eighty percent of IgG1 specific for larval antigens recognize a single shared epitope [76], now known to be the highly immunogenic carbohydrate, β-tyvelose [54]. The predominance of parasite-specific IgG1 and IgE during chronic infection is associated with the strong Th2 response in cervical lymph nodes [68].

EVALUATION OF THE HUMORAL IMMUNE RESPONSE FOR DIAGNOSTIC PURPOSES

The circulating antibody responses to *Trichinella* infection have been studied in infected persons. In general, specific IgG, IgA and IgM response accompanies trichinellosis; whereas specific IgE antibodies and increased levels of total IgE seem not to be obligatory findings in patients suffering from this infection, consequently its diagnostic value as single datum is limited. Generally, seroconversion takes place between the third and fifth week of infection and antibody levels do not correlate with the severity of the clinical course nor with a particular clinical course [77]. The sequential appearance of specific antibodies of the various IgG subclasses during the early stage of a *T. spiralis* infection has been studied during an outbreak in the West part of Poland. Sera were collected at various times after early infection and one year later and it was found that the peak response of IgG1 appeared before IgG4 and in about half of the patients simultaneously with IgG3. Specific IgG1 antibodies dominated the immune response. During the year following the infection, a statistically significant shift of specific antibodies to IgG4 was noted. In addition to specific IgG4 antibodies, specific IgG3 antibodies also appeared in high amounts. The authors conclude that the severity of illness is reflected in the IgG2 and IgG3 responses of the patients, while the IgG4 response seems to discriminate between an early and late infection with the parasite. The level of total IgE showed an inverse correlation to levels of specific IgG4 antibodies, the latter appearing late during infection. Specific IgE antibodies were not detected in any of the sera obtained during the early stage from infected patients at different times post infection [78].

In other studies, *Trichinella*-specific IgM, IgG, and IgA antibodies in sera from symptomatic and asymptomatic patients tested positive up to 15 years after infection [79]. The IgG4 antibody response to a 45 kDa *T. spiralis* antigen also persisted at least 18 months in *T. spiralis* infected patients [80] and up to15 years after *T. britovi* infection [79]. IgG specific antibodies can be detectable from 12 to 60 days post infection and may persist for more than 30 years after infection [81].

In late-stage trichinellosis patients (2-8 years from acute infection), involved in an outbreak occurred in Poland and presumably caused by *T. spiralis* the presence of

T. spiralis specific humoral response was evaluated by different methods: (i) indirect immunofluorescence assay (IFA), using muscle sections from mice, 30 days following synchronous infection by intramuscular injection with *T. spiralis* (NBL); (ii) enzyme immunoassay (EIA), employing a synthetic β-tyvelose antigen conjugated to bovine serum albumin; and (iii) western blot (WB) with both an "in house" and a commercial kit; iv) competitive inhibition assay (CIA) [82, 83].

By IFA and confocal laser microscopy all sera reacted against both surface and internal structures of L1 larvae, see Fig. (3), but at varying levels which correlated with the CIA results.

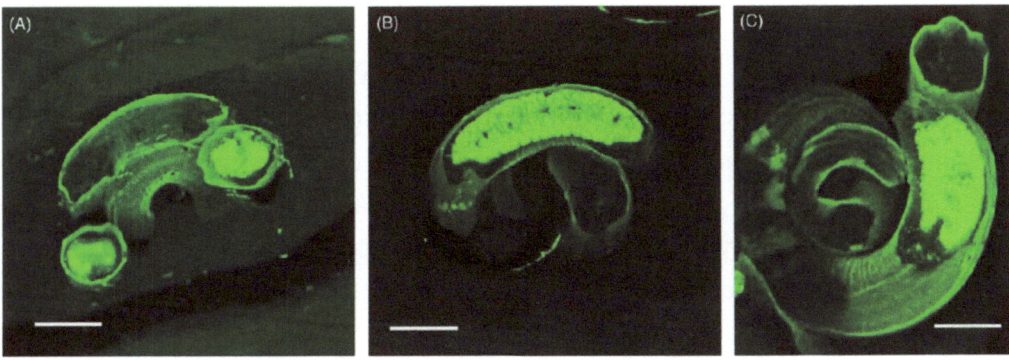

Figure 3: Confocal laser fluorescence microscope views of *Trichinella spiralis* L1 muscle larvae from infected mice at 32 days post synchronous infection, after reaction with serum from a trichinellosis patient. **A** and **C** show heavy staining at the cuticular level and **B** also in the stichosome (scale bar = 60 μm). From (Ref. [83]), with permission.

Fifty percent of sera from *Trichinella* infected persons tested positive for the presence of specific antibodies against β-tyvelose by EIA. By WB, all sera were reactive with the 45 kDa glycoprotein (45 gp). These data have suggested that reactivity against the β-tyvelosylated 45 gp persists even in very late stages of human trichinellosis. In patients, re-evaluated 15 years after acute infection with *T. britovi* 91.6% remained positive by WB (with reactivity against the 45 kDa protein) but only one of 13 was positive for antibodies specific for β-tyvelose [84].

Since there is not pathognomonic sign or symptom, the clinical diagnosis is difficult. Consequently, the diagnosis of trichinellosis should be based on three main criteria: anamnesis based on epidemiological data, clinical evaluation and laboratory tests including serology and/or the detection of *Trichinella* larvae in a muscle biopsy [85]. Because the collection of a muscle biopsy is invasive, painful, and not always gives the expected result, even if the suspected diagnosis is correct, the serological diagnosis, normally carried out by the detection of specific IgG in serum has a great and practical diagnostic value.

Although many tests for the detection of IgG antibodies have been developed, nowadays, the indirect enzyme linked immunosorbent assay (ELISA) is the most frequently used because its sensitivity [85-87], however sometimes the WB is used as the only test for humans [85]. ELISA has been first developed using the low specific crude worm extract (CWE) antigens prepared from the L1 larvae [88-92], and then has been used the more specific ESA, obtained from L1 larvae maintained in culture [93-105]. TSL antigens have been classified into eight groups (TSL-1 - TSL-8) according to their ability to react with different monoclonal and polyclonal antibodies. The antigenic pattern of all *Trichinella* species and genotypes recognized so far, is very similar, thus the antigen prepared with one species or genotype, can be used to detect specific antibodies in persons infected with different species [87, 106]. TSL-1 is stage specific, originates from the stichosome (a glandular structure consisting of 50-55 discoid cells, called stichocytes which occupies the anterior half of the L1 larva), it is present in the larval cuticular surface and thus in the CWE and it is the most abundant in the ESA. TSL-1 antigens share an immunodominant carbohydrate epitope (tyvelose, 3,6-dideoxy-D-arabinohexose) which is considered to be unique for parasites of the genus *Trichinella* [107]. Total soluble extracts from *T. spiralis* adult stage (AD-TSE) and NBL have been used to analyze by ELISA the class and subclass of the antibody response to *Trichinella,* AD-TSE antigens showed similar sensitivity that TSL-1 antigens but less specificity, whereas NBL antigens showed to be less sensitive than TSL-1 antigens [97, 108].

An important issue in serological diagnosis for parasitic infections, and especially for those caused by nematodes, is the cross-reactivity, especially when crude extracts and to a lesser extent excretory/secretory antigens are used. In fact, it has been largely reported the presence of shared antigens of *Trichinella* spp. in other parasites and pathogens [91, 104, 109-112]. For these reasons, different attempts to increase the specificity of ELISA have been done, thus the main components of ESA, which are the TSL-1 antigens, once purified by affinity chromatography with monoclonal antibodies have been used in an indirect and in a capture ELISA showing an improved specificity when compared to the CWE [101, 113]. The immunodominant carbohydrate tyvelose has been synthesized and used successfully to detect anti-*Trichinella* IgG in humans [114] and even if this antigen has the advantages of specificity, stability and standardization, its utility for diagnostic purposes is still not well known as there are contrasting results regarding sensitivity [87, 115-117] as well as specificity [118, 119]. Recently, it has been proposed to use ESA in a validated ELISA followed by WB to confirm positive results [120, 121].

In a glycan array containing over 250 different glycan antigens, a GalNAcβ1-4(Fucα1-3) GlcNAc-R (LDNF) was identified as an antigen that is recognized by antibodies from *Trichinella*-infected individuals Fig. (**4**). An ELISA based test using a glycan represented by 5 LDNF molecules linked to bovine serum albumin gave a 67% of specificity (false positive results were mainly obtained with cisticercosis and strongyloidosis sera) and 96% of sensitivity [122].

EVASION MECHANISMS AND IMMUNOMODULATION

Based on the continuous relationship between *Trichinella* spp. and its hosts during evolution, the parasites have developed several evasion mechanisms allowing the establishment of the infection with the minimum possible damage to the host, ensuring its own survival. The evasion mechanisms from the host's immune response have been classified in two types: i) antigen-dependent (including anatomic seclusion, antigen stage-specificity, shedding and renewal and molecular mimicry); ii) direct on the host immune response [63]. Among antigen-dependent mechanisms, anatomic seclusion and stage-specificity are the most important. *Trichinella* muscle larvae communicate with the host, releasing antigens that continuously stimulate the host immune response, even if the parasites are sequestered, inside the NC and thus protected from antibodies and effector cells. Regarding stage-specificity of the antigens, early antibodies specific for adult worms do not recognize the migrant stages. On the other hand, antibodies specific for surface antigens of NBL appear when the parasite is already established in the NC and cannot be attacked [123]. Furthermore, NBLs, during the first hours of life, undergo modifications of the surface proteins [124] and of the sensitivity to effector cells in both mice [125] and humans [126, 127]. In addition, the immunodominant antigens in the infective larvae are distinct from those in adult worms [128]. This antigenic variation, together with the brief period of time required for larvae to mature to adulthood (36-48 hours) and develop into fecund adults (4 to 5 days), allow intestinal worms to escape the immune response until they have reproduced [36].

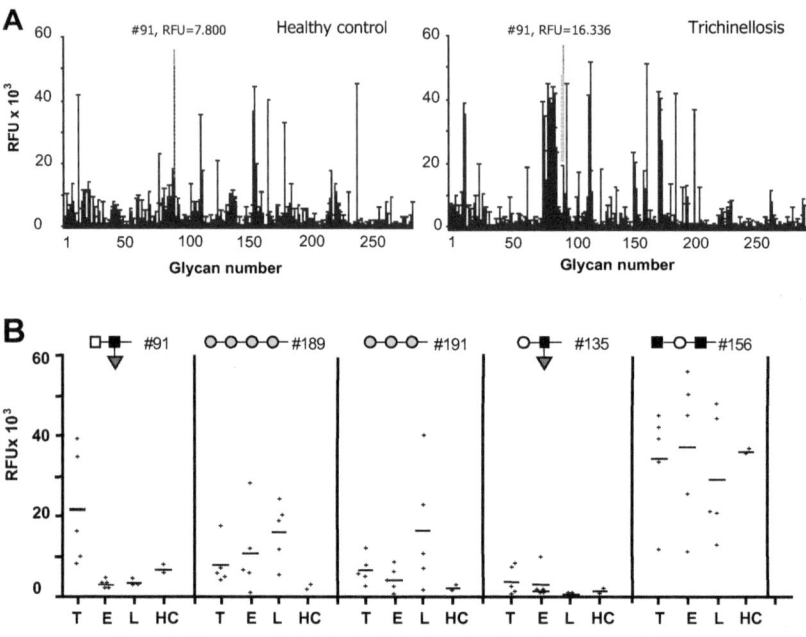

Figure 4: Glycan-array analysis of anti-glycan antibodies in the sera of parasite-infected individuals. Sera from individuals seropositive for trichinellosis (T, n = 5), leishmaniasis (L, n = 5) or echinococcosus (E, n = 5), as well as from healthy blood donors (HC, n = 2) were 1:100 diluted and analyzed for the presence of anti-glycan IgG antibodies using printed array Version 2.1 of the Consortium for Functional Glycomics. (**A**) Examples are shown of an array from an individual seropositive for trichinellosis and from a healthy blood donor. RFU = relative fluorescence units. The RFU for the LDNF glycan (#91) is indicated in both arrays. (**B**) Scatter plot of the RFU values for five selected glycan antigens, of all 17 sera analyzed. Three glycan antigens were selected that showed differential recognition by sera from parasite-infected individuals and healthy controls (#91, LDNF antigen, GalNAcb1 - 4(Fuca1-3) GlcNAc-R; #189, Mana1-2Mana1-2Mana1-3Man-R; #191, Mana1-2Mana1-3Man-R). In addition, one glycan antigen was selected that showed a very low binding, and one that showed high binding, respectively (#135, LeX antigen, Galb1-4(Fuca1-3)GlcNAc-R; #156, GlcNAca1-3Galb1 - 4GlcNAc-R). CFG monosaccharide symbols used are: green circle: Man; black square, GlcNAc; yellow square, GalNAc; yellow circle, Gal; red triangle, Fuc. From (Ref. [133]), with permission.

Recently, it has been observed that autoantibodies-containing human sera cross-reacts with *T. spiralis* antigens, in particular the human autoantibodies predominantly bound antigens belonging to the TSL1 group; more specifically, with the 53-kDa component [129].

The immunomodulation is one of the evasion mechanisms influencing the host immune response, and it can be exerted at the regulatory level and at the effector level of the immune response [63]. *Trichinella* modulates the host response by the induction of immune suppression, stimulating polyclonal lymphocyte activation and stimulating eosinophilia. Immune suppression during trichinellosis was observed in skin allograft rejection experiments. Furthermore, a depressed response was shown in infected mice to several unrelated parasite antigens such as goat red cell, Japanese encephalitis B virus and cholera toxin, in infected mice [130]. Since this depression is particularly evident during NBL production, the release of lymphocytotoxic factors by this stage could be the cause. However, these possible parasitic products have not been characterized so far.

Moreover, *T. spiralis* derived products, not yet identified, can suppress the response to thymus-dependent, but not to thymus independent parasite antigens. In particular, the suppression of host thymus-dependent response was shown to the *Trichinella* antigen FCp1, a molecule containing phosphorylcholine (PC) [131]. This remarkable fact occurs during the primary and secondary response to *Trichinella* infection, and it is directed exclusively to own antigens and not *versus* other parasite-derived PC bearing antigens.

T. spiralis muscle larvae ESA suppress *in vitro* DC maturation induced by both S- and R-form lipopolysaccharide (LPS) from enterobacteria. Using different toll-like receptor (TLR) agonists, was demonstrated that the suppressive effect of ESA on DC maturation is restricted to TLR4. Moreover, the presence of ESA resulted in the expansion of CD4+ CD25+ Foxp3+ T cells. These regulatory T (Treg) cells have suppressive activity and they produce TGF-β *in vitro* [132]. It has been also shown that DC treated with ESA induced the expansion of Treg cells *in vivo* [133].

As other helminths, *T. spiralis* infection influences the host immune system and the immune response to bystander antigens. Some authors have shown that

T. spiralis reduces the severity of colitis (Th1-mediated disease) in mice [134], in which besides the direct effect of the infection, the disorder can be modulated by rectal submucosal administration of *T. spiralis* CWE from ML [135]. *T. spiralis* infection also modifies the immune response responsible for the progression of autoimmune diabetes [136] and reduces the severity of the experimental autoimmune encephalomyelitis, the experimental model of multiple sclerosis, in a dose dependent fashion [137]. The development of new therapeutic approaches based on these studies would be the great importance for treatment of different autoimmune and allergic disorders.

IMMUNOPATHOLOGY

Enteral Phase of Infection

During experimental infection with nematodes, an enhanced hyperplasia (mastocytosis) and activation of mucosal mast cells occur [18, 19, 22, 23]. This observation was confirmed in the jejunum of patients infected with *T. spiralis* [20]. On twelve patients with trichinellosis studied, five did not underlie morphological changes at the jejunum level. In three patients, a focal small infiltrate with mononuclear cells and eosinophils was observed in the biopsy whereas in the remaining four patients, a typical chronic enteritis with a cellular infiltrate and fibrosis was observed. The number of mucosal mast cells in patients with *Trichinella* infection resulted markedly higher than the number of mast cells in the mucosa and the connective tissue from patients with other parasitic infections (teniosis and giardiosis).

Parenteral Phase of Infection

During this phase of infection allergic manifestations occur, which are caused by activation of sensitized mast cell, induced by parasitic antigens in an IgE dependent way [138]. The clinical manifestations which derive from this phenomenon is represented by facial and periorbital oedema [85].

Another characteristic of this phase is given by blood and tissue eosinophilia.

Blood eosinophilia is a typical response to nematode infections and this is particularly characteristic in human trichinellosis where eosinophil levels reach very high values, up to 19,000 cells/μl. The eosinophilia depends on the parasite inoculum size, on T cells, although a T cell-independent eosinophilia has been described, according to the results obtained in experimental models, and is under the control of genetic factors.

The control of eosinophil levels by T cells is exerted by activation of Th2 cells which, once activated, produce high amounts of IL-5, the cytokine responsible of the production and differentiation of this cell population in the bone marrow [139]. Moreover, IL-5, together with other factors, such as granulocyte-macrophage colony stimulating factor (GM-CSF) or IL-3, prevents the apoptosis in eosinophils, as shown in *Trichinella*-infected rats, especially in early period of infection [140].

In consideration of these results, it has been postulated that eosinophilia might be due also due to a reduced eosinophil apoptosis, favoured by increased levels of IL-5 and other protective cytokines such as IL-3, which would determine an accumulation of these cells in the blood and tissues [141].

A major question about eosinophils is whether they are protective or not against *Trichinella*. In *in vitro* antibody dependent cellular cytotoxicity (ADCC) experiments using NBL as target, many cell populations such as eosinophils, neutrophils in both experimental animals and humans are able to kill the parasites, using different cytotoxic mechanisms, oxygen-dependent (hydrogen peroxide, hypochlorite, *etc.*) and -independent (major basic protein, eosinophil peroxidase, *etc.*). Instead, results *in vivo* are controversial, depending on the experimental model used. Recently, it has been documented how eosinophils could support parasite growth and survival by promoting accumulation of Th2 cells and preventing induction of iNOS in macrophage and neutrophil NO-mediated killing which are characteristic of the Th1 cell response [69].

Whatever is the role of eosinophils *in vivo versus* helminthic parasites, the increase of the number of this cell population in the blood and tissues of infected hosts results in tissue damage to skeletal muscle cells, myocardium, lungs and central nervous system as well [139].

The invasion of the skeletal muscle cells by the migrating larvae during the parenteral or muscular phase is associated with inflammatory and allergic responses. The invading larvae can directly damage the muscle cells, or indirectly stimulate the infiltration of inflammatory cells, primarily eosinophils. A relationship between the eosinophil levels and serum muscle enzymes such as lactate dehydrogenase (LDH) and creatine phosphokinase (CPK), and between eosinophil levels and myalgic score in patients infected by *T. britovi*, previously considered *T. nelsoni*, was observed, see Fig. (**5**); this indicates a relationship between eosinophil levels, and tissue damage and pain suggesting that muscle damage and pain may be mediated indirectly by these activated granulocytes [142].

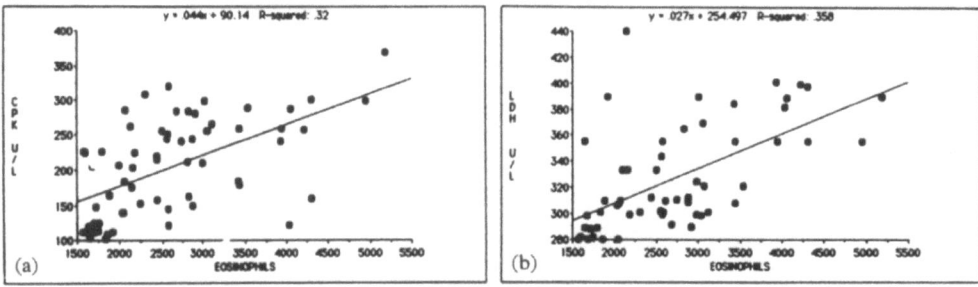

Figure 5: Correlation between severe eosinophilia, CPK (**a**) and LDH levels (**b**). From (Ref. [141]) with permission.

In late trichinellosis occurring some years from infection, antibodies specific for skeletal muscle, recognizing 28 and 41kDa proteins in this tissue extract were detected in patient sera, suggesting that muscle damage is caused in the early phase of infection by the invasion process by the NBL, but later is mediated by immunopathological processes [143].

Heart and Central Nervous System Involvement

Neurotrichinosis or better neurotrichinellosis, represents the major complication of trichinellosis in humans, and it is caused mainly by granulomatous inflammatory reactions and vasculitis. The NBL tend to wander, causing tissue damage before reentering the bloodstream, or remain trapped and destroyed by the following granulomatous reaction [144]. Eosinophil degranulation products such as eosinophil-derived neurotoxin (EDN) and major basic protein (MBP) can damage also neuronal cells [145, 146]. Neurotoxic activity was observed in eosinophils from three patients with eosinophilic syndromes. When cell preparations from the patients were injected into rabbits and guinea pigs, the animals developed a syndrome of muscular rigidity and ataxia, progressing to severe paralysis. These results were also obtained after injection with the purified eosinophil-derived protein, in particular clearance of Purkinje cells from the cerebellum by microscopy was always found among affected animals [145].

According to experimental results in rats [147] and histopathological observations [139], myocarditis is triggered initially by invasion of the migrating larvae, then the activated eosinophil infiltration and mast cell degranulation are involved. In the Fig. (**6**) the massive infiltration of eosinophils in the myocardium of a patient died for a severe trichinellosis is shown.

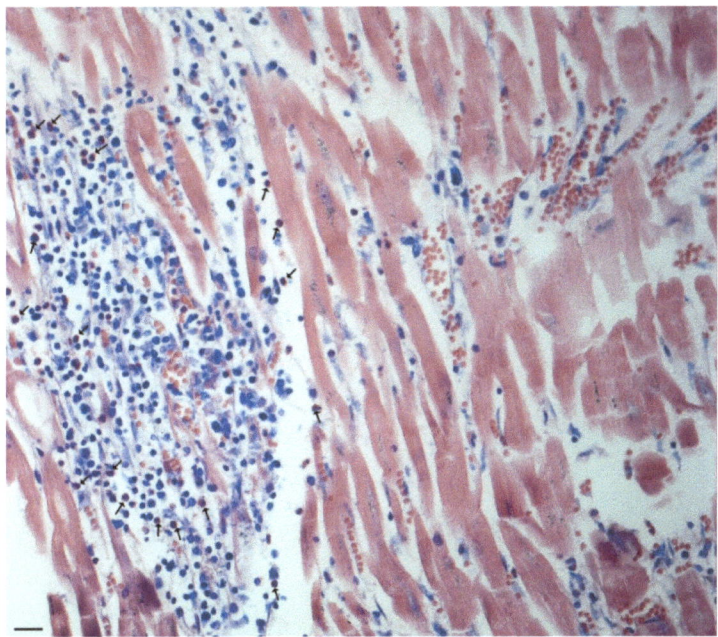

Figure 6: Eosinophils, indicated by arrows, infiltrating the myocardial tissue of a trichinellosis patient who died for the complications of a severe trichinellosis. Tissue samples provided by Prof. Wanda Kociecka. Sample stained with May-Grünwald-Giemsa. Scale bar represents 50 μm. From (Ref. [138]), with permission.

The mechanisms responsible for eosinophilia in trichinellosis as well as in other helmintic infections, are not yet fully elucidated. As already said, IL-5 plays a crucial role, but probably other factors can also be involved [139]. The role of IgE in the induction of eosinophilia is controversial [138].

Eosinophils are cytotoxic for NBL *in vitro* in both animal and human (ADCC) *in vitro* reactions; they release products such as the MBP, peroxidase, or products derived from oxidative metabolism [139]. However, their actual role *in vivo* is not clarified.

In a study performed on nineteen sera from late period trichinellosis patients, who acquired infection in Poland, it was shown that patients' sera recognized several antigens that were not recognized by normal sera. On rat and human heart ventricle wall, a high proportion of sera (42%) reacted with a protein of 68 kDa (Fig. 7). The reactivity with this antigen, however, was not significantly different in patients with or without cardiac involvement. The reactivity against the 68 kDa antigen and against the 27 and 41 kDa skeletal muscle antigens was not observed on kidney, placenta and spleen extracts, thus suggesting a high tissue specificity of the reactivity of trichinellosis sera [143].

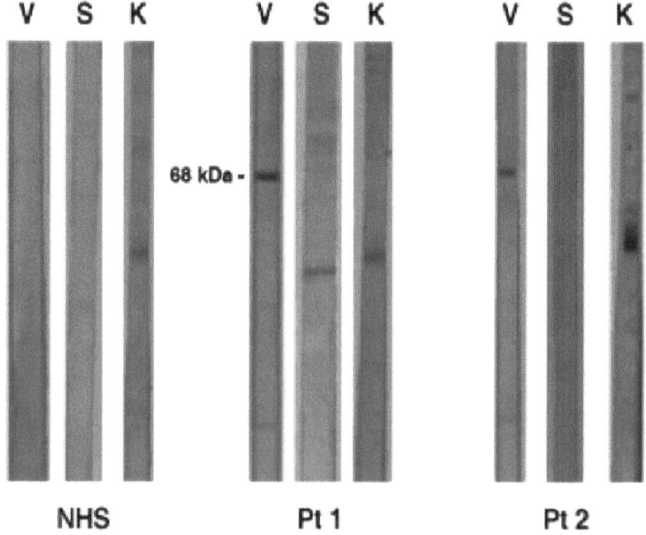

Figure 7: Reactivity of trichinellosis sera with tissue extracts: heart-specific antigen. Rat heart ventricle wall (V), spleen (S) and kidney (K) extracts were separated by SDS-PAGE, transferred to nitrocellulose and incubated with normal human sera (NHS) or sera from patients with trichinellosis (Pt). A band of 68 kDa was detected only in ventricular wall extracts and exclusively by trichinellosis sera. From (Ref. [142]) with permission.

PERSPECTIVES OF CONTROL

Control of trichinellosis in humans is mainly based on animal inspection at slaughterhouse as well as on well cooking meat before consumption [148, 149].

Vaccine development for this zoonosis is mainly focused on veterinary medicine. Unlike rodents, the typical experimental host, pigs do not develop strong intestinal immunity [150] hence, muscle larval L1 stage stichocyte antigens are insufficient for a vaccine. The antigens from the NBL have proved highly effective in pigs, and a first generation vaccine has been developed [151].

The major problem in the vaccine development for helminth parasites is represented by the complexity of these organisms, which is obviously much higher in comparison with bacteria and viruses [152].

Different strategies during the years have been employed with the aim to obtain a certain level of protection against *Trichinella* spp., using total crude extracts of larvae [153], recombinant proteins [154] such as the heat shock protein 70 [155] or paramyosin [156], synthetic peptides such as that derived from the 43 kDa. glycoprotein [153, 157], phage display [158] and DNA [159], even delivered by attenuated *Salmonella typhimurium* [160] or *Salmonella enterica* by intranasal route [161].

All these different approaches have resulted in variable levels of protection which however at present do not yet guarantee the availability of a reliable vaccine.

CONCLUSION

The study of this fascinating model of parasitic infection gives a major contribution to the understanding of the fine mechanisms which underlie the host-helminth relationship.

This will be of great value not only for the preparation of reliable vaccines but also for the progress of knowledge in the fields of Immunology as well as of Parasitology.

ACKNOWLEDGEMENT

Declared none.

CONFLICT OF INTEREST

The author(s) confirm that this chapter contents have no conflict of interest.

ABBREVIATIONS

L1	=	First larval stage
NBL	=	New born larva
NC	=	Nurse cell
AD	=	Adult
ML	=	Muscle larva
MC	=	Mast cell
mMCP	=	Mouse mast cell protease1
Abs	=	Antibodies
RMCP	=	Rat mast cell protease
HRMC	=	Rat mast cell line
Ig	=	Immunoglobulin
TSL	=	*T. spiralis* muscle larva
IL	=	Interleukin
TNF	=	Tumor necrosis factor
ADP	=	Adenosine diphosphate

UDP	=	Uridine diphosphate
ATP	=	Adenosine triphosphate
ENA	=	Epithelial cell-derived neutrophil-activating peptide
Stat	=	Signal transducer and activator of transcription
KO	=	Knock out
IFN	=	Interferon
Muc	=	Mucins
VEGF	=	Vascular endothelial growth factor
iNOS	=	Inducible NO synthase
ESA	=	Excretory-secretory antigens
TGF	=	Transforming growth factor
IFA	=	Indirect immunofluorescence assay
WB	=	Western blot
CIA	=	Competitive inhibition assay
EIA	=	Enzyme immunoassay
gp	=	Glycoprotein
ELISA	=	Enzyme linked immunosorbent assay
CWE	=	Crude worm extract
AD-TSE	=	Total soluble extracts from *T. spiralis* adult stage
LDNF	=	GalNAcβ1-4(Fucα1-3) GlcNAc-R

PC = Phosphorylcholine

DC = Dendritic cells

LPS = Lipopolysaccharide

TLR = Toll-like receptor

Treg = Regulatory T

GM-CSF = Granulocyte-macrophage colony stimulating factor

ADCC = Antibody dependent cellular cytotoxicity

LDH = Lactate dehydrogenase

CPK = Creatine phosphokinase

EDN = Eosinophil-derived neurotoxin

MBP = Major basic protein

RFU = Relative fluorescence units

V = Rat heart ventricle wall

S = Spleen

K = Kidney

NHS = Normal human sera

Pt = Patients with trichinellosis

REFERENCES

[1] Pozio E. World distribution of *Trichinella* spp. infections in animals and humans. Vet Parasitol 2007; 149: 3-21.
[2] Versillé N, Immunité anti-*Trichinella*: Etude de l'activation mastocytaire par les antigènes parasitaires et application à une stratégie vaccinale. PhD Thesis, Université Pierre et Marie Curie, Paris, France, 2012.

[3]   Krivokapich SJ, Pozio E, Gatti GM *et al*. *Trichinella patagoniensis* n. sp. (Nematoda), a new encapsulated species infecting carnivorous mammals in South America. Int J Parasitol 2012; 42: 903-10.

[4]   Pozio E. Trichinellosis in the European Union: epidemiology, ecology and economic impact. Parasitol Today 1998; 14: 35-8.

[5]   Pozio E, Murrell KD. Systematics and epidemiology of *Trichinella*. Adv Parasitol 2006; 63: 367-439.

[6]   Bruschi F. Trichinellosis in developing countries: is it neglected? J Infect Develop Ctries 2012; 12: 216-222.

[7]   Campbell WC. Epidemiology I: Modes of Transmission. In: Campbell WC, Ed. *Trichinella* and trichinosis. New York: Plenum Press 1983; pp. 425-44.

[8]   Stewart GL, Despommier DD, Burnham J *et al*. *Trichinella spiralis*: behavior, structure, and biochemistry of larvae following exposure to components of the host enteric environment. Exp Parasitol 1987; 63: 195-204.

[9]   Wright KA. *Trichinella spiralis*: an intracellular parasite in the intestinal phase. J Parasitol 1979; 65: 441-5.

[10] Despommier DD, Campbell WC. Synopsis of Morphology. In: Campbell WC Ed. *Trichinella and trichinosis"*. New York: Plenum Press1983; pp. 551-61.

[11] Capo V, Despommier DD. Clinical aspects of infection with *Trichinella* spp. Clin Microbiol Rev 1996; 9: 47-54.

[12] Wakelin D, Denham DA. The immune response. In: Campbell WC Ed. *Trichinella* and trichinosis. NewYork: Plenum Press; 1983; pp. 265-308.

[13] Walls RS, Leuchars E, Davies AJS *et al*. The immunopathology of trichiniasis in T-Cell deficient mice. Clin Exp Immunol 1973; 13: 231-42.

[14] Despommier DD. Biology. In: Campbell WC Ed. *Trichinella* and trichinosis. New York: Plenum Press; 1983; pp. 75-152.

[15] Despommier DD. How does *Trichinella spiralis* make itself at home? Parasitol Today 1998; 14: 318-23.

[16] Bell RG. The generation and expression of immunity to *Trichinella spiralis* in laboratory rodents. Adv Parasitol 1998; 41: 149-217.

[17] Wakelin D. *Trichinella spiralis*: immunity, ecology, and evolution. J Parasitol 1993; 79: 488-94.

[18] Woodbury RG, Miller HR, Huntley JF *et al*. Mucosal mast cells are functionally active during spontaneous expulsion of intestinal nematode infections in rat. Nature 1984; 312: 450-2.

[19] Lawrence CE, Paterson YY, Wright SH *et al*. Mouse mast cell protease-1 is required for the enteropathy induced by gastrointestinal helminth infection in the mouse. Gastroenterol 2004; 127: 155-65.

[20] Gustowska L, Ruitenberg EJ, Elgersma A *et al*. Increase of mucosal mast cells in the jejunum of patients infected with *Trichinella spiralis*. Int Arch Allergy Appl Immunol 1983;71: 304-8.

[21] Moqbel R, Wakelin D, MacDonald AJ *et al*. Release of leukotrienes during rapid expulsion of *Trichinella spiralis* from immune rats. Immunology 1987; 60: 425-30.

[22] Tuohy M, Lammas DA, Wakelin D *et al*. Functional correlations between mucosal mast cell activity and immunity to *Trichinella spiralis* in high and low responder mice. Parasite Immunol 1990; 12: 675-85.

[23] Ha TY, Reed ND, Crowle PK. Delayed expulsion of adult *Trichinella spiralis* by mast cell-deficient W/Wv mice. Infect Immun 1983;41: 445-7.

[24] Kamiya M, Oku Y, Itayama H *et al*. Prolonged expulsion of adult *Trichinella spiralis* and eosinophil infiltration in mast cell-deficient W/Wv mice. J Helminthol 1985; 59: 233-9.

[25] Oku Y, Itayama H, Kamiya M. Expulsion of *Trichinella spiralis* from the intestine of W/Wv mice reconstituted with haematopoietic and lymphopoietic cells and origin of mucosal mast cells. Immunology 1984; 53: 337-44.

[26] McDermott JR, Bartram RE, Knight PA *et al*. Mast cells disrupt epithelial barrier function during enteric nematode infection. Proc Natl Acad Sci (USA) 2003; 100: 7761-6.

[27] Patel N, Kreider T, Urban JF Jr *et al*. Characterisation of effector mechanisms at the host: parasite interface during the immune response to tissue-dwelling intestinal nematode parasites. Int J Parasitol 2009; 39: 13-21.

[28] Blum LK, Thrasher SM, Gagliardo LF *et al*. Expulsion of secondary *Trichinella spiralis* infection in rats occurs independently of mucosal mast cell release of mast cell protease II. J Immunol 2009; 183: 5816-22.

[29] MacLean JD, Viallet J, Law C *et al*. Trichinosis in the Canadian Arctic: report of five outbreaks and a new clinical syndrome. J Infect Dis 1989; 160: 513-20.

[30] Arizmendi N, Yépez-Mulia L, Cedillo-Rivera R *et al*. Interleukin mRNA changes in mast cells stimulated by TSL-1 antigens. Parasite 2001; 8: S114-6.

[31] Niborski V, Vallée I, Fonseca-Liñán R *et al*. *Trichinella spiralis*: stimulation of mast cells by TSL-1 antigens trigger cytokine mRNA expression and release of IL-4 and TNF through an Ig-independent pathway. Exp Parasitol 2004; 108: 101-8.

[32] Yépez-Mulia L, Montaño-Escalona C, Fonseca-Liñán R *et al*. Differential activation of mast cells by antigens from *Trichinella spiralis* muscle larvae, adults, and newborn larvae. Vet Parasitol 2009; 159: 253-7.

[33] Afferson HC, Eleftheriou E, Selkirk ME *et al*. *Trichinella spiralis* secreted enzymes regulate nucleotide-induced mast cell activation and release of mouse mast cell protease 1. Infect Immun 2012; 80: 3761-7.

[34] Vallance BA, Matthaei KI, Sanovic S *et al*. Interleukin-5 deficient mice exhibit impaired host defence against challenge *Trichinella spiralis* infections. Parasite Immunol 2000; 22: 487-92.

[35] Svensson-Frej M. Immunobiology of intestinal eosinophils - a dogma in the changing? J Innate Immun 2011; 3: 565-76.

[36] Fabre MV, Beiting DP, Bliss SK *et al*. Immunity to *Trichinella spiralis* muscle infection. Vet Parasitol 2009; 159: 245-248.

[37] Korenaga M, Wang CH, Bell RG *et al*. Intestinal immunity to *Trichinella spiralis* is a property of OX8- OX22- T-helper cells that are generated in the intestine. Immunology 1989; 66: 588-94.

[38] Li CK, Seth R, Gray T *et al*. Production of proinflammatory cytokines and inflammatory mediators in human intestinal epithelial cells after invasion by *Trichinella spiralis*. Infect Immun 1998; 66: 2200-6.

[39] Grencis RK, Lee TD, Wakelin D. Adoptive transfer of immunity to *Trichinella spiralis* in mice: generation of effective cells by different life cycle stages. Int J Parasitol 1985;15: 195-202.

[40] Riedlinger J, Grencis RK, Wakelin D. Antigen-specific T-cell lines transfer protective immunity against *Trichinella spiralis in vivo*. Immunology 1986; 58: 57-61.

[41] Grencis RK, Riedlinger J, Wakelin D. Lymphokine production by T cells generated during infection with *Trichinella spiralis*. Int Arch Allergy Appl Immunol 1987; 83: 92-5.

[42] Ramaswamy K, Negrao-Correa D, Bell R. Local intestinal immune responses to infections with *Trichinella spiralis*. Real-time, continuous assay of cytokines in the intestinal (afferent) and efferent thoracic duct lymph of rats. J Immunol 1996; 156: 4328-37.

[43] Finkelman FD, Shea-Donohue T, Morris SC *et al*. Interleukin-4- and interleukin-13-mediated host protection against intestinal nematode parasites. Immunol Rev 2004; 201: 139-55.

[44] Khan WI, Richard M, Akiho H *et al*. Modulation of intestinal muscle contraction by interleukin-9 (IL-9) or IL-9 neutralization: correlation with worm expulsion in murine nematode infections. Infect Immun 2003; 71: 2430-43.

[45] Vallance BA, Blennerhassett PA, Deng Y *et al*. IL-5 contributes to worm expulsion and muscle hypercontractility in a primary *T.spiralis* infection. Am J Physiol 1999; 277: G400-8.

[46] Lee TD. Helminthotoxic Responses of Intestinal Eosinophils to *Trichinella spiralis* Newborn Larvae. Infect Immun 1991; 59: 4405-11.

[47] Helmby H, Grencis RK. Contrasting roles for IL-10 in protective immunity to different life cycle stages of intestinal nematode parasites. Eur J Immunol 2003; 33: 2382-90.

[48] Helmby H, Grencis RK. IFN-gamma-independent effects of IL-12 during intestinal nematode infection. J Immunol 2003; 171: 3691-6.

[49] Chiumiento L, Del Prete G, Codolo G *et al*. Stimulation of TH1 response by *Helicobacter pylori* neutrophil activating protein decreases the protective role of IgE and eosinophils in experimental trichinellosis. Int J Immunopathol Pharmacol 2011; 24: 895-903.

[50] Fu Y, Wang W, Tong J *et al*. Th17 cells influence intestinal muscle contraction during *Trichinella spiralis* infection. Journal of Huazhong University Science and Technology Medical Sciences. 2009; 29: 481-5.

[51] Helmby H, Grencis RK. IL-18 regulates intestinal mastocytosis and Th2 cytokine production independently of IFN-gamma during *Trichinella spiralis* infection. J Immunol 2002; 169: 2553-60.

[52] Appleton JA, McGregor DD. Characterization of the immune mediator of rapid expulsion of *Trichinella spiralis* in suckling rats. Immunology 1987; 62: 477-84.

[53] Appleton JA, Schain SS, McGregor DD. Rapid expulsion of *Trichinella spiralis* in suckling rats: mediation by monoclonals antibodies. Immunology 1988; 65: 487-92.

[54] Reason AJ, Ellis LA, Appleton JA *et al*. Novel tyvelose-containing tri- and tetra-antennary N-glycans in the immunodominant antigens of the intracellular parasite *Trichinella spiralis*. Glycobiology 1994; 4: 593-603.

[55] McVay CS, Bracken P, Gagliardo LF *et al*. Antibodies to tyvelose exhibit multiple modes of interference with the epithelial niche of *Trichinella spiralis*. Infect Immun 2000; 68: 1912-8.

[56] Carlisle MS, McGregor DD, Appleton JA. The role of mucus in antibody-mediated rapid expulsion of *Trichinella spiralis* in suckling rats. Immunology 1990;70: 126-32.

[57] Knight PA, Brown JK, Pemberton AD. Innate immune response mechanisms in the intestinal epithelium: potential roles for mast cells and goblet cells in the expulsion of adult *Trichinella spiralis*. Parasitology. 2008; 135: 655-70.

[58] Jasmer D.P. *Trichinella spiralis* infected skeletal muscle cells arrest in G2/M and cease muscle genes expression. J Cell Biol, 1993; 121, 785-793.

[59] Beiting DP, Bliss SK, Schlafer DH et al. Interleukin-10 limits local and body cavity inflammation during infection with muscle-stage *Trichinella spiralis*. Infect Immun 2004; 72: 3129-37.

[60] Capo VA, Despommier DD, Polvere RI. *Trichinella spiralis*: vascular endothelial growth factor is up-regulated within the nurse cell during the early phase of its formation. J Parasitol 1998; 84, 209-14.

[61] Polvere RI, Kabbash CA, Capó VA et al. *Trichinella spiralis*: synthesis of type IV and type VI collagen during nurse cell formation. Exp Parasitol 1997; 86: 191-9.

[62] Purkerson M, Despommier DD. Fine structure of the muscle phase of *Trichinella spiralis* in the mouse. In: Trichinellosis. Educational Publishers; New York 1974; pp.7-23.

[63] Bruschi F, Chiumiento L. Immunomodulation in trichinellosis: does *Trichinella* really escape the host immune system? End Metabol Immun Disord Drug Targets 2012; 12: 4-15.

[64] Karmańska K, Houszka M, Widyma A et al. Macrophages during infection with *Trichinella spiralis* in mice. Wiad Parazytol 1997; 43: 245-9.

[65] Karmańska K, Houszka M, Widyma A et al. The cells observed inside capsules of larvae in the course of experimental trichinellosis in mice. Wiad Parazytol. 1997; 43: 251-6.

[66] Gerwel C, Kociecka W, Pawlowski Z. Parasitologic examination of muscles several years after trichinosis. Epidemiol Rev 1970; 24: 262-9.

[67] Shin K, Watts GF, Oettgen HC et al. Mouse mast cell tryptase mMCP-6 is a critical link between adaptive and innate immunity in the chronic phase of *Trichinella spiralis* infection. J Immunol 2008; 180: 4885-91.

[68] Beiting DP, Gagliardo LF, Hesse M et al. Coordinated control of immunity to muscle stage *Trichinella spiralis* by IL-10, regulatory T cells, and TGF-beta. J Immunol 2007; 178: 1039-47.

[69] Gebreselassie NG, Moorhead AR, Fabre V et al. Eosinophils preserve parasitic nematode larvae by regulating local immunity. J Immunol 2012; 188: 417-25.

[70] Li CK, Ko RC. Inflammatory response during the muscle phase of *Trichinella spiralis* and *T. pseudospiralis* infections. Parasitol Res 2001; 87: 708-14.

[71] Beiting DP, Park PW, Appleton JA. Synthesis of syndecan-1 by skeletal muscle cells is an early response to infection with *Trichinella spiralis* but is not essential for nurse cell development. Infect Immun 2006; 74: 1941-3.

[72] Zeller JC, Panoskaltsis-Mortari A, Murphy WJ et al. Induction of CD4+ T cell alloantigen-specific hyporesponsiveness by IL-10 and TGF-beta. J Immunol 1999; 163: 3684-91.

[73] Morales MA, Mele R, Sanchez M et al. Increased CD8(+)-T-cell expression and a type 2 cytokine pattern during the muscular phase of *Trichinella* infection in humans. Infect Immun 2002; 70: 233-9.

[74] Almond NM, Parkhouse RM. The Ig class distribution of anti-phosphoryl choline responses in mice infected with parasitic nematodes. Immunology 1986; 59: 633-5.

[75] Zakroff SG, Beck L, Platzer EG et al. The IgE and IgG subclass responses of mice to four helminth parasites. Cell Immunol 1989; 119: 193-201.

[76] Denkers EY, Wassom DL, Krco CJ et al. CE.The mouse antibody response to *Trichinella spiralis* defines a single, immunodominant epitope shared by multiple antigens. J Immunol 1990; 144: 3152-9.

[77] Bruschi F, Murrell KD. New aspects of human trichinellosis: the impact of new *Trichinella* species. Postgrad Medical J 2002;78: 15-22.

[78] Ljungström I, Hammarström L, Kociecka W et al. The sequential appearance of IgG subclasses and IgE during the course of Trichinella spiralis infection. Clin Exp Immunol 1988; 74: 230-5.

[79] Pinelli E, Mommers M, Kortbeek LM et al. Specific IgG4 response directed against the 45-kDa glycoprotein in trichinellosis: a re-evaluation of patients 15 years after infection. Eur J Clin Microbiol Infect Dis. 2007; 26: 641-5.

[80] Pinelli E, Mommers M, Homan W et al. Imported human trichinellosis: sequential IgG4 antibody response to Trichinella spiralis. Eur J Clin Microbiol Infect Dis 2004; 23: 57-60.

[81] Fröscher W, Gullotta F, Saathoff M et al. Chronic trichinosis. Clinical, bioptic, serological and electromyographic observations. Eur Neurol 1988; 28: 221-6.

[82] Kociecka W, Bruschi F, Marini C et al. Clinical appraisal of patients and detection of serum antibodies by ELISA and CIA tests in late periods of Trichinella sp. invasion. Parasite 2001; 8: S147-S51.

[83] Bruschi F, Locci MT, Cabaj W et al. Persistence of reactivity against the 45 k Da glycoprotein in late trichinellosis patients. Vet Parasitol 2005;132: 115-8.

[84] Piergili-Fioretti D, Castagna B, Frongillo RF et al. Re-evaluation of patients involved in a trichinellosis outbreak caused by Trichinella britovi 15 years after infection. Vet Parasitol 2005; 132: 119-23

[85] Dupouy-Camet J, Bruschi F. Management and diagnosis of human trichinellosis. In: Dupouy-Camet J, Murrell KD, Eds. FAO/WHO/OIE guidelines for the surveillance, management, prevention and control of trichinellosis, Paris: World Oganisation for Animal Health Press 2007, pp. 37-69.

[86] Dupouy-Camet J, Kociecka W, Bruschi F et al. Opinion on the diagnosis and treatment of human trichinellosis. Expert Opin on Pharmacother 2002; 3: 1117-30.

[87] Gamble HR, Pozio E, Bruschi F et al. International Commission on Trichinellosis: recommendations on the use of serological tests for the detection of Trichinella infection in animals and man. Parasite 2004; 11: 3-13.

[88] Van Knapen F, Franchimont JH, Verdonk AR et al. Detection of specific immunoglobulins (IgG, IgM, IgA, IgE) and total IgE levels in human trichinosis by means of the enzyme-linked immunosorbent assay (ELISA). Am J Trop Med Hyg 1982; 31: 973-6.

[89] Au AC, Ko RC, Simon JW et al. Study of acute trichinosis in Ghurkas: specificity and sensitivity of enzyme-linked immunosorbent assays for IgM and IgE antibodies to Trichinella larval antigens in diagnosis. Trans R Soc Trop Med Hyg 1983; 77: 412-5.

[90] Ruangkunaporn Y, Watt G, Karnasuta C et al. Immunodiagnosis of trichinellosis: efficacy of somatic antigen in early detection of human trichinellosis. Asian Pac J Allergy Immunol 1994; 12: 39-42.

[91] De la Rosa JL, Alcantara P, Correa D. Investigation of cross-reactions against Trichinella spiralis antigens by enzyme-linked immunosorbent assay and enzyme-linked immunoelectrotransfer blot assay in patients with various diseases. Clin Diagn Lab Immunol 1995; 2: 122-4.

[92] Contreras MC, Acevedo E, Aguilera S et al. Standardization of ELISA IgM and IgA for immunodiagnosis of human trichinosis. Bol Chil Parasitol 1999; 54: 104-9.

[93] Mahannop P, Chaicumpa W, Setasuban P et al. Immunodiagnosis of human trichinellosis using excretory-secretory (ES) antigen. J Helminthol 1992; 66: 297-304.

[94] Chen S, Li L, Wu C et al. Serological investigation on human trichinellosis spiralis in Hubei Province of PR China. Southeast Asian J Trop Med Public Health 1997; 28: 107-9.

[95] Gómez-Priego A, Crecencio-Rosales L, de-La-Rosa JL. Serological evaluation of thin-layer immunoassay-enzyme-linked immunosorbent assay for antibody detection in human trichinellosis. Clin Diagn Lab Immunol 2000; 7: 810-2.

[96] Tinoco-Velázquez I, Gómez-Priego A, Mendoza R et al. Searching for antibodies against *Trichinella spiralis* in the sera of patients with fever of unknown cause. Ann Trop Med Parasitol 2002; 96: 391-5.

[97] Chapa-Ruiz MR, González-Pantaleón D, Morales-Galán A et al. A follow-up study of the human class and subclass antibody response developed against the adult stage of *Trichinella spiralis*. Parasite 2001; 8: S163-7

[98] Andiva S, Yera H, Haeghebaert S et al. Evaluation comparative d'un test d'agglutination au latex, de deux tests ELISA et d'un test western blot pour le diagnostic sérologique de la trichinellose humaine. Ann Biol Clin 2002; 60: 79-83.

[99] Rodríguez-Osorio M, Gómez-Garcia V, Benito R et al. *Trichinella britovi* human infection in Spain: antibody response to surface, excretory/secretory and somatic antigens. Parasite 2003; 10: 159-64.

[100] Yera H, Andiva S, Perret C et al. Development and evaluation of a Western blot kit for diagnosis of human trichinellosis. Clin Diagn Lab Immunol 2003; 10: 793-6.

[101] Escalante M, Romarís F, Rodríguez M et al. Evaluation of *Trichinella spiralis* larva group 1 antigens for serodiagnosis of human trichinellosis. J Clin Microbiol 2004;42: 4060-6.

[102] Akisu C, Delibaş SB, Ozkoç S. Evaluation of three different ELISA kits for the diagnosis of trichinellosis. Mikrobiyol Bul 2005; 39: 325-33.

[103] Ozkoç S, Delıbaş SB, Akisü C. Use of the Western Blot assay in the diagnosis of trichinosis. Turkiye Parazitol Derg2005; 29: 26-30.

[104] Møller LN, Krause TG, Koch A et al. Human antibody recognition of *Anisakidae* and *Trichinella* spp. in Greenland. Clin Microbiol Infect 2007; 13: 702-8.

[105] Barennes H, Sayasone S, Odermatt P et al. A major trichinellosis outbreak suggesting a high endemicity of *Trichinella* infection in northern Laos. Am J Trop Med Hyg 2008; 78: 40-4.

[106] Ortega-Pierres MG, Yepez-Mulia L, Homan W et al. Workshop on a detailed characterization of *Trichinella spiralis* antigens: a platform for future studies on antigens and antibodies to this parasite. Parasite Immunol 1996; 18: 273-84.

[107] Ellis LA, McVay CS, Probert MA et al. Terminal beta-linked tyvelose creates unique epitopes in *Trichinella spiralis* glycan antigens. Glycobiology 1997; 7: 383-90.

[108] Mendez-Loredo B, Martínez Y, Zamora R et al. The stage-specificity of the IgA response to newborn larva and TSL-1 antigens of *Trichinella spiralis* in humans infected with the parasite. Parasite 2001; 8: S158-62.

[109] Aronstein WS, Lewis SA, Norden AP et al. Molecular identity of a major antigen of *Schistosoma mansoni* wich cross reacts with *Trichinella spiralis* and *Fasciola hepatica*. Parasitology 1986; 92: 133-51.

[110] Linder E, Thors C, Lundin L et al. *Schistosome* antigen gp50 is responsible for serological cross-reactivity with *Trichinella spiralis*. J Parasitol 1992; 78: 999-1005.

[111] Roach TI, Wakelin D, Else KJ et al. Antigenic cross-reactivity between the human whipworm, *Trichuris trichiura*, and the mouse trichuroids *Trichuris muris* and *Trichinella spiralis*. Parasite Immunol 1988; 10: 279-91.

[112] Intapan PM, Maleewong W, Sukeepaisarnjaroen W *et al*. Potential use of *Trichinella spiralis* antigen for serodiagnosis of human capillariasis philippinensis by immunoblot analysis. Parasitol Res 2006; 98: 227-31.

[113] Srimanote P, Ittiprasert W, Sermsart B *et al*. *Trichinella spiralis*-specific monoclonal antibodies and affinity-purified antigen-based diagnosis. Asian Pac J Allergy Immunol 2000; 18: 37-45.

[114] Bruschi F, Moretti A, Wassom D *et al*. The use of a synthetic antigen for the serological diagnosis of human trichinellosis. Parasite. 2001; 8: S141-43.

[115] Pozio E, Gomez Morales MA, Dupouy-Camet J. Clinical aspects, diagnosis and treatment of trichinellosis. Expert Rev Anti Infect Ther 2003; 1: 471-82.

[116] Owen IL, Pozio E, Tamburrini A *et al*. Focus of human trichinellosis in Papua New Guinea. Am J Trop Med Hyg 2001; 65: 553-7.

[117] Owen IL, Gómez Morales MA, Pezzotti P *et al*. *Trichinella* infection in a hunting population of Papua New Guinea suggests an ancient relationship between *Trichinella* and human beings. Trans R Soc Trop Med Hyg 2005; 99: 618-24.

[118] Van Die I, Cummings RD. Glycans modulate immune responses in helminth infections and allergies. Chem. Immunol. Allergy 2006; 90: 91-112.

[119] Van Die I, Cummings RD. Glycan gimmickry by parasitic helminths: a strategy for modulating the host immune response? Glycobiology 2010; 20: 2-12.

[120] Gómez-Morales MA, Ludovisi A, Amati M *et al*. Validation of an enzyme-linked immunosorbent assay for diagnosis of human trichinellosis. Clin Vaccine Immunol 2008; 15: 1723-29.

[121] Gómez-Morales MA, Ludovisi A, Amati M *et al*. A distinctive Western blot pattern to recognize *Trichinella* infections in humans and pigs. Int J Parasitol 2012; 42: 1017-23.

[122] Aranzamendi C, Tefsen B, Jansen M *et al*. Glycan microarray profiling of parasite infection sera identifies the LDNF glycan as a potential antigen for serodiagnosis of trichinellosis. Exp Parasitol 2011; 129: 221-6.

[123] McKenzie CD, Preston PM, Ogilvie BM. Immunological properties of the surface of parasite nematodes. Nature 1978; 276: 826-828

[124] Jungery M, Clark NWT, Parkhouse RME. A major change in surface antigens during the maturation of newborn larvae of *Trichinella spiralis*. Mol Biochem Parasitol 1983; 7: 101-9.

[125] Gansmüller A, Anteunis A, Venturiello SM *et al*. Antibody-dependent in-vitro cytotoxicity of newborn *Trichinella spiralis* larvae: nature of the cells involved. Parasite Immunol 1987; 9: 281-92

[126] Venturiello SM, Giambartolomei GH, Costantino SN. Immune killing of newborn *Trichinella* larvae by human leucocytes. Parasite Immunol 1993; 15: 559-64.

[127] Venturiello SM, Giambartolomei GH, Costantino SN. Immune cytotoxic activity of human eosinophils against *Trichinella spiralis* newborn larvae. Parasite Immunol. 1995; 17: 555-9.

[128] Philipp M, Parkhouse RM, Ogilvie BM. Changing proteins on the surface of a parasitic nematode. Nature 1980; 287: 538-40.

[129] Radovic I, Gruden-Movsesijan A, Ilic N *et al*. *Trichinella spiralis* shares epitopes with human autoantigens. Mem Inst Oswaldo Cruz 2012; 107: 503-9.

[130] Bruschi F. The immune response to the parasitic nematode *Trichinella* and the ways to escape it. From experimental studies to implications for human infection. Curr Drug Targets Immune Endocr Metabol Disord 2002; 2: 269-78.

[131] Leiro J, Santamarina MT, Sernández L *et al*. Immunomodulation by *Trichinella spiralis*: primary *versus* secondary response to phosphorylcholine-containing antigens. Med Microbiol Immunol 1988; 177: 161-7.

[132] Aranzamendi C, Fransen F, Langelaar M *et al*. *Trichinella spiralis*-secreted products modulate DC functionality and expand regulatory T cells *in vitro*. Parasite Immunol 2012; 34: 210-23.

[133] Gruden-Movsesijan A, Ilic N, Colic M. *et al*. The impact of *Trichinella spiralis* excretory-secretory products on dendritic cells. Comp Immunol Microbiol Infect Dis 2011; 34: 429-39.

[134] Khan WI, Blennerhasset PA, Varghese AK *et al*. Intestinal nematode infection ameliorates experimental colitis in mice. Infect Immun, 2002; 70: 5931-7.

[135] Motomura Y, Wang H, Deng Y *et al*. Helminth antigen-based strategy to ameliorate inflammation in an experimental model of colitis. Clin Exp Immunol 2009; 155: 88-95.

[136] Saunders KA, Raine T, Cooke A *et al*. Inhibition of autoimmune type 1 diabetes by gastrointestinal helminth infection. Infect Immun 2007; 75: 397-407.

[137] Ilic N, Gruden-Movsesijan A, Sofronic-Milosavljevic L. *Trichinella spiralis*: shaping the immune response. Immunol Res 2012; 52: .111-9.

[138] Watanabe N, Bruschi F, Korenaga M. IgE: a question of protective immunity in *Trichinella spiralis* infection. Trends Parasitol, 2005; 21: 175-8.

[139] Bruschi F, Korenaga M, Watanabe N. Eosinophils and *Trichinella* infection: toxic for the parasite and the host? Trends Parasitol 2008; 24: 462-7.

[140] Gon S, Saito S, TakedaY *et al*. Apoptosis and *in vivo* distribution and clearance of eosinophils in normal and *Trichinella spiralis*-infected rats. J Leukoc Biol 1997; 62: 309-17.

[141] Simon HU, Blaser K. Inhibition of programmed eosinophil death: a key pathogenic event for eosinophilia? Immunol Today 1995; 16: 53-5.

[142] Ferraccioli G, Mercadanti M, Salaffi F *et al*. Prospective rheumatological study of muscle and joint symptons during *Trichinella nelsoni* infection. Q J Med 1988; 69: 973-84.

[143] Pratesi F, Bongiorni F, Kociecka W *et al*. Heart and skeletal muscle specific antigens recognized by trichinellosis patient sera. Parasite Immunol 2006; 28: 447-51.

[144] Katz M, Despommier DD, Gwadz RW. *Trichinella spiralis* In: Parasitic Diseases Katz M, Despommier DD, Gwadz RW, Eds. New York: Springer-Verlag. 1989, p. 28.

[145] Durack DT, Sumi SM, Klebanoff SJ. Neurotoxicity of human eosinophils. Proc Natl Acad Sci U.S.A. 1979; 76: 1443-7.

[146] Mawhorter ST, Kazura JW. Trichinosis of the central nervous system. Sem. Neurol 1993; 13: 148-9

[147.] Paolocci N, Sironi M, Bettini M *et al*. Immunopathological mechanisms underlying the time course of *Trichinella spiralis* cardiomyopathy in rats. Virchows Arch 1998; 432: 261-6.

[148] Nöckler K, Kapel CMO. Detection and surveillance for *Trichinella*: meat inspection and hygiene, and legislation. In: Dupouy-Camet J, Murrell KD, Eds. FAO/WHO/OIE guidelines for the surveillance, management, prevention and control of trichinellosis, Paris: World Oganisation for Animal Health Press 2007, p. 69.

[149] Gamble HR, Boireau P, Nöckler K *et al*. Prevention of *Trichinella* infection in the domestic pig. In: Dupouy-Camet J, Murrell KD, Eds. FAO/WHO/OIE guidelines for the

surveillance, management, prevention and control of trichinellosis, Paris: World Oganisation for Animal Health Press 2007, p. 69.

[150] Murrell KD. *Trichinella spiralis*: Acquired immunity in swine. Exp Parasitol 1985; 59: 347-54.

[151] Marti HP, Murrell KD, Gamble HR. *Trichinella spiralis*: Immunization of pigs with newborn larval antigens. Exp Parasitol 1987; 63: 68-73.

[152] Meeusen EN, Piedrafita D. Exploiting natural immunity to helminth parasites for the development of veterinary vaccines. Int J Parasitol 2003; 33: 1285-90.

[153] McGuire C, Chan WC, Wakelin D. Nasal immunization with homogenate and peptide antigens induces protective immunity against *Trichinella spiralis*. Infect Immun 2002; 70: 7149-52.

[154] Sun S, Xu W, He N *et al*. An antigenic recombinant fusion protein from *Trichinella spiralis* induces a protective response in BALB/c mice. J Helminthol 1994; 68: 89-91.

[155] Wang S, Zhu X, Yang Y *et al*. Molecular cloning and characterization of heat shock protein 70 from *Trichinella spiralis*. Acta Tropica 2009; 110: 46-51.

[156] Yang J, Gu Y, Yang Y *et al*. *Trichinella spiralis:* Immune response and protective immunity elicited by recombinant paramyosin formulated with different adjuvants. Exp Parasitol 2010; 124: 403-8

[157] Robinson K, Bellaby T, Chan WC *et al*. High levels of protection induced by a 40-mer synthetic peptide vaccine against the intestinal nematode parasite *Trichinella spiralis*. Immunology 1995; 86: 495-8.

[158] Gu Y, Li J, Zhu X *et al*. *Trichinella spiralis*: characterization of phage-displayed specific epitopes and their protective immunity in BALB/c mice. Exp Parasitol 2008; 118: 66-74.

[159] Wang ZQ, Cui J, Wei HY *et al*. Vaccination of mice with DNA vaccine induces the immune response and partial protection against *T. spiralis* infection. Vaccine. 2006; 24: 1205-12.

[160] Yang Y, Zhang Z, Yang J *et al*. Oral vaccination with Ts87 DNA vaccine delivered by attenuated *Salmonella typhimurium* elicits a protective immune response against *Trichinella spiralis* larval challenge. Vaccine 2010; 28: 2735-42

[161] Pompa-Mera EN, Yépez-Mulia L, Ocaña-Mondragón A *et al*. *Trichinella spiralis*: Intranasal immunization with attenuated *Salmonella enterica* carrying a gp43 antigen-derived 30mer epitope elicits protection in BALB/c mice. Exp Parasitol 2011; 129: 393-401.

[162] Bruschi F, Murrell KD. Trichinellosis. In: Guerrant RL, Walker DH, Weller PF, Eds. Tropical Infectious Diseases: Principles, Pathogens and Practice 3th ed. New York: Elsevier 2012, pp.768-73.

Chapter 7: Anisakis Simplex Infestation and Immune-Mediated Responses

CHAPTER 7

Anisakis Simplex Infestation and Immune-Mediated Responses

Ventura M. Teresa[1,*], Buquicchio Rosalba[2], F. Gatti[3], F.L. Traetta[4] and G. Iadarola[5]

[1]*Interdisciplinary Department of Medicine, University of Bari Medical School, Polyclinic, Bari, Italy;* [2]*Unit of Dermatology, University of Bari Medical School, Polyclinic, Bari, Italy;* [3]*Unit of Gastroenterology and Digestive Endoscopy, S. Camillo De Lellis Hospital, Manfredonia, Foggia, Italy;* [4]*Unit of Clinical Immunology and Allergology, "Miulli" Hospital, Acquaviva delle Fonti, Bari, Italy and* [5]*Department of Internal Medicine, Clinical Immunology and Allergology of Foggia General Hospital, University Medical School, Foggia, Italy*

Abstract: Nowadays *Anisakis simplex (A.s.)* infestation is underestimated and under-diagnosis, as the correlated clinical pictures suggest differential diagnosis of the majority of gastrointestinal internal pathologies and of various symptoms of allergic diseases, including the most severe and potentially fatal form represented by the anaphylactic shock. However we must cope with a pervasive and emerging disease which causes public serious health problems.

A. is a zoonotic disease caused by parasitic nematodes of the marine Anisakidae family; the infection is caused by consuming raw parasitized fish. The experimental data in our possession suggest that *A.* can determine different kinds of immunopathogenesis, in particular the I, III and IV type. From the immunophlogistic point of view a conspicuous eosinophilic infiltration is realized around the implant site tissue of the *A.* larva, as a result of the action of chemotactic factors released by T lymphocytes, mast cells, basophils, and also by the same *A.* It usually does not result into a blood eosinophilia.

Keywords: Allergens, allergic diseases, anaphylactic shock, acute gastric anisakiasis, acute intestinal anisakiasis, *Anisakis simplex*, basophil activation test, chronic intestinal anisakiasis, eosinophils, eosinophilic granuloma, immunopathogenesis, infestation, *larvae*, mast cells, nematodes, proteolytic enzymes, T lymphocytes, tropomyosin, urticaria, zoonotic diseases.

*Corresponding author M. T. Ventura: Interdisciplinary Department of Medicine, University of Bari Medical School, Polyclinic, Bari, Italy, Piazza G. Cesare, 70124 Bari, Italy; Tel: +390805478793; E-Mail: mt.ventura@allergy.uniba.it

Emilio Jirillo, Thea Magrone and Giuseppe Miragliotta (Eds)
All rights reserved-© 2014 Bentham Science Publishers

INTRODUCTION

Anisakiasis is a zoonotic disease caused by parasitic nematodes of the Anisakidae family. Among them the most frequently involved causative agent is the *Anisakis simplex* (*A.s.*) (Fig. **1**). The first report in the literature of *A.s.* infestation dates back to about 50 years ago, when Van Thiel [1] described the case of a patient complaining acute abdominal pain with the presence of an intestinal eosinophilic phlegmon, inside which the nematode was isolated.

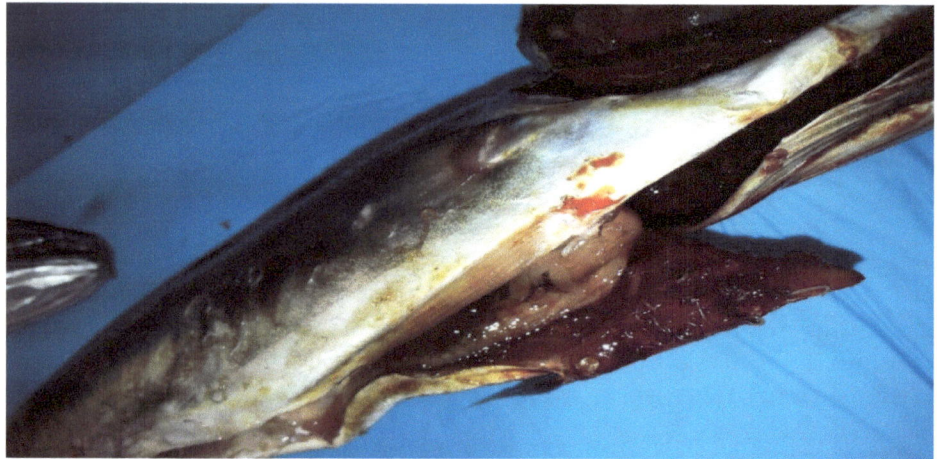

Figure 1: Larvae of *Anisakis simplex* in the celomic cavity of a fish.

The parasites of the Anisakidae family are marine nematodes that during their adult stage live in the gastrointestinal tract of many marine mammals (dolphins, seals, whales). The pairing of the nematode takes place inside these mammals and its fertilized eggs are passed in the feces. The larvae develop from the eggs that are ingested from small crustaceans and small fish (intermediate hosts). Larger fish (tuna, salmon, mackerel, hake, anchovy, sardine, alice, *etcetera*) and cephalopods (cuttlefish, squid, *etc.*) that eat these crustaceans and small fish can get the larvae of the nematode and transfer them to the human who eats them (accidental host). The larvae are about two inches long and have a whitish appearance (Fig. **2**). They are generally found in the bowels of fish, very rarely in its muscles. However the passage in the muscles almost always takes place when the fish is not promptly gutted or not stored at temperatures lower than the refrigeration value because of the alive motility of the larvae [2]. When a person ingests raw or undercooked parasitized fish or inadequately maintained or unproperly gutted fish, the larvae can implant themselves in the gastrointestinal mucosa (from the stomach to the colon) causing the Anisakiasis, which can develop in different clinical pictures [3].

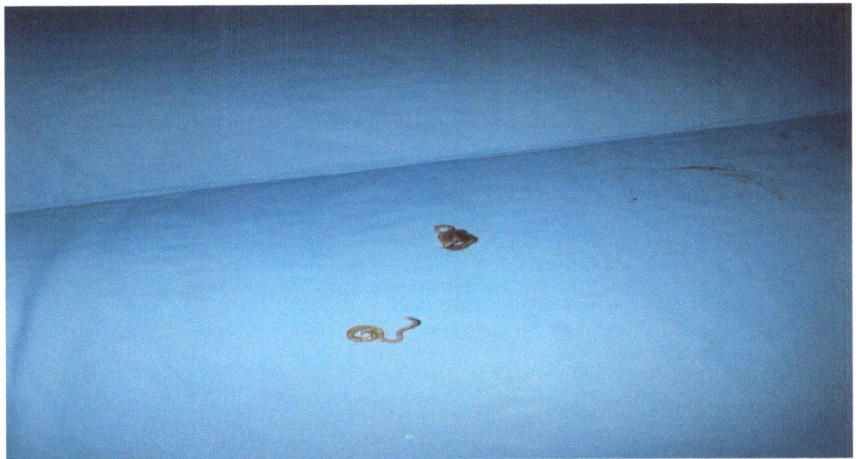

Figure 2: *A.s.* larvae.

The prevalence of this parasite is related to man eating habits and it is particularly linked to the culinary traditions of certain locations. Several recipes of fish are considered to be at high risk for infestation with *A.* [4]. These include sushi and sashimi in Japan, smoked and salted herring in the Dutch tradition; Italian and Spanish anchovies and marinated anchovies [5]. On the contrary it seems that anisakiasis is uncommon in China, where traditional vegetable seasonings used for food preparation exert a toxic effect on *A*.

CLINICAL MANIFESTATIONS

A. infestation can cause gastrointestinal symptoms that may be associated with allergic-type events. More frequently patients show hypersensitivity reactions without associated digestive disorders. *A.* can attack directly human gastrointestinal mucosa causing acute or chronic clinical pictures (acute gastric anisakiasis, acute intestinal anisakiasis and chronic intestinal anisakiasis) [6] or escape to the detrimental action of the gastric juices and give rise to immunoallergic manifestations inducing IgE-mediated reactions (asthma and also chronic-relapsing urticaria, as it has been recently suggested by some authors, or angioedema and anaphylactic shock) [7-9]. Delayed hypersensitivity reactions such as allergic contact dermatitis, especially for the professional categories (fishmongers, fishermen, or housewives) who handle infected fish that is not yet gutted are also possible [10, 11]. Generally the symptoms disappear after the estrangement of the causative agent.

The symptoms of *A.* infestation occur acutely a few hours after the ingestion of parasitized fish. The clinical picture is like an acute gastroenteritis with intense abdominal pain, which is often associated with nausea and vomiting [12]. It is possible to locate and remove the parasite by an early gastroscopy. Generally the larvae die after a short period of stay in the gastrointestinal tract. Sometimes it does not happen: the so-called "syndrome of the larva migrant" clinical picture, in which the parasite can localize in various organs (liver, spleen, lungs, pancreas, myocardium, blood vessels) configuring multiform and severe clinical diseases [13]. Moreover the *A.* can determine an inflammatory chronic reaction at the level of the gastrointestinal mucosa with the formation of an eosinophilic granuloma, which can lead to intestinal obstruction or even perforation of the bowel and consequent peritonitis. Rheumatic symptoms may occur in the course of infection, but they are extremely rare. More recent cases of bronchial hyperactivity can be correlated to the *A.*

Cases of sensitivity to *A.s.* arising from the consumption of chicken fed with fish meal contaminated with the parasite material have also been described [14].

GASTROINTESTINAL PATHOGENICITY OF *A.S.*

During the last few years it has been demonstrated that the changes occurring within the gastrointestinal tract during *A.s.* infection are the result of the direct action of the larva on the tissues and the interaction between the host immune system and the released substances [15]. Humans can be exposed to the antigens of *A.s.* from different sources: from living larvae and somatic and from cuticular antigens of dead larvae disintegrated in food [12]. The epithelial cells of the gastrointestinal mucous membranes secrete cytotoxic molecules such as nitric oxide (NO), chemokines and cytokines, which in turn perform a chemotactic action on the polymorphonuclear leukocytes, tissue macrophages and dendritic cells [16]. Protective responses to intestinal nematodes are associated with the production of T helper (h)2 cytokines, resulting in immunoglobulin (Ig)E-mediated response, and eosinophilia. Besides promoting Th2 responses, helminth infections have shown they can modulate the immune responses involved in immunological tolerance, unmasking autoimmune diseases and thus resulting in an increased susceptibility to infections. Th1-type cytokines (IFN-γ, TNF-β, IL-2 and IL-3) can induce the production of IgG2a, antibody-dependent cytotoxicity and delayed hypersensitivity. Mastocytosis and eosinophilia are induced by a Th2 response and basophils are crucial for the starting of a Th2 response. The eosinophilia may be due to the releasing of numerous chemotactic factors by the epithelial cells: T lymphocytes, mast cells, basophils and factors directly derived from the parasites.

INVASIVE MECHANISMS

The invasion of gastrointestinal mucosa by the *A.s. larvae* occurs through the mechanical destruction of the tissue by the release of powerful proteolytic enzymes that can degrade the extracellular matrix. These proteases are secreted from the dorsal esophageal gland of the larva of *A.s.* [17]. The invasive capacity of the larvae, along with the presence of anticoagulant substances in the excretion products explains the existence of multiple, erosive and hemorrhagic lesions detected near the main lesion within the gastric mucosa of patients with anisakiasis. The metabolic products released by the larva are also important from the immunological point of view, as they can induce immunopatogenetic responses both of immediate and delayed type [18]. These metabolites have also immunosuppressive capacities (associated with the thermolabile components), mutagenic properties, anticoagulant activity and can induce eosinophil chemotaxis.

IMMUNE RESPONSE

Eosinophilia

One of the main features of the local inflammatory lesions produced by *A.s.* larvae is the presence of a large eosinophilic infiltration into the tissues surrounding the parasite. The concentration of eosinophils in the damaged areas can not only be due to the release of chemotactic factors by T lymphocytes, mast cells and basophils, but also to the secretion of chemotactic substances by the parasite. The presence of these cells may reflect the late stage of hypersensitivity response. The response of the eosinophils occurs mainly at a local level (digestive tract), instead of a systemic level [19].

Main Innate Immune Mechanisms

The first cells involved in the response to the immunophlogistic stimulus due to the parasite are the epithelial cells of the gastro-enteric mucosa. They lead in turn to the activation and recruitment of other inflammatory cells, including neutrophils, eosinophils, monocytes, tissue macrophages [20], dendritic cells and basophils. It has been shown that *A.s.* larvae can induce the production of nitric oxide which has an effective microbicidal activity and plays an important role in the defense response against such nematode. At the same time basophils are also activated by both nonspecific and specific mechanisms, releasing proinflammatory cytokines. Actually they play a crucial role both in the innate and in the acquired immunity, being the main source of early production of IL-4, which is required for the polarization in the Th2 sense of the immunophlogistic response [21].

Main Acquired Immune Mechanisms

The granulomatous lesion observed in chronic forms of gastrointestinal anisakiasis or parenchymal organs can be attributed to a typical cell-mediated (type IV Gell and Coombs) immune response [22]. In these cases the inflammatory infiltrate is rich in lymphocytes and eosinophils, that are relevant for the killing of the parasites thanks to the substances they produce: MBP, ECP, EPX and NO. *A.s.* can stimulate effectively the immune system, inducing a simultaneous polarized response both in the sense of Th1 and Th2. In fact at the entry of the parasite in the body, it is elicited the typical early humoral response with the production of IgM antibodies. After about a month the isotype switching can take place simultaneously in the sense of IgG, IgA and IgE. However such an intense response usually occurs only when the antigen power, especially the somatic antigen component, is very high.

Allergens

A.s. has got various kinds of antigens, that are responsible for the immune response in the parasitized host: somatic antigens, obtained by the homogenization of the whole larvae, that are responsible for the cross-reactivity of *A.s.* with other nematodes; ES antigens (excretion-secretion) that are enzymes with a proteolytic and ialuronidasica activity. In addition to them there are surface antigens expressed in the cuticle of the parasite. These molecules play an important role in the formation of granuloma.

In particular it should be mentioned the ' Ani s 1 (between the main ES antigens), the Ani s 2 or somatic antigen so called paramiosina; the Ani s 3 also called tropiomiosina; the Ani s 4, a somatic antigen resistant to heat-pepsin, the Ani s 5, a heat-resistant antigen (excretory glands), the' Ani s 6 and the 'Ani s 7, the latter is identified as the "real" *Anisakis* allergen, present in 100% of patients with infestation by *A*. Ani s 8 and 9, as Ani s 5, belong to the SXP/RAL-2 protein family. The last allergenic epitopes to be identified and coded, thanks to the technology of the recombinant allergens, are Ani s 10 (21 kDa), Ani s 11 (27 kDa) and Ani s 12 (31 kDa) [23]. They are protein molecules whose functionality is still unknown (Table 1).

Table 1: Anisakis Simplex allergens nomenclature

Allergen	Biochemical name	MW(SDS-PAGE)	Food Allergen
Ani s 1	unknown function, similar to Kunitz serine protease inhibitors	24	Yes
Ani s 2	Paramyosin	97	Yes
Ani s 3	Tropomyosin	41	Yes
Ani s 4	Cysteine protease inhibitor	9	Yes
Ani s 5	SXP/RAL-2 family protein	15	Yes
Ani s 6	Serine protease inhibitor	unknown	Yes
Ani s 7	Protein with unknown function	139	Yes
Ani s 8	SXP/RAL-2 family protein	15	Yes
Ani s 9	SXP/RAL-2 family protein	14	Yes
Ani s 10	Protein with unknown function	21 kDa	Yes
Ani s 11	Protein with unknown function	27 kDa	Yes
Ani s 12	Protein with unknown function	31 kDa	Yes
Ani s 13	Hemoglobin	37 kD	Yes

Cross-Reactivity

Anisakis tropomyosin (Ani s 3) is one of the major allergens; it is a protein that regulates muscle contraction and is present in shrimps, oysters, lobsters but also in insects, nematodes, mites [24]. It can induce pulmonary or gastric manifestations according to the way of penetration of the antigen. The cross-reactivity induced by tropomyosin is also responsible for the so-called "Acari-Shellfish-Snails syndrom" (Fig. **3**). In addition to it Ani s 1 (the main antigens), Ani s 2, called paramyosin, and Ani s 3, also known as tropomyosin, are the main allergens responsible for cross-reactivity. In fact it has recently been proved an association between sensitization to *A.* and the sensitization to many kinds of dust mites such as *Dermatophagoides pteronyssinus* [25].

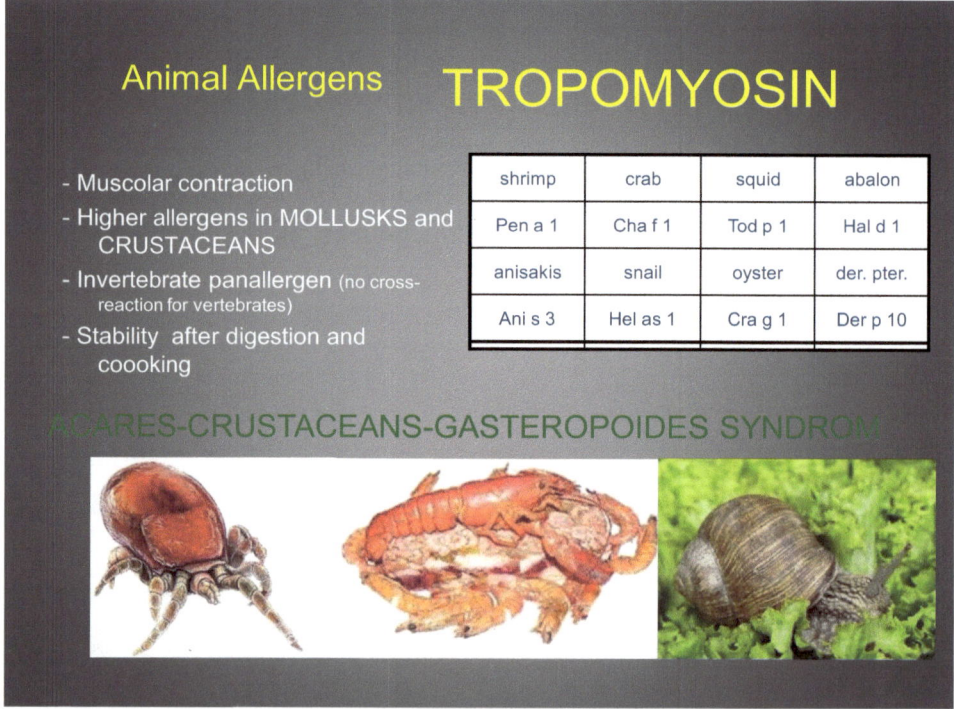

Figure 3: Cross-reactivity induced by tropomyosin.

Diagnosis

The commonly used tests (both *in vivo* and *in vitro*): Skin Prick Test with a panel of inhalant allergens and food, including *A.*; RadioAllergoSorbent Test: to identify the presence in serum of specific IgE to the antigens of *A.s.* Patch test for the evaluation of delayed reactions; gastrointestinal permeability testing; endoscopy to visualize the presence of the nematode immobilized or encysted in the intestinal wall – are useful for the diagnosis. Basophil Activation Test is a new useful tool in the diagnosis of *A.* allergy [26]. The test seems to have a better correlation with clinical response to the parasite compared with specific IgE levels [27]. Its usefulness is also in the ability to discriminate patients with *A.* sensitization without clinical symptoms from patients with hypersensitivity reactions after parasite intake [28].

Prevention

Some authors propose not to consume small fish (such as anchovies) as for them it is more difficult to recognize the parasite. Other authors believe that aquaculture may have advantages over the traditional fishing for the supply of fish free from *A.s.* and related parasites. However, despite the currently world wide preventive measures such as fish cooking and freezing, the incidence of A. has significantly increased, so as to convince EC to issue guidelines for the production and marketing of fish products. The real problem is that the A. antigens are resistant to cooking, due to the presence of thermostable allergenic epitopes [29]. Therefore, in order to avoid sensitization to *A.s.*, actually the most appropriate way is the compliance with the European standard that recommends freezing at -20 ° C the fish intended for raw consumption for 48 hours as a prophylactic measure. Otherwise it is advisable to follow American Food and drug Administration recommending to freeze it at -35° for at least 5 hours. For the consumer it is essential to buy only fresh fish and to gut it at the time of the purchase, so that the larvae do not move from the coelomic cavity to the muscle fibers and to avoid buying fish of unknown origin which may be contaminated.

ACKNOWLEDGEMENT

Declared none.

CONFLICT OF INTEREST

The author(s) confirm that this chapter contents have no conflict of interest.

ABBREVIATIONS

Anisakis = (*A.*)

Anisakis simplex = (*A.s.*)

Ig = Immunoglobulin

Th = T helper cell

REFERENCES

[1] Van Thiel PH. Anisakiasis. Parasitology 1962; 52: 16-7.
[2] Audicana MT, Ansotegui IJ, Fernández de Corres L, *et al*. *Anisakis simplex*: dangerous dead and alive? Trends Parasitol 2002; 18: 20-5.
[3] Ventura MT, Tummolo RA, Di Leo E, *et al*. Immediate and cell-mediated reactions in parasitic infections by *Anisakis simplex*. J Investig Allergol Clin Immunol 2008; 18: 253-9.
[4] Alonso A, Moreno-Ancillo A, Daschner A, *et al*. Dietary assesment in five cases of allergic reactions due to gastroallergic anisakiasis. Allergy 1999; 54: 517-20.
[5] Añibarro B, Seoane FJ, Múgica MV. Involvement of hidden allergens on food allergic reactions. J Invest Allergol Clin Immunol 2007; 17: 168-72.
[6] Daschner A, Alonso-Gomez A, Barranco P, *et al*. Gastric anisakiasis: an underestimated cause of acute urticaria and angio-oedema. Br J Dermatol 1998; 139: 822-8.
[7] Armentia A, Lombardero M, Callejo A, *et al*. Occupational asthma by *Anisakis simplex*. J Allergy Clin Immunol 1998; 102: 831-4.
[8] Daschner A, Vega de la Osada F, Pascual C. Allergy and parasites reevaluated: wide-scale induction of chronic urticaria by the ubiquitous fish-nematode *Anisakis simplex* in an endemic region. Allergol Immunopathol 2005; 33: 31-7.
[9] Del Pozo MD, Audicana MT, Diez J, *et al*. *Anisakis simplex*, a relevant etiologic factor in acute urticaria. Allergy1997; 52: 576-9.
[10] Añibarro B, Seoane FJ. Occupational conjunctivitis caused by sensitization to *Anisakis simplex*. J Allergy Clin Immunol 1998; 102: 331-2.
[11] Scala E, Giani M, Pirrotta L, *et al*. Occupational generalised urticaria and allergic airborne asthma due to *Anisakis simplex*. Eur J Dermatol 2001; 11: 249-50.
[12] Alonso-Gomez A, Moreno-Ancillo A, López-Serrano MC, *et al*. *Anisakis simplex* only provokes allergic symptoms when the worm parasitises the gastrointestinal tract. Parasitol Res 2004; 93: 378-84.
[13] Asaishi K, Nishino C, Ebata TT, *et al*. Studies on the etiologic mechanism of anisakiasi. I. Immunological reactions of digestive tract induced by *Anisakis* larva. Gastroenterol Jpn 1980; 15: 120-7.
[14] Armentia A, Callejo A, Vega JM, *et al*. *Anisakis* allergy after eateing chicken meat. J Investig Allergol Clin Immunol 2006; 16: 258-63.
[15] Daschner A, Cuellar C, Sánchez-Pastor S, *et al*. Gastro-allergic anisakiasis as a consequence of simultaneous primary and secondary immune response. Parasite Immunol 2002; 24: 243-51.

[16] Shea-Donohue T, Urban JF. Gastrointestinal parasite and host interactions. Curr Opin Gastroenterol 2004; 20: 3-9.

[17] Caballero ML, Moneo I. Several allergens from *Anisakis simplex* are highly resistant to heat and pepsin treatments. Parasitol Res 2004; 93: 248-51.

[18] Polimeno L, Loiacono M, Pesetti B, *et al.* Anisakiasis, an understimated infection: effect on intestinal permeability of Anisakis simplex-sensitized patients. Foodborne Pathog Dis 2010; 7: 809-14.

[19] Audicana MT, Kennedy M W. *Anisakis simplex*: from obscure infectious worm to inducer of immune hypersensitivity. Clin Microbiol Rev 2008; 21: 360-79.

[20] Cuellar C, Perteguer MJ, De Las Heras B. Effects of *Anisakis simplex* on nitric oxide production in J774 macrophages. Scand J Infect Dis 1998; 30: 603-6.

[21] Falcone FH, Zillikens D, Gibbs B F. The 21st century renaissance of the basophil? Current insight into its role in allergic responses and innate immunity. Exp Dermatol 2006; 15: 855-64.

[22] Kikuchi Y, Saeki H, Ishikura H. Detection of cellular immnunity by migration inhibition test on rabbits and guinea pigs immunized with *Anisakis* larval antigens, p. 191-198. Intestinal anisakiasis in Japan. Infected fish, sero-immunological diagnosis, and prevention. 1990; Springer-Verlag, Tokyo, Japan.

[23] Caballero ML, Moneo I. Specific IgE determination to Ani s 1, a major allergen from *Anisakis simplex*, is a useful tool for diagnosis. Ann Allergy Asthma Immunol 2002; 89: 74-77.

[24] Johansson E, Aponno M, Lundber M, *et al.* Allergenic cross-reactivity between the nematode *Anisakis simplex* and the dust mites *Acarus siro*, *Lepidoglyphus destructor*, *Tyrophagus putrescentiae*, and *Dermatophagoides pteronyssinus*. Allergy 2001; 56: 660-6.

[25] Ventura MT, D'Erasmo M, Di Gioia R, *et al.* Adverse reaction to specific immunotherapy for house-dust mite in a patient with *Anisakis* allergy. J Eur Acad Dermatol Venereol 2008; 22: 259-60.

[26] Gonzales-Munoz M, Luque R, Nauwelaers F *et al.* Detection of *Anisakis simplex* induced basophil activation by flow cytometry. Cytometry B Clin Cytom 2005; 68: 31-6.

[27] Frezzolini A, Cadoni S, De Pità O. Usefulness of the CD63 basophil activation test in detecting *Anisakis* hypersensitivity in patients with chronic urticaria: diagnosis and follow up. Clin Exp Dermatol 2009; 35: 765-70.

[28] Maietta G, Arsieni A, De Donno M, *et al.* Urticaria and angioedema associated with *Anisakis simplex*: usefulness of the basophil activation test in discriminating sensitization from allergy. EAACI Skin Allergy Meeting 2012; 29 nov-1 dec, Berlin (Germany).

[29] Audicana L, Audicana MT, Fernández de Corres L, *et al.* Cooking and freezing may not protect against allergic reactions to ingested *Anisakis simplex* antigens in humans. Vet Rec 1997; 140: 235.

Chapter 8: Immunomodulation by Parasitic Helminths and its Therapeutic Exploitation

CHAPTER 8

Immunomodulation by Parasitic Helminths and its Therapeutic Exploitation

Miguel Angel Pineda[1] and William Harnett[2],*

[1]*Division of Immunology, Infection and Inflammation, University of Glasgow, Glasgow, G12 8TA and* [2]*Strathclyde Institute of Pharmacy and Biomedical Sciences, University of Strathclyde, Glasgow, G4 ORE, United Kingdom*

Abstract: Parasitic worms are able to survive in their mammalian hosts for many years due to their ability to manipulate the immune response by secreting immunomodulatory products. These products differ between species of helminths, but they share common mechanisms of action such as modulation of Toll-like receptor pathways and induction of regulatory immune responses along with pro-inflammatory Th2 responses, what is often termed as a 'modified Th2 response'. Interestingly, it is increasingly clear that, reflecting the anti-inflammatory actions of such worm-derived immunomodulators, there is an inverse correlation between helminth infection and autoimmune diseases in the developing world. As the decrease in helminth infections due to increased sanitation has correlated with an alarming increase in prevalence of such disorders in industrialised countries, this "Hygiene Hypothesis" has led to the proposal that worms and their secreted products offer a novel platform for the development of safe and effective strategies for the treatment of allergic and autoimmune disorders. We summarize here, the current understanding of helminth-derived molecules with immunomodulatory activity and their associated cellular and molecular mechanisms that act in the host to modulate the immune response. In addition, we reveal how these findings have been applied in the clinic and in research to develop novel therapies for allergy and autoimmune diseases, like asthma, rheumatoid arthritis, inflammatory bowel disease and multiple sclerosis.

Keywords: Allergy, antigen presenting cell, autoimmunity, cystatin, dendritic cell, ES-62, FOXP3, helminth, helminth-based therapy, hygiene hypothesis, IL-10, immunomodulation, modified Th2 response, NFκB, regulatory T cell, Soluble Egg Antigen, TGFβ, Th1/Th2 responses, Th17 responses, Toll-like receptors.

---

*Corresponding author **William Harnett**: Strathclyde Institute of Pharmacy and Biomedical Sciences, University of Strathclyde, 161 Cathedral Street, Glasgow G4 0RE, United Kingdom; Tel: 0044-141-548-3725; Fax: 0044-141-552-2562; E-mail: W.Harnett@strath.ac.uk

Emilio Jirillo, Thea Magrone and Giuseppe Miragliotta (Eds)
All rights reserved-© 2014 Bentham Science Publishers

INTRODUCTION

Parasitic worms have co-evolved with their mammalian hosts for millions of years. When worms, perhaps accidentally, had the opportunity of including a vertebrate host as part of their life cycle, natural selection made them adapt to this new environment due to a number of evolutionary advantages. Compared to the outside world, the new environment offered stable conditions in terms of temperature, humidity or access to nutrients. From the worm's perspective, there is only one major problem, the presence of an active immune system with one goal: to kill or expel the worm from the host. However, worms have developed numerous survival strategies, including the ability of producing molecules with the ability of being immunomodulators in the host. This was an evolutionary adaptation because, in fact, some of the molecules able to regulate immune system cells in the host are produced not only by parasitic worms, but also by free-living worms, suggesting that these organisms adapted this capacity to turn their life cycle into a parasitic one. Thanks to the immunomodulatory products, helminths are able to escape from the host immune response, allowing them to survive for years, as parasitic worms usually produce long-term infections. Immunomodulation by helminths is so specific and sophisticated that it dampens down the response elicited against the worm, but it does not completely switch off the host immune system. Indeed, the host is forced to develop an immune system that works effectively in the presence of worms, but avoiding exaggerated responses against the parasite and therefore, self-damage. Hence, parasitic helminths must be master regulators of immune responses in order to ensure their prolonged persistence in the host without compromising immunity against other infections. This fine balance achieved between helminth and host has been optimised only after many millennia of mutual evolutionary pressure on both sites.

Parasitic worms form a very heterogeneous group that is found within two phyla and within each phylum parasitism is also found in different orders, Trematoda and Cestoda in the phylum Platyhelminthes and Ascaridiata and Filariata in the phylum Nematoda. Even within an order, parasitic worms show differences in structure, mode of transmission and location in the host. However, remarkably, as if natural selection had directed each of them to the right strategy to ensure persistence, they generally seem to share common mechanisms to avoid the host immune system. Therefore, despite the biological diversity found in helminths, the concept of 'immunomodulation by helminths' is often found and accepted in the literature and the mechanisms associated with this process will be discussed throughout the text.

Helminths induce very different immune responses compared to other pathogens like bacteria, fungi, viruses or protozoa and they are known to skew the immune response towards a Th2-like phenotype [1]. The question is, why worms could take advantage of the Th2, and hence pro-inflammatory, responses that they are able to induce in the host to regulate the immune system? This would not seem to be the right strategy for survival, but it is important to bear in mind at this point that helminths do not suppress the immune response activated to eliminate them, but as alluded to earlier, they modulate, modify and ameliorate this response. To recall, immunomodulation is hypothesized to be beneficial to both the vertebrate host and the parasite, as it protects helminths from being eradicated, and at the same time protects the host from excessive pro-inflammatory responses that may lead to self-damage. According to this idea of modulation but not suppression, some authors define the Th2 response against helminths as a 'modified Th2 immune response' [2, 3], the unique scenario where pro-inflammatory Th2 responses occur along with enhanced regulatory T cell responses. Particular immune responses have been selected by the host in order to tolerate the presence of the parasite, preventing any potential self-damage [4]. In other words, immunoregulatory pathways would have been selected that work well in the presence of worm infections.

The concept of a modified Th2 response is a very appealing premise that could explain why helminths specifically drive Th2 immunity. One simple hypothesis is that the resulting Th2 response is just a default mechanism reduced in the absence of a Th1-induced system [5]. On the other hand, Th2-type immune responses are involved in mediating acute wound healing during helminth infection [6], an important role in this context where skin and gut epithelia are often damaged, compromising the host.

These facts can explain why helminths are strong inducers of modulated Th2 responses upon infection and also explain another important and unique feature associated with immune regulation by helminths, their ability to inhibit Th1 and

Th17 responses. Th1/Th17 responses are completely different to Th2 responses, and are induced in response to other types of pathogens like bacteria or fungi. Indeed, Th1/Th17 responses inhibit Th2 responses, in the same way that a Th2 response can block Th1 and Th17 responses. Therefore, helminth products that induce Th2 immune responses also down-regulate Th1 and Th17 responses as has been seen in a number of animal models [7-10]. Although much more work must be done to fully understand the mechanisms associated with helminth immunomodulation, there is a related obvious and appealing hypothesis. If helminths have co-evolved with human beings to develop the perfect anti-inflammatory compound, could we not take advantage of such a molecule to treat inflammatory diseases? Of relevance, compared to developing countries, the prevalence of allergic and autoimmune diseases is recently increased in developed countries, where the improvement in sanitation has eradicated parasite worms. Epidemiological and experimental evidence supports the 'hygiene hypothesis', proposed by D.P. Strachan in 1989 [11]. According to this theory, atopic disorders are due to a reduced exposure to microorganisms in childhood as an inverse relationship between the incidence of hay fever and co-infection between siblings was observed, suggesting that children with more siblings were more prone to getting infections and that this was somehow able to protect them from hay fever. Nowadays there is accumulative evidence not only for allergic diseases but also with respect to autoimmune diseases that supports the protective role of parasites against these conditions. An inverse correlation between multiple sclerosis, asthma, type 1 diabetes, arthritis and inflammatory bowel disease with increased hygiene conditions is observed [12-16], and an increasing number of experimental studies shows that mechanisms of helminth-induced immunomodulation can contribute to this protection against autoimmune inflammatory diseases in developing countries. In this context, parasitic helminths and their secreted products are now important candidates for the development of novel anti-inflammatory and anti-allergic agents. Despite this, we are still at a very early stage and much more research needs to be done in order to develop effective drugs. Nevertheless, as will be seen, work to date has shown promising results and suggests that helminths are truly a potential source of new drugs.

Many inflammatory diseases are associated with an excessive Th1 response that turns into a double-edged sword, causing as much tissue destruction as pathogen eradication. Aberrant Th17 responses have been proposed to be the cause of many autoimmune diseases that affect millions of people, like rheumatoid arthritis (RA), and many allergies and airway diseases depend on the Th2 response triggered by non-pathogenic molecules. Although some other factors could induce autoimmunity (diet, obesity, psychological stress), a number of studies in animal models and also clinical trials have shown that lack of helminth infections correlates with a higher incidence of chronic auto-inflammatory disease. Therefore, it has been hypothesised that helminths can be used successfully to treat some of these clinical conditions, like RA, asthma and IBD [17]. It seems that the protective mechanism is associated with down-regulation of Th1/Th17 responses and enhanced Th2-dependent mechanisms. In addition, and perhaps unexpectedly, Th2-driven pathologies, such as asthma or allergic reactions, are also abrogated by helminth infections, due to the capacity of worms to activate some regulatory pathways to control a potential excessive inflammatory process of this type. Some of these mechanisms include activation of regulatory B and T cells, and alternatively activated macrophages that often lead to the production of IL-10.

We will summarize the recent findings in this field showing the molecular and cellular mechanisms responsible for the protective effects of helminth-based therapy in allergic and autoimmune disorders.

CELLULAR MECHANISMS ACTIVATED BY HELMINTHS AND IMMUNE SYSTEM MODULATION

Immunity against worms involves a rapid and transient Th1 response that is replaced by a Th2/Treg response. This activates many cell types in the host, including dendritic cells, CD4 T cells and B cells, which during chronic infections leads to a state of balance between the parasite and the host that allows the latter to tolerate the chronic infection. We will describe briefly the mechanisms triggered by individual cell types, but it is worth bearing in mind that the infection is more complex than the dissected components. For example, cells, molecules and receptors change dramatically in different sites of infection, like the gut, skin or lungs. It is also very different at early stages, resembling an acute infection, to late stages when the infection becomes chronic. The main events occurring during helminth infection are described below, where effector cell types are analyzed separately. Nevertheless, specific information is required to understand the immunomodulation achieved by different helminth species at different infection stages.

Up-Regulation of Th2 Responses by Helminths

Helminth infections are unique in the sense that initially they develop Th1 responses [18], which convert over time to Th2 responses. Indeed, some clinical conditions associated with schistosomiasis result in exacerbated granuloma inflammation causing substantial liver damage because the parasite fails to skew the original Th1 response to a Th2 phenotype [19]. Th1 responses against helminths are often driven by acute infections, but helminths usually establish chronic infections that induce Th2 responses in the long-term scenario and define the immune response elicited against them. Infections with parasitic worms induce Type 2 responses in the host that are characterized by the expansion of CD4 Th2 cells, activated lymphocytes that secrete cytokines such as IL-4, IL-5, IL-13 and IL-9. Th2 cells promote IgE and IgG4 production by B cells and IgE binds to high affinity IgE receptors (FcεR1) on basophils and mast cells, leading to their activation and release of pro-inflammatory molecules such as cytokines (IL-33), histamine, heparin and serotonin [5, 20, 21]. The combination of these molecules triggers an unstoppable inflammatory process characterized by recruitment of alternatively activated macrophages and granulocytes [22].

Type 2, Th2 or Th2-like responses are terms often used in the literature to define this whole process that starts with the polarization of naive T cells towards Th2 cells and it includes not only Th2 lymphocytes but also other cell types like basophils, mast cells or granulocytes. Th2 cell responses are only a subgroup belonging to a larger spectrum of Th responses that have evolved to face a great diversity of pathogens. Therefore, different types of Th subsets are defined by specific production of cytokines and transcription factors profiles as well as by the different kind of pathogens that they can control. Infection with intracellular bacteria or viruses typically induces strong Th1 responses, with high levels of IFNγ and CD8 cytotoxic T cells that ultimately kill infected cells preventing pathogen replication. Other Th subsets include Th17 cells that produce IL-17 and express the transcription factor RORγt and are directed against extracellular bacteria and fungi.

Compared to the relatively well-studied Th1/Th17 responses, much less is understood about Th2 responses, the kind of immune response triggered by helminths. There is an apparent heterogeneity of cytokine profiles within the Th2 cells, probably as a consequence of the great diversity of stimuli that are able to induce them. Th2 responses have been most explored in the context of helminth infections, but a large number of different stimuli also induce type 2 immunity, both microbial stimuli like viruses, bacteria or lipopolysaccharides and non microbial stimuli such as pollen allergens, food allergens (*e.g.* peanuts, shellfish), venoms (*e.g.* bee) and vaccine adjuvants like Alum [23]. Importantly, based on T cell skewing patterns, disorders associated with excessive immune responses have been classified as Th1-dependent and Th2-dependent according to the Th1/Th2 paradigm. Also, more recently, the discovery of Th17 responses led to the concept of Th17-dependent diseases, where we can include a significant number of diseases that were originally thought to be Th1-driven pathologies and where it has now been reported that the leading pathological pathway could be mediated by the IL-23/IL-17 axis.

Helminths have been shown to suppress Th1, Th2 and Th17 responses in different animal models of inflammatory and autoimmune diseases. As mentioned earlier, it is well known that Th2-like cytokines inhibit both Th1 and Th17 immune responses in the same way that Th1 and Th17 pathways inhibit the Th2 ones. Therefore, it is not surprising to find out that helminth-induced Th2-skewing along with down-regulation of Th1 responses results in attenuation of Th1-associated diseases, for example, experimental diabetes and colitis [24-28]. In the same way, given the role of IL-17 in autoimmunity, it has been shown that helminths are able to down-regulate IL-17-mediated diseases by skewing the immune response to a Th2 phenotype, as IL-4 has been shown to inhibit Th17 differentiation and IL-17 expression by committed Th17 cells, even in the presence of TGFβ, IL-6 and IL-23 [29], cytokines involved in Th17 differentiation pathways and maintenance of activated Th17 cells. This shows that IL-4 is a deactivation signal for IL-17 pathways that prevails over other cytokines and explains why helminth infections are so protective in the context of Th17-driven diseases like RA [10, 30] or experimental autoimmune encephalomyelitis [31].

IL-10 and Regulatory T Cells

It has been extensively demonstrated that the increased expression of the regulatory cytokine IL-10 is a common effect of helminth immunomodulation, and it can provide an answer to a less obvious question based on the Th1 and Th17 regulation by Th2 helminth-induced cytokines. We have previously said that helminths have been shown to down-regulate Th1 and Th17 responses in a number of animal models of inflammatory diseases, by skewing the global immune response to a type 2 phenotype, but some other studies show that they can also down-regulate Th2 inflammatory responses and in fact, some helminth infections are protective against asthma or airway hypersensitivity [32-34]. Surprisingly, mechanisms protective against hypersensitivity associated with helminth infections involve down-regulation of IL-4 and IL-5, crucial cytokines in the Type 2 immune response.

The helminth-induced suppression of these Th2 diseases is difficult to explain in terms of the Th1/Th2 paradigm, suggesting that other mechanisms of immunomodulation may be involved. After infection by parasitic worms, a Th2 response is induced by the immune system and potentially the resultant production of IL-4/IL-5, IgE and hypereosinophilia, which would be expected to cause an exacerbation of allergic reactions. Indeed, helminth infections do not always protect against Th2 disorders or allergies and some helminth infections have been reported to promote allergic reactions. Thus, a number of studies performed in South America, Europe and Asia report a positive correlation between *A. lumbricoides* infections and the prevalence of asthma [35-37] and exacerbation of allergic airway inflammation was observed in *Toxocara*-infected mice [38]. The inconsistencies observed with respect to decreased, *versus* increased allergy might be explained by a number of factors. In the case of epidemiological studies we have to take into account that the age and genetic background of the studied population can lead to a different outcome, as well as the helminth species studied. Also, environmental changes can affect the resulting immune response dramatically. For example, infection with a nematode parasite in protein-malnourished mice produced less IL-4 and more IFNγ than observed in the control cohort, leading to reduced Th2 effector responses in a model where the genetic background of the mice and the nematode species were conserved through the study [39]. Also, the intensity of infection is thought to be important because heavy, chronic helminth infections are associated with protection from Th2 diseases, whereas low parasite burden enhances Th2 responses, without inducing any immune regulation [16, 40]. However, keeping in mind the great variability present both in parasite and host, studies to gain insight into the suppression of Th2 diseases by helminths have led to the discovery of a number of mechanisms triggered by worms to modulate the immune response that are independent of the reciprocal Th1/Th2 inhibition. This proposes an interesting explanation for the observed anti-allergic effects of helminths and as an example, it has been described that helminths induce up-regulation of the regulatory cytokine IL-10 from different cell sources.

Furthermore, studies in animal models showed an expansion of certain regulatory immune cell types, such as alternatively activated macrophages, regulatory T cells (Treg) and regulatory B cells (Breg). It does not seem to be likely that the expansion of these cells is only a consequence of the initiated immune response in a homeostatic attempt to control it, because the parasite *H. polygyrus* actively releases a product that mimics mammalian TGFβ, a cytokine that is required to convert naive T cells into suppressive FOXP3+ Tregs [41].

The up-regulation of TGFβ activity is also observed in other helminth species like *S. mansoni*, but using a different strategy. Soluble egg antigen (SEA) from *S. mansoni* acts on DCs to enhance their ability of inducing Tregs from naive T cells [28]. Either way, the overall effect is an increased Treg activity during helminth infections. We will use the term Treg, although it is rather simplistic; Treg cells are a very heterogeneous population, not fully understood as yet [42-44]. The best described Treg subpopulations in the literature are 'natural' nTregs and 'induced' iTregs, both with regulatory ability but phenotypically different regarding mRNA transcripts, epigenetic modification and stability, although it has been only recently that specific surface markers have been found to distinguish subtypes [45, 46]. This will allow further studies on Treg biology and indeed, some work on helminth regulation of different Tregs has been shown already [47], opening a new exciting research field.

The cellular mechanisms that mediate suppression of allergic responses by helminths often result in expansion and/or activation of Tregs [28, 41, 48-52] and it is well accepted that Tregs play an essential role in helminth-induced protection in inflammatory diseases. Adoptive transfer of CD4+CD25+ T cells (markers expressed by Tregs) from mice infected with *H. polygyrus* was shown to suppress allergic inflammation in recipient mice, although IL-10 activity was not essential for the regulatory activity in this model, since adoptive transfer of Tregs from IL-10 deficient mice still confers protection [53]. Supporting these data, the anti-allergic effect of *A. lumbricoides* infection in humans is associated with Treg activity, but not IL-10 [54]. Hence, despite it being clear that protective responses induced by helminths lead to an increased IL-10 production, the importance of IL-10 in helminth-mediated suppression of Th2 diseases is not fully established. Further research must be undertaken in order to fully understand the mechanisms underlying Treg-mediated protection induced by helminths, including studies on different Treg subtypes and perhaps new mediators produced by these cells. For example, IL-10 is not always the main effector cytokine and perhaps other cytokines produced by Treg cells can show us other potential targets for clinical use. IL-35 is a cytokine recently described that is secreted by Tregs and it has been shown to be essential for the regulatory activity of these cells [55]. Interestingly, IL-35 suppresses some diseases of autoimmune or allergic origin [56] raising the question as to whether helminths can manipulate Treg biology *via* IL-35.

Modulation of Effector and Regulatory B Cells

Tregs can also interact with B cells, down-regulating effector B cell responses and increasing their IgG4 production in an IL-10-dependent manner in a mechanism that also involves GITR-GITR-L interactions and TGFβ [57]. This contributes to skewing of the attenuated immune response to a Th2 phenotype. However, B cells are not limited to being immunoglobulin producers, they exert some antibody-independent activities like antigen presentation, co-stimulation and regulatory/effector functions.

Regarding B cell activity, a new cell type within the B cell compartment has attracted a lot of attention recently, the regulatory B cell (Breg). Bregs constitute a subpopulation of B cells that are able to down-regulate immune responses and produce IL-10. Interestingly, IL-10-producing Bregs are also up-regulated upon helminth infections, protecting against allergic diseases [58], thereby suggesting that Bregs might play a relevant role in the cellular networks that are affected by helminths [59]. However, little is known yet regarding the effects of helminth infection on innate and regulatory B cell responses. Recent studies have shown a certain parallelism between Tregs and Bregs in the sense that IL-10 is not always essential for their regulatory activity. Using a murine model of airway inflammatory reaction, Bregs induced during *H. polygyrus* infection were able to prevent disease progression independently of IL-10 [53]. Interestingly, these Bregs were characterized by high expression of CD23 in addition to classical pan markers. On the other hand, *S. mansoni*-mediated protection against experimental induced allergic airway inflammation was specifically dependent on IL-10-producing CD1d(+) splenic regulatory B cells, a finding that was recently confirmed in epidemiological studies with *Schistosoma haematobium*-infected Gabonese children [60].

The diversity of regulatory lymphocytes expanded upon helminth infection, both T and B cells, might explain some contradictory data regarding IL-10 in helminth infections and its relevance to the ability of parasitic worms to manipulate host immune responses, since there have been described regulatory effects on T and B cells with respect to both dependent and independent IL-10 mechanisms. This possibly depends on particular diseases, parasite burden or helminth species and therefore further elucidation of these helminth induced regulatory B cells may identify new strategies to treat chronic inflammatory disorders.

Alternative Macrophage Activation

Macrophages play a crucial role in initiating and modulating the host immune response to pathogen infections. The classically known macrophage activation is induced by IFNγ, which triggers a proinflammatory response that is required to kill intracellular pathogens. However, helminths do not induce this type of macrophage activation and these cells become a target for immunoregulation by the worm. During helminth infection macrophages assume a distinct state of alternative activation [61-63] induced by Th2-like cytokines, IL-4 and IL-13, which mediate expression of some specific markers (arginase I, mannose receptor, RELM-α, Ym-1) along with changes in metabolic pathways [64]. Alternatively activated macrophages (AAMφ) play a role in immune regulation and also contribute to maintenance of physiological homeostasis and tissue repair [22], essential for helminth and host survival during helminth infection.

MOLECULAR BASIS OF IMMUNE MODULATION BY HELMINTHS

In 1989 Janeway proposed the pattern recognition theory [65] and in many ways it revolutionized our understanding of the immune system, providing a conceptual framework for the integration of the innate and adaptive arms. This theory proposed that the signals required for co-stimulation of APCs were inducible by conserved microbial products. To sense such products, the innate immune system possessed a set of germline-encoded pattern recognition receptors (PRRs) that detected conserved products of microbial origin, what we call today pathogen-associated molecular patters (PAMPs). More than 20 years later, this theory has been confirmed and a large number of PRRs have been defined and characterized, C-type lectins, NOD-like Receptors (NLRs), pentraxins, mannan-binding lectins (MBLs) but the most studied and perhaps the most relevant ones are the Toll Like Receptors (TLRs). PRRs are expressed by immune and non-immune cells, but most research has focused on the response of classical innate cells such as dendritic cells (DCs) and macrophages and it has been observed that the immunomodulatory activity of worms can be dependent on interaction with specific PRRs on the cells of the host immune system. Through manipulation of PRRs and their associated pathways, helminths down-regulate the host immune response leading to a hyporesponsive status, the main hallmark of helminth infections. As alluded to earlier, this immunoregulation is of outstanding importance because it allows the parasite to escape from the host immune system and it also controls excessive responses that could damage tissues and organs. Helminths express a large mixture of compounds with immunoregulatory potential, both proteins and lipids that are in many cases heavily glycosylated. In addition, they actively secrete products with strong immunomodulatory actions to attenuate and control the host immune system. These secreted products are key elements in helminth immunomodulation, and many clinical cases of elephantiasis, a condition characterized by the thickening of the skin and underlying tissues after an uncontrolled inflammatory process, occur when filarial nematode-infected patients receive anti-helminth treatment, leading to a situation where dead parasites induce a strong inflammation, but the lack of secreted regulatory products by the dead parasite leads to an inflammatory process that cannot be controlled [66]. The exceptional capacity of these products synthesized by helminths to regulate inflammatory responses offers growing opportunities for the discovery of novel drugs from parasitic helminths. Although we are still at a very early stage, some functional molecules have been isolated and studied both *in vitro* and *in vivo*, showing the great potential of helminths as a depository for new therapeutics.

Molecules Which Immunomodulate

The interest in the area of drug development against autoimmune and allergic diseases has facilitated the investigation of a significant number of worms and worm-derived molecules with strong immunomodulatory properties. Helminth infections utilize a complex mixture of products resulting in the observed ameliorated Th2-skewed immune response. Some worms have been used in clinical trials already, *e.g.*, the use of *Trichuris suis* ova in patients with immune-mediated diseases [67]. These studies have demonstrated the safety and efficacy of helminth-treatment [68], but some other clinical trials showed some significant adverse effects associated to the ingestion of *T. suis* eggs [69]. Therefore, the use of live worms in the clinic has shown promising results, but it can present important drawbacks. An alternative to this could be to use crude parasite extracts, but these might be highly immunogenic, limiting their use in clinic. To get around this problem, some isolated products with high anti-inflammatory potential have been tested in animal models, although none of these compounds have been tested in clinical trials to date. We will focus here on some of the isolated molecules produced by helminths that have been shown to mimic the immunoregulation induced by worms (summarized in Table **1**), and therefore, they could provide the first step towards the discovery of safe and efficient drugs based on helminth-derived products.

ES-62

ES-62 is a glycosylated protein secreted by the filarial nematode *Acanthocheilonema viteae* and it is probably one of the best-characterized helminth-derived immunomodulators. It has been shown to possess a plethora of immunomodulatory activities that have been successfully tested in a number of animal models like asthma and RA. The glycoconjugates present in ES-62 express an unusual modification, a PC moiety attached to the terminal N-acetylglucosamine. The PC is largely responsible for its anti-inflammatory action and this small molecule attached to a non-specific protein like bovine serum albumin (BSA) is able to down-regulate immune responses in the same way as the parental ES-62 [70]. This PC-containing glycoprotein modulates DCs to induce Th2 responses, inhibits proinflammatory cytokine production by macrophages, and generation of IL-10 by B1 cells [71]. It has been shown that ES-62 down-regulates TLR4-mediated responses affecting MyD88-dependent pathways to reduce NFκB activation and the subsequent synthesis of pro-inflammatory cytokines such as IL-12, IL-6 and TNFα [72]. Also, ES-62 is able to inhibit the IL-17/IL-23 inflammatory axis in an animal model of RA, protecting against disease progression though modulating a complex cellular network of DCs, Th17/Th1 cells and gamma-delta T cells [10].

CYSTATINS

Cystatins play a major role in the modulation of the immune response by helminths. They are reversible inhibitors of cysteine proteases that are wide spread in all living organisms, including mammals and nematodes. In mammals they are involved in proteolysis and in immune cells, cystatins regulate antigen processing and presentation, phagocytosis, cytokine expression and nitric oxide production. Helminth cystatins are secreted proteins that have been shown to inhibit macrophage-dependent responses. Early studies showed that cystatin from the rodent filarial nematode *A. viteae* down-regulated mitogen-induced T cell proliferation and up-regulated IL-10 production [73], and this was reproduced by recombinant cystatin produced in *E. coli*. Further research indicated that macrophages were the main target of helminth cystatins. Cystatins inhibit antigen presentation and cytokine responses in macrophages, up-regulating IL-10 production [74]. Interestingly, cystatins from the non-parasitic worm *C. elegans* induced IL-12 production but not IL-10, suggesting the importance of cystatins in parasitic helminth-derived immunomodulation. In contrast, cystatins from both filarial nematodes and *C. elegans* induce NO production [75], a well-known immune mediator whose relevance in immune responses against helminths is not clear. The mechanisms underlying macrophage regulation have been well characterized, although the receptor or molecules targeted by nematode cystatins remain elusive. Cystatins exploit modulation of the MAP kinases ERK1/2 and p38 pathways to induce IL-10-producing regulatory macrophages [76, 77]. Recently, filarial cystatins have shown their potential in the treatment of inflammatory diseases using animal models. Cystatin purified from *Clonorchis sinensis* inhibited dextran sodium sulfate-induced intestinal inflammation by recruiting IL-10-producing macrophages [78] and a recombinant form of *Angiostrongylus cantonensis* cystatin was protective in a model of grass pollen allergic responses, where Th2 responses like eosinophil recruitment or IgE, IL-5 and IL-13 production were inhibited, meanwhile the production of IL-10 was induced [79].

PRODUCTS ISOLATED FROM SOLUBLE EGG ANTIGEN (SEA) OF SCHISTOSOMA: LNFPIII AND OMEGA-1

Soluble egg antigens (SEA) from *Schistosoma ssp.* are among the strongest natural stimuli of Th2 responses [80] and are composed of a complex mixture of highly glycosylated molecules. Two individual products from this mixture have been isolated and shown to exert immunomodulatory actions similar to SEA, the carbohydrate Lacto-N-fucopentaose III (LFNPIII) and the glycoprotein Omega-1, and both drive immune biasing towards Th2 responses, in the same way that SEA does. Both Omega-1 and LFNPIII contain glycans in their structure, as shown by the presence of the Lewis X motifs (Le^x). The Le^x antigen, Galβ1-4(Fucα1-3)GlcNAc, is found mainly in schistosomes [81] and it seems to cooperate with other sugars to induce Th2-like responses.

LFNPIII modulates DC responses to induce a polarized Th2 immune response using several receptors. It has been reported that LFNPIII utilizes TLR4, dendritic cell-specific ICAM-3-grabbing protein (DC-SIGN) and some other C-type lectin receptors like the mannose receptor and macrophage galactose lectin-1 (MGL-1) [82-84]. LFNPIII affects macrophages to drive them towards an alternative phenotype associated with elevated arginase I activity and IL-10 production [85, 86]. The up-regulation of IL-10 production has been shown to be responsible for an improved glucose tolerance and insulin sensitivity in diet-induced obese mice

[86], and this represents the first application of helminth products to treating metabolic disorders. However, the potential of LFNPIII in the clinic is even more fascinating, since LFNPIII accumulates FoxP3+ regulatory T cells to extend median graft survival in a murine model of heart transplantation [87].

The glycoprotein Omega-1 also targets DCs to initiate Th2 responses like SEA [88], but contrary to LFNPIII, it does not manipulate MyD88/TRIFF signalling pathways and therefore, it is unlikely that this protein targets TLR4 [89]. As an alternative explanation, it has been suggested that Omega-1 polarizes DCs towards a Th2-inducing phenotype due to cytoskeletal changes that avoid cell-cell interactions during T cell priming. However, the fact that Omega-1 is still able to down-regulate IL-12 production by LPS-activated DCs indicated that other receptors different to TLRs might be involved and in fact, it has been recently discovered that omega-1 is bound and internalized by the mannose receptor impairing protein synthesis by degrading both ribosomal and messenger RNA [90]. Like LFPNIII, Omega-1 is able to induce FoxP3+ T cells and IL-4 production, and some groups have proposed the potential of this glycoprotein to treat autoimmune diabetes [91].

OTHER HELMINTH-DERIVED PRODUCTS

There are some other examples in the literature of products produced by helminths with immunomodulatory ability, some of them have been only recently discovered and some others have not been studied in great detail yet. Doubtless, further work with these molecules will contribute to gain insight into some of the mechanisms that currently remain unknown.

Calreticulin of *H. polygyrus* (HpCRT) is a secreted protein that interacts with the murine scavenger receptor A and induces a Th2-skewed response along with an up-regulation of IL-4 production by CD4 T cells [92]. A schistosomal phosphatidylserine (PS) fraction contained the lipid, Lyso-PS. Lyso-PS activated TLR2 in DCs to induce the expansion of IL-10+ regulatory T cells [93]. The activity of Lyso-PS seems to depend on specific acyl chains. However, the presence of (PC) in this molecule may be important as it has been established that certain immunomodulatory activity of nematode glycolipids relies on the presence of PC [94]. In fact as alluded to earlier, the biological activity of ES-62, a filarial PC-containing glycoprotein whose mechanism of action has been described in detail, depends largely on the PC moiety attached to the glycans [70]. Antigen B (AgB) is an excretory-secreted product of larval stage Echinococcus granulosus, which is encoded by a multigene family and seems to be involved in evasion of host immunesurveillance. AgB inhibits polymorphonuclear cell recruitment, skews the Th1/Th2 ratio towards a Th2 polarized response and modulates co-stimulatory ability of DCs, down-modulating CD1a and CD83 expression but up-regulating CD86 [95, 96]. Inhibition of the recruitment of effector cells such as neutrophils has been also observed after administration of the purified recombinant *S. mansoni* chemokine binding protein (smCKBP) in a mechanism that depends on the chemokine CXCL-8 [97].

Contrary to the products already commented on that exert their biological activity by modulating specific receptors, some helminth products have evolved to achieve the same effect by employing a completely different strategy, such as mimicking endogenous inflammatory mediators. This is the case with *B. malayi* and *H. polygyrus* that secrete a TGFβ functional homolog capable of inducing IL-10 production and Treg development [41, 98]. Nematodes also express galectin-like proteins that are highly conserved between species [99]. It was suggested that based on the high degree of homology with the mammalian proteins, helminth galectins might be involved in immune regulation but only recently was this hypothesis confirmed. Galectins are carbohydrate-binding proteins that play important roles in innate and adaptive immune response. In particular, galectin-9 induces apoptosis of activated T cells and it is also an important eosinophil chemoattractor. A galectin-9 homolog from *Toxascaris leonina* termed Tl-gal has been identified and cloned, and the recombinant protein has been shown to retain the ability to bind to galactosides and inhibit Th1 and Th2 cytokine production in a murine model of intestinal inflammation by increasing the production of TGFβ and IL-10 [100].

dsRNA from *S. mansoni* acts also as an inducer of the innate immune system through TLR3, increasing IFNα production by DCs and inducing a dominant Th1 response [101].

Table 1: Isolated products derived from helminths that exert immunomodulatory actions. ↑ and ↓ represent enhanced and down-regulated responses respectively. ND = non-determined

Helminth product	Species	Nature	Receptor	Mechanism	Ref
ES-62	Filarial nematode Acanthocheilonema viteae	secreted PC-containing glycoprotein	TLR4	↓ IL-12, TNFα, IL-6 in APCs ↓ Th1/Th17 responses ↑ IL-10 in B1 cells	[10, 72, 102, 103]
Cystatin	Multiple, mainly filarial nematodes	protein, cysteine protease	ND	↑ Erk/p38-dependent-IL-10 production in macrophages	[73, 74, 77, 79]
LFNPIII	Schistosoma eggs	carbohydrate	TLR4, DC-SIGN, mannose recpetor, MGP-1	↑ Th2 responses ↑ IL-10 by macrophages and DCs ↑ FoxP3+ T cells	[82-84, 86, 87]
Omega-1	Schistossoma eggs	glycoprotein	Mannose receptor	↑ Th2 response ↑ FoxP3+ T cells ↑ IL-4 ↓ IL-12	[88, 90, 91]
TGFβ homolog	Brugia malayi	protein	ND	↑ IL-10 ↑ FoxP3+ T Cells	[98]
TI-gal	Toxascaris leonina	recombinant protein	ND	↑ TGFβ and IL-10 ↓ Th1/Th2 responses	[100]
Lyso-PS	Schistosoma mansoni	glycolipid	TLR2	↑ IL-10-producing T cells	[93]
Calreticulin	Heligmosomoides polygyrus	secreted protein	scavenger receptor A	↑ Th2 response ↑ IL-4+ CD4 T cells	[92]
Antigen B	Echinococcus granulosus	secreted protein	TLRs?	↑ Th2 response DC modulation (CD1a, CD83, CD86) ↓ PMN cells recruitment	[95, 96]

Molecular Mechanisms of DC Modulation by Helminths

As described above, effects of helminths on the host immune response have been studied extensively and it is well known that helminth parasites skew immune reactions towards a Th2 phenotype and also promote IL-10-dependent and independent regulatory responses. Despite the recent advances in the field, the exact mechanism of how the worms achieve this has yet to be elucidated. However, parasite products and their interaction with dendritic cells seem to play a central role. Indeed, instructions for development of specific T cell responses are mediated by DCs and therefore, the immunomodulation achieved by parasitic worms may affect DC maturation. DCs play an essential role in providing information on the nature of the pathogen that the immune system must face, and helminths have designed specific molecules to regulate DC-mediated responses. This allows parasites to skew immunity toward a modulated Th2 phenotype that enables parasite survival without compromising the host immune system to fight other infections. This is so important for the parasite's survival that many of the immunoregulatory compounds are actively secreted during infection [104]. The term 'excretory-secretory' (ES) describes the mixture of products released by helminths into their mammalian host and this ES fraction includes immune regulators but also components that are released as a consequence of other biological processes. Individual characterization of the products that are responsible for the immunomodulation is a key step in order to develop new therapeutics from helminths and as alluded to earlier, some of them have been isolated and studied (Table **1**), raising great expectation in the field of drug discovery.

Helminths affect maturation of DCs, so it can be said that DCs reach an 'attenuated activation status' [105-108]. Different stimuli, both exogenous and endogenous, can activate DCs and depending on the nature of such stimuli DCs will polarize naive T cells towards the production of specific cytokines (via specific transcription factors) that will define the subsequent T cell response. Intracellular bacteria infections will result in cells exposing antigens to DCs to induce expression of activation markers and co-stimulatory molecules like MHC class II, CD40, CD83, CD80 and CD86 that will induce IFNγ-producing T cells and Th1 immunity. However, helminths work in a very subtle way on DCs, even when they target the same PRRs employed by Th1 antigens like TLRs. Compared to Th1 stimuli, helminths induce Th2 T cell responses that are characterized by a mild DC activation, or in other words, they are less strong inducers of DC maturation. For example, SEA from *S. mansoni* does not activate murine DCs *in vitro*, but they are still able to expand Th2 lymphocytes *in vivo* [109]. Even when helminths do not affect the maturation status of DCs like Th1-inducing antigens, helminth products usually induce hyporesponsiveness, in the sense that DCs exposed to worm-derived products show a reduced response against pro-inflammatory stimuli like LPS, IL-1 or TNFα. ES of the cestode *Taenia crassiceps* (TcES) represent a good example. TcES do not induce the maturation of DCs, in light of the lack of increment in the expression of activation markers like CD83, HLA-DR, CD80 and CD86, but TcES-treated cells showed a reduced expression of pro-inflammatory cytokines (IL-1β, IL-6, TNFα and IL-12) after LPS stimulation [110].

Something similar to the regulation mediated by TcES occurs in the case of many others molecules secreted by helminths, where usually these ES products reduce the response of DCs to LPS without maturing DCs, but some products induce a partial up-regulation of some activation markers. The PC-containing glycoprotein ES-62, although it does not significantly modulate expression of co-activation markers, initially induces antigen presenting cells to produce low levels of IL-12 and TNFα [72]. The ES products of *N. brasilensis* up-regulate CD86, CD40 and OX40L [105] but no increase in CD80 or MHCII is observed and products secreted by schistosome larvae induced MHCII, CD40 and CD86 whereas CD80 and OX40L were not affected [111]. However, it is relevant to highlight that a common hallmark of DC activation by different helminth products is that even when they induce expression of a variable number of maturation markers it is always to a lower degree than what is seen when cells are incubated with classical Th1 stimuli.

Thus, helminth infections usually do not induce full activation of DCs and only transient or minor up-regulation of some activation markers can be observed. However, these partially matured DCs are still strong inducers of Th2 differentiation when they encounter naive T cells, the main effector mechanism of helminth immunomodulation, showing that immature DCs are not inactive cells. Nevertheless, the process of DC modulation by parasitic worms is not fully understood yet, but it has been suggested that the attenuated status of DCs after exposure to helminth products can be a consequence of a mild or partial cell activation and/or a selective expression of certain activation markers.

Therefore, helminths modulate DCs to initiate Th2 responses, but this must be subsequently controlled to avoid any over-response that might lead to tissue damage or parasite killing. This is achieved by the induction of Tregs, but whether the modulation of DC activation status by worms is responsible for the helminth-induced Treg expansion is still unknown. Induction of Treg activity is another important pathway triggered by helminths to modulate the host immune response and it has been shown that immature DCs can promote a tolerogenic response stimulating naive T cells to become regulatory T cells. Recently, a wide array of helminth ES products from *Echinococcus multilocularis* and *Trichinella spiralis* have been shown to promote the expansion of CD25+FoxP3+ Treg cells [112-114]. As alluded to earlier, the lipid LysoPS isolated from *S. mansoni* triggers TLR2 signalling in DCs making them gain the ability to induce the development of IL-10-producing regulatory T cells [93] although the role of TLRs in Treg induction remains controversial. However, some worm-derived products have failed to induce IL-10-producing Treg *in vitro*, despite the fact that during *in vivo* infection there is a general expansion of regulatory T cells. This could be explained by local differences and requirements for Treg development. For example, IL-6 produced by DCs can suppress Treg function [115], whereas the combination of IL-1 and IL-6 can enhance their suppressive activity [116]. There are also some effector mechanisms independent of DC activity that may contribute to Treg expansion *in vivo*. ES products from *H. polygyrus* and *Teladorsagia circumcincta* are able to induce *de novo* FoxP3 expression in spleen cells by using helminth-derived TGFβ homologs [41, 98]. Fig. (**1**) summarizes all the potential mechanisms employed by helminth-derived products to achieve successful modulation of the host immune system, from the molecular to the cellular level. TLRs, the best characterized PPRs targeted by helminths are also shown in the illustration and due to the relevance of TLR signaling in helminth-dependent immunoregulation, this family of receptors is discussed in detail below.

Modulation of Toll-Like Receptors by Helminth Derived Molecules

Toll receptor was originally identified in Drosophila in 1988 [117], but it was in 1996 when studies performed by Hoffmann and colleagues changed the current understanding of innate immunology, demonstrating that Toll-mutant flies were highly susceptible to fungal infection [118]. This finding made us aware that the innate immune system has a skillful means of detecting invasion by microorganisms by using specialized receptors able to detect specific pathogen products, which are known today as PRRs. TLRs, are transmembrane proteins that belong to the Toll/IL-1R (TIR) superfamily. They consist of extracellular leucine-rich repeats, a transmembrane domain and an intracellular domain containing a TIR domain that is conserved between all TLRs (reviewed in [119]). TLRs are probably the best characterized PRRs to date and are expressed in many cells of the immune system like antigen presenting cells, neutrophils and lymphocytes, and also in non-immune cells like endothelial cells and fibroblasts. Mammalian species typically have 10 to 13 TLR members that recognize conserved PAMPs like LPS, CpG sequences, double stranded RNA or flagellin, for example. The binding of these PAMPs to TLRs triggers activation and recruitment of intracellular proteins that lead to NFkB nuclear translocation and, as result, induction of inflammatory responses. The first event after ligand binding is the recruitment of the adaptor protein MyD88, a molecule involved in the signalling pathways for all TLRs except TLR3. MyD88 induces MAP kinase activation before activating NFkB. TRIF is the sole adaptor protein for TLR3, but it can also signal for all the TLRs in a MyD88-independent fashion.

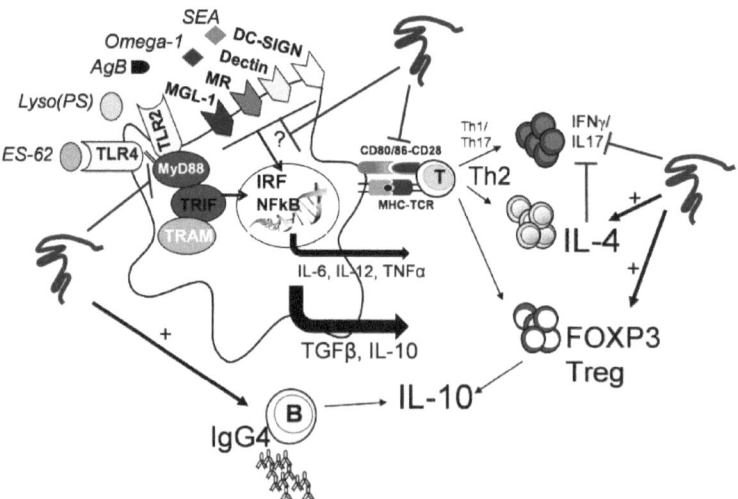

Figure 1: The illustration summarizes the mechanisms used by immunoregulatory helminth products in the host immune system, where the dendritic cell is the main target of the parasite. Products synthesized by helminths (ES-62, LysoPS, AgB, Omega-1, SEA) are shown together with the immune receptors (TLR2, TLR4, MGL-1, MR, Dectin, DC-SIGN). The immune pathways that are enhanced or inhibited after parasite products and receptors are shown.

TLRs are best known for their interaction with potent Th1 agents such as bacterial LPS, where most of the current knowledge about TLR signaling pathways has been obtained. It is accepted that TLRs are important targets of helminth immunoregulators, since pretreatment of DCs with helminth ES has been shown to inhibit classical LPS cell activation [120, 121]. Since the interaction between helminth products and TLRs does not lead to full DC maturation or any major pro-inflammatory response, it may be better to define the outcome of this interaction as a modulation rather than an activation, but this process is often found in the literature as TLR activation by helminths. The mechanism employed by the secreted glycoprotein ES-62 from *A. viteae* has been studied in great detail and indicates that ES-62 triggers TLR4 signaling but in a very different way to the bacterial LPS. ES-62 is ineffective against DCs from TLR4 or MyD88 deficient mice, but surprisingly, DCs from C3H/HeJ mice are fully responsive to ES-62 [72]. This shows that the mechanism underlying TLR4-ES-62 interaction has to be unconventional, because C3H/HeJ mice present a TLR4 molecule that carries a point mutation in the intracellular TIR domain that makes this TLR4 incapable of signaling in response to LPS. By interacting with TLR4, ES-62 is able to induce a DC2 phenotype using TLR4/MyD88 pathways, affecting the balance between the activation of p38 MAP Kinase, essential for induction of IL-6, IL-12 and TNFα, and Erk MAP kinase activity, whose activation promotes negative feedback inhibition of IL-12p40 [122, 123]. Perhaps as a consequence of this example, further work was done to investigate whether some other helminths and secreted immunoregulators with a similar phenotype to ES-62 were also modulating TLR4/MyD88 responses in DCs. However, this was not observed with other helminth-derived molecules like SEA from *S. mansoni* that was shown to attenuate TLR-induced activation independently of TLR4 and MyD88 [124] and it has been only recently described that SEA targets TLR2 instead [125]. On the other hand, some molecules, like ES-62, do utilise TLR4 to exert immunomodulation of DCs, for example, Lex-containing carbohydrates, similar to LFNPIII, that was able to drive DC responses in a TLR4-dependent manner [126]. Interestingly, the difference between LPS interaction with TLR4 and LFPNIII interaction with TLR4 in DCs relates to the strength and duration of the subsequent signal. LPS induces a persistent NFkB activation whereas LFPNIII only triggers a rapid and transient one.

Helminth-Based Therapy in Disease

We are still at a very early stage in fully understanding how helminths regulate the immune system response. Indeed, it could be said that we are still crawling and some attempts have been made to achieve the first steps, but what we do know is that helminths are able to manipulate the immune response in a way that the host has become 'dependent' on. A significant association between the lack of helminths and the appearance of inflammatory and autoimmune diseases has been observed. Based on this observation, it was hypothesized that helminths could be used to treat chronic inflammatory disease. In order to test this theory, a number of helminth species or their secreted products have been used to treat some clinical conditions both in experimental models in the laboratory and in human patients in some clinical trials and studies. Exciting progress has been achieved in this field and some recent findings regarding helminth-based therapy in multiple sclerosis, RA, allergy and inflammatory bowel disease are presented below.

Multiple Sclerosis (MS)

Multiple sclerosis is thought to be a Th1/Th17-mediated inflammatory autoimmune demyelinating disease, although the exact etiology remains unknown. MS affects the Central Nervous System (CNS) and, after post-traumatic injuries, it is the most common cause of neurological disabilities in young adults in developed countries [127]. The disease induces episodes that include clinical manifestations such as loss of vision, weakness, numbness or incoordination. After some years suffering these attacks, disease changes to a steady progression that may be mild or incapacitating in some patients. Although there are available drugs to treat early symptoms, more effective and safer treatments are needed. Some studies examining the geoepidemiological distribution of helminths and MS suggest that helminths are a protective factor in the MS development [12] and therefore a suitable context in which to find new drugs.

The animal model most accepted to study MS is experimental autoimmune encephalitis (EAE), which mimics the paralysis and demyelination observed in the human disorder. Studies in the EAE model have shown that helminths can protect mice against EAE mainly when employed as a prophylactic treatment. When helminths or related products were administered in effector phases there was no benefit, most likely because some irreversible damage had occurred in the CNS. Two different approaches have been employed with animal models, administration of either live helminths or derived products. *S. mansoni* eggs and cercariae have been reported to be protective against a mouse model of EAE [128, 129], likewise larvae from *Fasciola hepatica, T. spiralis, H. polygirus* and *T. crassicepts* [9, 130, 131] have exerted the same effect in a number of mouse and rat models. The protective effects of these helminths in animals undergoing EAE have been reproduced by administration of some of their products, such as SEA from *Schistosoma* and *Trichuris* ssp. Interestingly, the molecule LFNPIII isolated from SEA is able to protect animals against EAE [132]. The protective mechanisms reported in animal models have been also observed in humans patients [133] and have encouraged some groups to perform some clinical trials in order to optimize the use of helminths in humans based on administration of the parasite *T. suis*, that is not able to establish a permanent infection in humans [68, 134]. Results show that treatment is safe and worms provided a beneficial trend in immunological assessments.

Rheumatoid Arthritis

RA is a chronic, systemic inflammatory disorder that principally attacks flexible synovial joints although it may affect many tissues and organs. RA was thought to be a Th1-dependent disease, but recently it has been shown that the Th17/IL-23 pathways might be of greater importance than Th1 responses, but the exact etiology remains uncertain. A recent study show a correlation between the lack of lymphatic filariasis and a high prevalence of RA in endemic areas [13] but there are no reports of helminth-based therapy in human RA. Nevertheless, promising results have been published in animal models. Indeed, a first study in 1975 showed that helminths could reduce the incidence and severity of experimental arthritis in rats using the nematode *Syphacia oblevata* [135]. This was observed again in the murine model of collagen-induced arthritis (CIA), where a number of helminth species, *Schistosoma japonicum, S. mansoni* and *Hymenoleptis diminuta* [30, 136-138] were able to protect mice against CIA. Remarkably, expression of receptor activator of NFkB ligand (RANKL), a molecule involved in osteoclast formation and bone degradation, was down-regulated in inflamed paws of *S. mansoni* infected mice [30], probably as a consequence of the inhibition of IL-17 production, a proinflamatory cytokine that in CIA drives autoimmunity, recruits neutrophils to the joint and induces osteoclast formation. In fact, the parasite product ES-62 has been shown to reduce CIA severity using a mechanism that is largely dependent on the downregulation of IL-17 production [10]. Noteworthy, ES-62 does not target a single cell type or molecule, but it affects a complex network of cells, including γδ T cells, conventional CD4 T cells and DCs to achieve its protective effect. ES-62 is not the only isolated helminth product tested in animal models of RA. A recombinant protein of *S. japonicum* named rSj16 is able to reduce CFA-induced arthritis in rats [139]. Both ES-62 and rSj16 modulate DC activity to exert their anti-arthritic effects and in fact, adoptive transfer of DCs treated with *Fasciola hepatica* extracts to CIA mice attenuated disease severity [140].

Allergic Diseases

Allergies in Westernised countries are emerging increasingly in the last decades along with a decrease in helminth infections. The possibility of a direct correlation between both has been extensively studied, and results often show negative associations. However, other studies show the opposite, probably due to the Th2 nature of allergic diseases and different mechanisms of protection triggered by helminths compared to Th1/Th17-based disorders, as has been previously discussed. There are many studies published supporting both cases and only a few examples will be mentioned here. Epidemiological studies show that schistosiomiasis and filariasis in African and South-American countries present negative associations between helminth infections and allergies [40, 141-145] suggesting that helminths could protect against allergic responses. In an attempt to link helminth immunoregulation and protection against allergy some studies were conducted by depleting parasites with anti-helminth drugs like albendazol, but these gave contradictory results. For example, treatment of schistosomiasis increases skin reactivity to house dust mite [146] but no effect on clinical allergy was observed after one year of anti-helminth treatment in an epidemiological study conducted in Ecuador [147]. Differences in the treatment and helminth species might explain these discrepancies. Nevertheless, helminths have been shown to protect animals against allergic response in experimental models of allergic diseases. Experimental infection with *S. mansoni*, *H. polygirus* and *A.*

suum can suppress asthma symptoms, allergic airway inflammation, lung inflammation and anaphylaxis [32, 33, 50, 53, 148]. Secreted products of helminths have also the ability to impair allergic inflammation in experimental allergic inflammation and interestingly, the same effect was observed when mice were immunised with a crude extract of the non-parasitic worm *C. elegans* [149], showing again that the immunoregulation exerted by helminths is an adaptation of a common feature of worms. Regarding individual parasite products, a recent study shows that filarial cystatin has a modulatory effect on grass pollen-specific responses in a murine model [79].

Trichuris suis ova (TSO) have been used as a therapeutic agent in some clinical trials with different outcomes. Evidence of safety comes from studies performed in multiple sclerosis and inflammatory bowel disease and it was tested in a clinical trial in 100 adults with allergic rhinitis [150], Although the results were not conclusive, the study shows that TSO might be beneficial in seasonal rhinitis.

Inflammatory Bowel Disease

Inflammatory bowel disease (IBD) is a chronic autoimmune disease of the gastrointestinal tract associated with a strong inflammatory response. The origin of the inflammation is not fully understood, but it is thought to be caused by an inappropriate immune response to the commensal bacteria. There are two major types of IBD, Chohn's disease (CD) and ulcerative colitis (UC). Clinical manifestations of both diseases are similar, patients suffer from diarrhea, bloody stool, abdominal pain and fever, but the immunological events underlying both types of disease are quite different. CD seems to be a Th1-driven pathology, whereas UC is driven by the Th2 cytokine IL-13 [151]. Interestingly, available treatment for IBD is not as effective as natural worm infections, as it has been reported as being a successful treatment in a number of studies performed in animal models [48, 152]. *S. mansoni*, *S. japonicum*, *H. diminuta* and *T. spiralis* are examples of parasitic worms that ameliorate experimental induced colitis [48, 153-156]. These results correlate with some studies undertaken in humans. There are good examples reported in the literature, like the case of a patient who suffered aggravation of ulcerative colitis after being treated for infection with the parasite *Enterobius vernicularis* [157]. Moreover, there are some reports on helminth therapy in humans, where IBD patients went into remission after ingestion of eggs of *T. suis* [15]. Effective and safer treatments than *T. suis* infection have been reported in animal models for products secreted by *S. mansoni*, *T. spiralis* or *Ancylostoma ceylanicum* [7, 27, 158, 159]. These studies used a mixture of secreted products, and although they show very promising results, isolation and characterization of individual molecules is still needed.

CONCLUSION

The increase in understanding of how helminths interact with their hosts over the past 10-20 years has been striking. We now realise that these organisms not only immunoregulate that ensure their own survival, but have evolved strategies to ensure the survival of their hosts. The range of mechanisms they employ is extensive, targeting many immune system components, and the molecular events underlying helminth immunoregulation are increasingly being unravelled. The identification of helminth molecules involved in immunoregulation has been an important contributor to this but ironically the possibility of using them for the benefit of the human host may assume even greater importance.

ACKNOWLEDGEMENT

Declared none.

CONFLICT OF INTEREST

The author(s) confirm that this chapter contents have no conflict of interest.

ABBREVIATIONS

Breg = Regulatory B cell,

CIA = Collagen-induced arthritis,

DC = Dendritic cell,

DC-SIGN = Dendritic cell-specific intracellular adhesion molecule 3 (ICAM-3)-grabbing nonintegrin,

EAE	=	Experimental autoimmune encephalomyelitis,
ES	=	Excreted-secreted,
LPS	=	Lipopolysaccharide,
IBD	=	Inflammatory bowel disease,
IFN	=	Interferon,
IgE	=	Immunoglobulin E,
IgG	=	Immunoglobulin G,
IL	=	Interleukin,
MGL	=	Macrophage galactose lectin-1,
MR	=	Mannose receptor,
MHC	=	Major histocompatibility complex,
MS	=	Multiple sclerosis,
NFkB	=	Nuclear factor kappa-light-chain-enhancer of activated B cells,
PAMP	=	Pathogen-associated molecular pattern,
PRR	=	Pattern recognition receptor,
RA	=	Rheumatoid arthritis,
SEA	=	Soluble egg antigen,
TGFβ	=	Transforming growth factor beta,
TLR	=	Toll-like receptor,
TNF	=	Tumor necrosis factors,
Treg	=	Regulatory T cell,

REFERENCES

[1] Allen JE, Maizels RM. Diversity and dialogue in immunity to helminths. Nat Rev Immunol 2011; 11: 375-88.

[2] Jackson JA, Friberg IM, Little S, et al. Review series on helminths, immune modulation and the hygiene hypothesis: immunity against helminths and immunological phenomena in modern human populations: coevolutionary legacies? Immunology 2009; 126: 18-27.

[3] Hewitson JP, Grainger JR, Maizels RM. Helminth immunoregulation: the role of parasite secreted proteins in modulating host immunity. Mol Biochem Parasitol 2009; 167: 1-11.

[4] Medzhitov R, Schneider DS, Soares MP. Disease tolerance as a defense strategy. Science 2012; 335: 936-41.

[5] Pulendran B, Tang H, Manicassamy S. Programming dendritic cells to induce T(H)2 and tolerogenic responses. Nat Immunol 2010; 11: 647-55.

[6] Che, F, Liu Z, Wu W, Rozo C, et al. An essential role for TH2-type responses in limiting acute tissue damage during experimental helminth infection. Nat Med 2012; 18: 260-6.

[7] Ruyssers NE, De Winter BY, De Man JG, et al. Therapeutic potential of helminth soluble proteins in TNBS-induced colitis in mice. Inflamm Bowel Dis 2009; 15: 491-500.

[8] Elliott DE, Metwali A, Leung J, et al. Colonization with Heligmosomoides polygyrus suppresses mucosal IL-17 production. J Immunol 2008; 181: 2414-9.

[9] Walsh KP, Brady MT, Finlay CM, et al. Infection with a helminth parasite attenuates autoimmunity through TGF-beta-mediated suppression of Th17 and Th1 responses. J Immunol 2009; 183: 1577-86.

[10] Pineda MA, McGrath MA, Smith PC, et al. The parasitic helminth product ES-62 suppresses pathogenesis in collagen-induced arthritis by targeting the interleukin-17-producing cellular network at multiple sites. Arthritis Rheum 2012; 64: 3168-78.

[11] Strachan DP. Hay fever, hygiene, and household size. BMJ 1989; 299: 1259-60.

[12] Fleming JO, Cook TD. Multiple sclerosis and the hygiene hypothesis. Neurology 2006; 67: 2085-6.

[13] Panda AK, Ravindran B, Das BK. Rheumatoid arthritis patients are free of filarial infection in an area where filariasis is endemic: comment on the article by Pineda et al. Arthritis Rheum 2013; 65: 1402-3.

[14] Saunders KA, Raine T, Cooke A, et al. Inhibition of autoimmune type 1 diabetes by gastrointestinal helminth infection. Infect Immun 2007; 75: 397-407.

[15] Summers RW, Elliott DE, Urban JF Jr, et al. Trichuris suis therapy in Crohn's disease. Gut 2005; 54: 87-90.

[16] Yazdanbakhsh M, van den Biggelaar A, Maizels RM. Th2 responses without atopy: immunoregulation in chronic helminth infections and reduced allergic disease. Trends Immunol 2001; 22: 372-7.

[17] Osada Y, Kanazawa T. Parasitic helminths: new weapons against immunological disorders. J Biomed Biotechnol 2010; 743758.

[18] Babu S, Nutman TB. Proinflammatory cytokines dominate the early immune response to filarial parasites. J Immunol 2003; 171: 6723-32.

[19] Pearce EJ, M Kane C, Sun J, et al. Th2 response polarization during infection with the helminth parasite Schistosoma mansoni. Immunol Rev 2004; 201: 117-26.

[20] Paul WE, Zhu J. How are T(H)2-type immune responses initiated and amplified? Nat Rev Immunol 2010; 10: 225-35.

[21] Zhu J, Yamane H, Paul WE. Differentiation of effector CD4 T cell populations (*). Annu Rev Immunol 2010; 28: 445-89.
[22] Van Dyken SJ, Locksley RM. Interleukin-4- and Interleukin-13-Mediated Alternatively Activated Macrophages: Roles in Homeostasis and Disease. Annu Rev Immunol 2013.
[23] Pulendran B, Artis D. New paradigms in type 2 immunity. Science 2012; 337: 431-5.
[24] Bogers J, Moreels T, De Man J, et al. Schistosoma mansoni infection causing diffuse enteric inflammation and damage of the enteric nervous system in the mouse small intestine. Neurogastroenterol Motil 2000; 12: 431-40.
[25] Elliott DE, Li J, Blum A, et al. Exposure to schistosome eggs protects mice from TNBS-induced colitis. Am J Physiol Gastrointest Liver Physiol 2003; 284: G385-91.
[26] Espinoza-Jimenez A, Rivera-Montoya I, Cárdenas-Arreola R, et al. Taenia crassiceps infection attenuates multiple low-dose streptozotocin-induced diabetes. J Biomed Biotechnol 2010; 2010: 850541.
[27] Ruyssers NE, De Winter BY, De Man JG, et al. Schistosoma mansoni proteins attenuate gastrointestinal motility disturbances during experimental colitis in mice. World J Gastroenterol 2010; 16: 703-12.
[28] Zaccone P, Burton O, Miller N, et al. Schistosoma mansoni egg antigens induce Treg that participate in diabetes prevention in NOD mice. Eur J Immunol 2009; 39: 1098-107.
[29] Cooney LA, Towery K, Endres J, et al. Sensitivity and resistance to regulation by IL-4 during Th17 maturation. J Immunol 2011; 187: 4440-50.
[30] Osada Y, Shimizu S, Kumagai T, et al. Schistosoma mansoni infection reduces severity of collagen-induced arthritis via down-regulation of pro-inflammatory mediators. Int J Parasitol 2009; 39: 457-64.
[31] Zheng X, Hu X, Zhou G, et al. Soluble egg antigen from Schistosoma japonicum modulates the progression of chronic progressive experimental autoimmune encephalomyelitis via Th2-shift response. J Neuroimmunol 2008; 194: 107-14.
[32] Itami DM, Oshiro TM, Araujo CA, et al. Modulation of murine experimental asthma by Ascaris suum components. Clin Exp Allergy 2005; 35: 873-9.
[33] Lima C, Perini A, Garcia ML, et al. Eosinophilic inflammation and airway hyper-responsiveness are profoundly inhibited by a helminth (Ascaris suum) extract in a murine model of asthma. Clin Exp Allergy 2002; 32: 1659-66.
[34] Mangan NE, van Rooijen N, McKenzie AN, et al. Helminth-modified pulmonary immune response protects mice from allergen-induced airway hyperresponsiveness. J Immunol 2006; 176: 138-47.
[35] Dold S, Heinrich J, Wichmann HE, et al. Ascaris-specific IgE and allergic sensitization in a cohort of school children in the former East Germany. J Allergy Clin Immunol 1998; 102: 414-20.
[36] Joubert JR, van Schalkwyk DJ, Turner KJ. Ascaris lumbricoides and the human immunogenic response: enhanced IgE-mediated reactivity to common inhaled allergens. S Afr Med J 1980; 57: 409-12.
[37] Palmer LJ, Celedón JC, Weiss ST, et al. Ascaris lumbricoides infection is associated with increased risk of childhood asthma and atopy in rural China. Am J Respir Crit Care Med 2002; 165: 1489-93.
[38] Pinelli E, Brandes S, Dormans J, et al. Infection with the roundworm Toxocara canis leads to exacerbation of experimental allergic airway inflammation. Clin Exp Allergy 2008; 38: 649-58.

[39] Ing R, Su Z, Scott ME, et al. Suppressed T helper 2 immunity and prolonged survival of a nematode parasite in protein-malnourished mice. Proc Natl Acad Sci U S A 2000; 97: 7078-83.

[40] Cooper PJ. Intestinal worms and human allergy. Parasite Immunol 2004; 26: 455-67.

[41] Grainger JR, Smith KA, Hewitson JP, et al. Helminth secretions induce *de novo* T cell Foxp3 expression and regulatory function through the TGF-beta pathway. J Exp Med 2010; 207: 2331-41.

[42] Lin X, Chen M, Liu Y, et al. Advances in distinguishing natural from induced Foxp3(+) regulatory T cells. Int J Clin Exp Pathol 2013; 6: 116-23.

[43] Okamura T, Fujio K, Sumitomo S, et al. Roles of LAG3 and EGR2 in regulatory T cells. Ann Rheum Dis 2011; 71 Suppl 2: i96-100.

[44] Schmitt EG, Williams CB. Generation and function of induced regulatory T cells. Front Immunol 2013; 4: 152.

[45] Sugimoto N, Oida T, Hirota K, et al. Foxp3-dependent and -independent molecules specific for CD25+CD4+ natural regulatory T cells revealed by DNA microarray analysis. Int Immunol 2006; 18: 1197-209.

[46] Yadav M, Louvet C, Davini D, et al. Neuropilin-1 distinguishes natural and inducible regulatory T cells among regulatory T cell subsets *in vivo*. J Exp Med 2012; 209: 1713-22, S1-19.

[47] Metenou S, Dembele B, Konate S, et al. At homeostasis filarial infections have expanded adaptive T regulatory but not classical Th2 cells. J Immunol 2010; 184: 5375-82.

[48] Mo HM, Liu WQ, Lei JH, et al. Schistosoma japonicum eggs modulate the activity of CD4+ CD25+ Tregs and prevent development of colitis in mice. Exp Parasitol 2007; 116: 385-9.

[49] Yang J, Zhao J, Yang Y, et al. Schistosoma japonicum egg antigens stimulate CD4 CD25 T cells and modulate airway inflammation in a murine model of asthma. Immunology 2007; 120: 8-18.

[50] Wilson MS, Taylor MD, Balic A, et al. Suppression of allergic airway inflammation by helminth-induced regulatory T cells. J Exp Med 2005; 202: 1199-212.

[51] McKee AS, Pearce EJ. CD25+CD4+ cells contribute to Th2 polarization during helminth infection by suppressing Th1 response development. J Immunol 2004; 173: 1224-31.

[52] Blankenhaus B, Klemm U, Eschbach ML, et al. Strongyloides ratti infection induces expansion of Foxp3+ regulatory T cells that interfere with immune response and parasite clearance in BALB/c mice. J Immunol 2011; 186: 4295-305.

[53] Wilson MS, Taylor MD, O'Gorman MT, et al. Helminth-induced CD19+CD23hi B cells modulate experimental allergic and autoimmune inflammation. Eur J Immunol 2010; 40: 1682-96.

[54] Matera G, Giancotti A, Scalise S, et al. Ascaris lumbricoides-induced suppression of total and specific IgE responses in atopic subjects is interleukin 10-independent and associated with an increase of CD25(+) cells. Diagn Microbiol Infect Dis 2008; 62: 280-6.

[55] Collison LW, Workman CJ, Kuo TT, et al. The inhibitory cytokine IL-35 contributes to regulatory T-cell function. Nature 2007; 450: 566-9.

[56] Niedbala W, Wei XQ, Cai B, et al. IL-35 is a novel cytokine with therapeutic effects against collagen-induced arthritis through the expansion of regulatory T cells and suppression of Th17 cells. Eur J Immunol 2007; 37: 3021-9.

[57] Satoguina JS, Adjobimey T, Arndts K, et al. Tr1 and naturally occurring regulatory T cells induce IgG4 in B cells through GITR/GITR-L interaction, IL-10 and TGF-beta. Eur J Immunol 2008; 38: 3101-13.

[58] Smits HH, Everts B, Hartgers FC, et al. Chronic helminth infections protect against allergic diseases by active regulatory processes. Curr Allergy Asthma Rep 2010; 10: 3-12.

[59] Correale J, Farez M, Razzitte G. Helminth infections associated with multiple sclerosis induce regulatory B cells. Ann Neurol 2008; 64: 187-99.

[60] van der Vlugt LE, Labuda LA, Ozir-Fazalalikhan A, et al. Schistosomes induce regulatory features in human and mouse CD1d(hi) B cells: inhibition of allergic inflammation by IL-10 and regulatory T cells. PLoS One 2012; 7: e30883.

[61] Anthony RM, Urban JF Jr, Alem F, et al. Memory T(H)2 cells induce alternatively activated macrophages to mediate protection against nematode parasites. Nat Med 2006; 12: 955-60.

[62] Herbert DR, Hölscher C, Mohrs M, et al. Alternative macrophage activation is essential for survival during schistosomiasis and downmodulates T helper 1 responses and immunopathology. Immunity 2004; 20: 623-35.

[63] Semnani RT, Mahapatra L, Moore V, et al. Functional and phenotypic characteristics of alternative activation induced in human monocytes by interleukin-4 or the parasitic nematode Brugia malayi. Infect Immun 2011; 79: 3957-65.

[64] Martinez FO, Helming L, Gordon S. Alternative activation of macrophages: an immunologic functional perspective. Annu Rev Immunol 2009; 27: 451-83.

[65] Janeway CA Jr. Approaching the asymptote? Evolution and revolution in immunology. Cold Spring Harb Symp Quant Biol 1989; 54 Pt 1: 1-13.

[66] Dreyer G, Medeiros Z, Netto MJ, et al. Acute attacks in the extremities of persons living in an area endemic for bancroftian filariasis: differentiation of two syndromes. Trans R Soc Trop Med Hyg 1999; 93: 413-7.

[67] Jouvin MH, Kinet JP. Trichuris suis ova: testing a helminth-based therapy as an extension of the hygiene hypothesis. J Allergy Clin Immunol 2012; 130: 3-10; quiz 11-2.

[68] Fleming J, Isaak A, Lee JE, et al. Probiotic helminth administration in relapsing-remitting multiple sclerosis: a phase 1 study. Mult Scler 2011; 17: 743-54.

[69] Bager P, Danzeisen JL, Trampel D, et al. Symptoms after ingestion of pig whipworm Trichuris suis eggs in a randomized placebo-controlled double-blind clinical trial. PLoS One 2013; 6: e22346.

[70] Goodridge HS, McGuiness S, Houston KM, et al. Phosphorylcholine mimics the effects of ES-62 on macrophages and dendritic cells. Parasite Immunol 2007; 29: 127-37.

[71] Harnett MM, Melendez AJ, Harnett W. The therapeutic potential of the filarial nematode-derived immunodulator, ES-62 in inflammatory disease. Clin Exp Immunol 2009; 159: 256-67.

[72] Goodridge HS, Marshall FA, Else KJ, et al. Immunomodulation via novel use of TLR4 by the filarial nematode phosphorylcholine-containing secreted product, ES-62. J Immunol 2005; 174: 284-93.

[73] Hartmann S, Kyewski B, Sonnenburg B, et al. A filarial cysteine protease inhibitor down-regulates T cell proliferation and enhances interleukin-10 production. Eur J Immunol 1997; 27: 2253-60.

[74] Hartmann S, Lucius R. Modulation of host immune responses by nematode cystatins. Int J Parasitol 2003; 33: 1291-302.

[75] Hartmann S, Schönemeyer A, Sonnenburg B, et al. Cystatins of filarial nematodes up-regulate the nitric oxide production of interferon-gamma-activated murine macrophages. Parasite Immunol 2002; 24: 253-62.

[76] Figueiredo AS, Höfer T, Klotz C, et al. Modelling and simulating interleukin-10 production and regulation by macrophages after stimulation with an immunomodulator of parasitic nematodes. FEBS J 2009; 276: 3454-69.

[77] Klotz C, Ziegler T, Figueiredo AS, et al. A helminth immunomodulator exploits host signaling events to regulate cytokine production in macrophages. PLoS Pathog 2011; 7: e1001248.

[78] Jang SW, Cho MK, Park MK, et al. Parasitic helminth cystatin inhibits DSS-induced intestinal inflammation via IL-10(+)F4/80(+) macrophage recruitment. Korean J Parasitol 2011; 49: 245-54.

[79] Danilowicz-Luebert E, Steinfelder S, Kühl AA, et al. A nematode immunomodulator suppresses grass pollen-specific allergic responses by controlling excessive Th2 inflammation. Int J Parasitol 2013; 43: 2012-10.

[80] Grzych JM, Pearce E, Cheever A, et al. Egg deposition is the major stimulus for the production of Th2 cytokines in murine schistosomiasis mansoni. J Immunol 1991; 146: 1322-7.

[81] Nyame AK, Debose-Boyd R, Long TD, et al. Expression of Lex antigen in Schistosoma japonicum and S.haematobium and immune responses to Lex in infected animals: lack of Lex expression in other trematodes and nematodes. Glycobiology 1998; 8: 615-24.

[82] Harn DA, McDonald J, Atochina O, et al. Modulation of host immune responses by helminth glycans. Immunol Rev 2009; 230: 247-57.

[83] Thomas PG, Carter MR, Atochina O, et al. Maturation of dendritic cell 2 phenotype by a helminth glycan uses a Toll-like receptor 4-dependent mechanism. J Immunol 2003; 171: 5837-41.

[84] van Liempt E, van Vliet SJ, Engering A, et al. Schistosoma mansoni soluble egg antigens are internalized by human dendritic cells through multiple C-type lectins and suppress TLR-induced dendritic cell activation. Mol Immunol 2007; 44: 2605-15.

[85] Atochina O, Da'dara AA, Walker M, et al. The immunomodulatory glycan LNFPIII initiates alternative activation of murine macrophages in vivo. Immunology 2008; 125: 111-21.

[86] Bhargava P, Li C, Stanya KJ, et al. Immunomodulatory glycan LNFPIII alleviates hepatosteatosis and insulin resistance through direct and indirect control of metabolic pathways. Nat Med 2012; 18: 1665-72.

[87] Dutta P, Hullett DA, Roenneburg DA, et al. Lacto-N-fucopentaose III, a pentasaccharide, prolongs heart transplant survival. Transplantation 2010; 90: 1071-8.

[88] Everts B, Perona-Wright G, Smits HH, et al. Omega-1, a glycoprotein secreted by Schistosoma mansoni eggs, drives Th2 responses. J Exp Med 2009; 206: 1673-80.

[89] Steinfelder S, Andersen JF, Cannons JL, et al. The major component in schistosome eggs responsible for conditioning dendritic cells for Th2 polarization is a T2 ribonuclease (omega-1). J Exp Med 2009; 206: 1681-90.

[90] Everts B, Hussaarts L, Driessen NN, et al. Schistosome-derived omega-1 drives Th2 polarization by suppressing protein synthesis following internalization by the mannose receptor. J Exp Med 2012; 209: 1753-67, S1.

[91]   Zaccone P, Burton OT, Gibbs SE, *et al.* The S. mansoni glycoprotein omega-1 induces Foxp3 expression in NOD mouse CD4(+) T cells. Eur J Immunol 2011; 41: 2709-18.

[92]   Rzepecka J, Rausch S, Klotz C, *et al.* Calreticulin from the intestinal nematode Heligmosomoides polygyrus is a Th2-skewing protein and interacts with murine scavenger receptor-A. Mol Immunol 2009; 46: 1109-19.

[93]   van der Kleij D, Latz E, Brouwers JF, *et al.* A novel host-parasite lipid cross-talk. Schistosomal lyso-phosphatidylserine activates toll-like receptor 2 and affects immune polarization. J Biol Chem 2002; 277: 48122-9.

[94]   Deehan MR, Goodridge HS, Blair D, *et al.* Immunomodulatory properties of Ascaris suum glycosphingolipids - phosphorylcholine and non-phosphorylcholine-dependent effects. Parasite Immunol 2002; 24: 463-9.

[95]   Riganò R, Buttari B, Profumo E, *et al.* Echinococcus granulosus antigen B impairs human dendritic cell differentiation and polarizes immature dendritic cell maturation towards a Th2 cell response. Infect Immun 2007; 75: 1667-78.

[96]   Riganò R, Profumo E, Bruschi F, *et al.* Modulation of human immune response by Echinococcus granulosus antigen B and its possible role in evading host defenses. Infect Immun 2001; 69: 288-96.

[97]   Smith P, Fallon RE, Mangan NE, *et al.* Schistosoma mansoni secretes a chemokine binding protein with antiinflammatory activity. J Exp Med 2005; 202: 1319-25.

[98]   Gomez-Escobar N, Gregory WF, Maizels RM. Identification of tgh-2, a filarial nematode homolog of Caenorhabditis elegans daf-7 and human transforming growth factor beta, expressed in microfilarial and adult stages of Brugia malayi. Infect Immun 2000; 68: 6402-10.

[99]   Meeusen EN, Balic A, Bowles V. Cells, cytokines and other molecules associated with rejection of gastrointestinal nematode parasites. Vet Immunol Immunopathol 2005; 108: 121-5.

[100] Kim JY, Cho MK, Choi SH, *et al.* Inhibition of dextran sulfate sodium (DSS)-induced intestinal inflammation *via* enhanced IL-10 and TGF-beta production by galectin-9 homologues isolated from intestinal parasites. Mol Biochem Parasitol 2010; 174: 53-61.

[101] Aksoy E, Zouain CS, Vanhoutte F, *et al.* Double-stranded RNAs from the helminth parasite Schistosoma activate TLR3 in dendritic cells. J Biol Chem 2005; 280: 277-83.

[102] Goodridge HS, Marshall FA, Wilson EH, *et al. In vivo* exposure of murine dendritic cell and macrophage bone marrow progenitors to the phosphorylcholine-containing filarial nematode glycoprotein ES-62 polarizes their differentiation to an anti-inflammatory phenotype. Immunology 2004; 113: 491-8.

[103] Harnett W, Harnett MM. Filarial nematode secreted product ES-62 is an anti-inflammatory agent: therapeutic potential of small molecule derivatives and ES-62 peptide mimetics. Clin Exp Pharmacol Physiol 2006; 33: 511-8.

[104] Segura M, Su Z, Piccirillo C, *et al.* Impairment of dendritic cell function by excretory-secretory products: a potential mechanism for nematode-induced immunosuppression. Eur J Immunol 2007; 37: 1887-904.

[105] Balic A, Harcus Y, Holland MJ, *et al.* Selective maturation of dendritic cells by Nippostrongylus brasiliensis-secreted proteins drives Th2 immune responses. Eur J Immunol 2004; 34: 3047-59.

[106] Fujiwara RT, Cançado GG, Freitas PA, *et al.* Necator americanus infection: a possible cause of altered dendritic cell differentiation and eosinophil profile in chronically infected individuals. PLoS Negl Trop Dis 2009; 3: e399.

[107] Silva SR, Jacysyn JF, Macedo MS, *et al.* Immunosuppressive components of Ascaris suum down-regulate expression of costimulatory molecules and function of antigen-presenting cells *via* an IL-10-mediated mechanism. Eur J Immunol 2006; 36: 3227-37.

[108] Vignali DA, Crocker P, Bickle QD, *et al.* A role for CD4+ but not CD8+ T cells in immunity to Schistosoma mansoni induced by 20 krad-irradiated and Ro 11-3128- terminated infections. Immunology 1989; 67: 466-72.

[109] Cervi L, MacDonald AS, Kane C, *et al.* Cutting edge: dendritic cells copulsed with microbial and helminth antigens undergo modified maturation, segregate the antigens to distinct intracellular compartments, and concurrently induce microbe-specific Th1 and helminth-specific Th2 responses. J Immunol 2004; 172: 2016-20.

[110] Terrazas CA, Sánchez-Muñoz F, Mejía-Domínguez AM, *et al.* Cestode antigens induce a tolerogenic-like phenotype and inhibit LPS inflammatory responses in human dendritic cells. Int J Biol Sci 2011; 7: 1391-400.

[111] Jenkins SJ, Mountford AP. Dendritic cells activated with products released by schistosome larvae drive Th2-type immune responses, which can be inhibited by manipulation of CD40 costimulation. Infect Immun 2005; 73: 395-402.

[112] Aranzamendi C, Fransen F, Langelaar M, *et al.* Trichinella spiralis-secreted products modulate DC functionality and expand regulatory T cells *in vitro*. Parasite Immunol 2012; 34: 210-23.

[113] Gruden-Movsesijan A, Ilic N, Colic M, *et al.* The impact of Trichinella spiralis excretory-secretory products on dendritic cells. Comp Immunol Microbiol Infect Dis 2011; 34: 429-39.

[114] Nono JK, Pletinckx K, Lutz MB, *et al.* Excretory/secretory-products of Echinococcus multilocularis larvae induce apoptosis and tolerogenic properties in dendritic cells *in vitro*. PLoS Negl Trop Dis 2012; 6: e1516.

[115] Pasare C, Medzhitov R. Control of B-cell responses by Toll-like receptors. Nature 2005; 438: 364-8.

[116] Kubo T, Hatton RD, Oliver J, *et al.* Regulatory T cell suppression and anergy are differentially regulated by proinflammatory cytokines produced by TLR-activated dendritic cells. J Immunol 2004; 173: 7249-58.

[117] Hashimoto C, Hudson KL, Anderson KV. The Toll gene of Drosophila, required for dorsal-ventral embryonic polarity, appears to encode a transmembrane protein. Cell 1988; 52: 269-79.

[118] Lemaitre B, Nicolas E, Michaut L, *et al.* The dorsoventral regulatory gene cassette spatzle/Toll/cactus controls the potent antifungal response in Drosophila adults. Cell 1996; 86: 973-83.

[119] Beutler B. Inferences, questions and possibilities in Toll-like receptor signalling. Nature 2004; 430: 257-63.

[120] Falcon C, Carranza F, Martínez FF, *et al.* Excretory-secretory products (ESP) from Fasciola hepatica induce tolerogenic properties in myeloid dendritic cells. Vet Immunol Immunopathol 2010; 137: 36-46.

[121] Langelaar M, Aranzamendi C, Franssen F, *et al.* Suppression of dendritic cell maturation by Trichinella spiralis excretory/secretory products. Parasite Immunol 2009; 31: 641-5.

[122] Goodridge HS, Harnett W, Liew FY, *et al.* Differential regulation of interleukin-12 p40 and p35 induction *via* Erk mitogen-activated protein kinase-dependent and -independent

mechanisms and the implications for bioactive IL-12 and IL-23 responses. Immunology 2003; 109: 415-25.

[123] Harnett W, Goodridge HS, Harnett MM. Subversion of immune cell signal transduction pathways by the secreted filarial nematode product, ES-62. Parasitology 2005; 130 Suppl: S63-8.

[124] Kane CM, Jung E, Pearce EJ. Schistosoma mansoni egg antigen-mediated modulation of Toll-like receptor (TLR)-induced activation occurs independently of TLR2, TLR4, and MyD88. Infect Immun 2008; 76: 5754-9.

[125] Gao Y, Zhang M, Chen L, et al. Deficiency in TLR2 but not in TLR4 impairs dendritic cells derived IL-10 responses to schistosome antigens. Cell Immunol 2012; 272: 242-50.

[126] Thomas PG, Carter MR, Da'dara AA, et al. A helminth glycan induces APC maturation via alternative NF-kappa B activation independent of I kappa B alpha degradation. J Immunol 2005; 175: 2082-90.

[127] Goldenberg MM. Multiple sclerosis review. P T 2012; 37: 175-84.

[128] Sewell D, Qing Z, Reinke E, et al. Immunomodulation of experimental autoimmune encephalomyelitis by helminth ova immunization. Int Immunol 2003; 15: 59-69.

[129] La Flamme AC, Canagasabey K, Harvie M, et al. Schistosomiasis protects against multiple sclerosis. Mem Inst Oswaldo Cruz 2004; 99: 33-6.

[130] Reyes JL, Espinoza-Jiménez AF, González MI, et al. Taenia crassiceps infection abrogates experimental autoimmune encephalomyelitis. Cell Immunol 2011; 267: 77-87.

[131] Gruden-Movsesijan A, Ilic N, Mostarica-Stojkovic M, et al. Mechanisms of modulation of experimental autoimmune encephalomyelitis by chronic Trichinella spiralis infection in Dark Agouti rats. Parasite Immunol 2010; 32: 450-9.

[132] Zhu B, Trikudanathan S, Zozulya AL, et al. Immune modulation by Lacto-N-fucopentaose III in experimental autoimmune encephalomyelitis. Clin Immunol 2012; 142: 351-61.

[133] Correale J, Farez MF. Does helminth activation of toll-like receptors modulate immune response in multiple sclerosis patients? Front Cell Infect Microbiol 2012; 2: 112.

[134] Benzel F, Erdur H, Kohler S, et al. Immune monitoring of Trichuris suis egg therapy in multiple sclerosis patients. J Helminthol 2012; 86: 339-47.

[135] Pearson DJ, Taylor G. The influence of the nematode Syphacia oblevata on adjuvant arthritis in the rat. Immunology 1975; 29: 391-6.

[136] He Y, Li J, Zhuang W, et al. The inhibitory effect against collagen-induced arthritis by Schistosoma japonicum infection is infection stage-dependent. BMC Immunol 2010; 11: 28.

[137] Shi M, Wang A, Prescott D, et al. Infection with an intestinal helminth parasite reduces Freund's complete adjuvant-induced monoarthritis in mice. Arthritis Rheum 2011; 63: 434-44.

[138] Song X, Jilong Shen, Huiqin Wen, et al. Impact of Schistosoma japonicum infection on collagen-induced arthritis in DBA/1 mice: a murine model of human rheumatoid arthritis. PLoS One 2010; 6: e23453.

[139] Sun X, Liu YH, Lv ZY, et al. rSj16, a recombinant protein of Schistosoma japonicum-derived molecule, reduces severity of the complete Freund's adjuvant-induced adjuvant arthritis in rats' model. Parasite Immunol 2010; 32: 739-48.

[140] Carranza F, Falcón CR, Nuñez N, et al. Helminth antigens enable CpG-activated dendritic cells to inhibit the symptoms of collagen-induced arthritis through Foxp3+ regulatory T cells. PLoS One 2012; 7: e40356.

[141] Hagel I, Lynch NR, Pérez M, et al. Modulation of the allergic reactivity of slum children by helminthic infection. Parasite Immunol 1993; 15: 311-5.

[142] Araujo MI, Lopes AA, Medeiros M, et al. Inverse association between skin response to aeroallergens and Schistosoma mansoni infection. Int Arch Allergy Immunol 2000; 123: 145-8.

[143] van den Biggelaar AH, van Ree R, Rodrigues LC, et al. Decreased atopy in children infected with Schistosoma haematobium: a role for parasite-induced interleukin-10. Lancet 2000; 356: 1723-7.

[144] Medeiros M Jr, Figueiredo JP, Almeida MC, et al. Schistosoma mansoni infection is associated with a reduced course of asthma. J Allergy Clin Immunol 2003; 111: 947-51.

[145] Dagoye D, Bekele Z, Woldemichael K, et al. Wheezing, allergy, and parasite infection in children in urban and rural Ethiopia. Am J Respir Crit Care Med 2003; 167: 1369-73.

[146] van den Biggelaar AH, Rodrigues LC, van Ree R, et al. Long-term treatment of intestinal helminths increases mite skin-test reactivity in Gabonese schoolchildren. J Infect Dis 2004; 189: 892-900.

[147] Cooper PJ, Chico ME, Vaca MG, et al. Effect of albendazole treatments on the prevalence of atopy in children living in communities endemic for geohelminth parasites: a cluster-randomised trial. Lancet 2006; 367: 1598-603.

[148] Mangan NE, Fallon RE, Smith P, et al. Helminth infection protects mice from anaphylaxis via IL-10-producing B cells. J Immunol 2004; 173: 6346-56.

[149] Kim SE, Kim J-H, Min B-H, et al. Crude extracts of Caenorhabditis elegans suppress airway inflammation in a murine model of allergic asthma. PLoS One 2011; 7: e35447.

[150] Bager P, Kapel C, Roepstorff A, et al. Symptoms after ingestion of pig whipworm Trichuris suis eggs in a randomized placebo-controlled double-blind clinical trial. PLoS One 2011; 6: e22346.

[151] Bouma G, Strober W. The immunological and genetic basis of inflammatory bowel disease. Nat Rev Immunol 2003; 3: 521-33.

[152] Melon A, Wang A, Phan V, et al. Infection with Hymenolepis diminuta is more effective than daily corticosteroids in blocking chemically induced colitis in mice. J Biomed Biotechnol 2010; 2010: 384523.

[153] Bodammer P, Waitz G, Loebermann M, et al. Schistosoma mansoni infection but not egg antigen promotes recovery from colitis in outbred NMRI mice. Dig Dis Sci 2011; 56: 70-8.

[154] Hang L, Setiawan T, Blum AM, et al. Heligmosomoides polygyrus infection can inhibit colitis through direct interaction with innate immunity. J Immunol 2010; 185: 3184-9.

[155] Khan WI, Blennerhasset PA, Varghese AK, et al. Intestinal nematode infection ameliorates experimental colitis in mice. Infect Immun 2002; 70: 5931-7.

[156] Leung J, Hang L, Blum A, et al. Heligmosomoides polygyrus abrogates antigen-specific gut injury in a murine model of inflammatory bowel disease. Inflamm Bowel Dis 2012; 18: 1447-55.

[157] Buning J, Homann N, von Smolinski D, et al. Helminths as governors of inflammatory bowel disease. Gut 2008; 57: 1182-3.

[158] Cancado GG, Fiuza JA, de Paiva NC, et al. Hookworm products ameliorate dextran sodium sulfate-induced colitis in BALB/c mice. Inflamm Bowel Dis 2011; 17: 2275-86.

[159] Motomura Y, Wang H, Deng Y, et al. Helminth antigen-based strategy to ameliorate inflammation in an experimental model of colitis. Clin Exp Immunol 2009; 155: 88-95.

CHAPTER 9

Parasites-Based Immunotherapy to Treat Allergies and Autoimmune Diseases

Camila Alexandrina Figueiredo[1,*], Valdirene Leão Carneiro[2], Ryan Santos Costa[1], Leonardo Nascimento Santos[1], Raimon Rios[1] and Neuza M Alcantara Neves[1]

[1]*Institute of Health Sciences, Federal University of Bahia, Brazil* and [2]*Department of Life Sciences, Statal University of Bahia, Brazil*

Abstract: It is postulated that helminth infections are able to protect their hosts from immune mediated diseases such as allergies and autoimmune diseases, due to strong parasite-driven immune regulatory processes. The development of helminth-based therapies is very attractive to treat those pathologies. In this chapter, we will be reviewing some epidemiological and experimental evidences whereby helminth infection could protects from immune-mediated diseases, the mechanisms that are behind this phenomenon as well as the main strategies that have been used by research groups to develop biological products for treatment and prophylaxis of these immunopathologies based in mild infection by worms or, more importantly, their molecules.

Keywords: Allergy, *Ascaris lumbricoides*, asthma, autoimmune diseases, Cronh's disease, diabetes, Foxp3, helminthes, helminth-derived molecules, IgE, IL-10, immune mechanisms, immune modulation, immune regulation, immunotherapy, multiple sclerosis, TGF-β, *Trichuris trichiura*, ulcerative colitis, worms.

1. INTRODUCTION

Allergy and autoimmunity are immune-mediated diseases in which the host genetics and environmental factors play a complex, and not complete understood, role in the etiology and pathogenesis of these diseases [1-3]. Over the last few decades, it has been observed an increased prevalence of allergies in large cities of

---

*Corresponding author Camila Alexandrina Figueiredo: Institute of Health Sciences, Federal University of Bahia, Av. Rector Miguel Calmon, s/n, Vale do Canela, Salvador, Bahia, Brazil, CEP: 41.110-100; Tel/Fax: +557132838348. cavfigueiredo@gmail.com.

Emilio Jirillo, Thea Magrone and Giuseppe Miragliotta (Eds)
All rights reserved-© 2014 Bentham Science Publishers

developed countries [4,7], particularly during childhood. An international asthma survey found in the literature shows that the prevalence of such disease ranges from 1.6 to 36% [7]. Improvements in hygiene, modern health care services, and a westernized way of life have brought a decline of infectious diseases during the childhood, but according to the hygiene hypothesis, such factors have also contributed to the increased prevalence of allergic diseases [8,9]. Similarly, autoimmune diseases are also increasing in many affluent and developing countries and an inverse association between infections and these diseases have been reported as well [10]. In those countries, infectious diseases are in decline, which compromises the chance of people develop a regulatory immune system capable of acting efficiently [11,12] leading to inflammatory conditions such as diabetes and asthma.

Immunotherapy for allergic and autoimmune diseases, based on helminth molecules, has been significantly investigated in the last few years. Geohelminth infections afflict 25% of the world population [13] most of them are children from developing countries supported by families with low income and without access to sanitation and clean water. Parasites such as *Ascaris lumbricoides*, *Toxocara* spp., *Trichuris trichiura*, *Ancylostoma duodenale*, and *Necator americanus* are the most frequent geohelminths present in those populations in addition to *Schistossoma* spp. and round worms Filarioidea type, where these last two are present in limited endemic areas only but also may play an important role in the immune modulation of atopic disorders [13].

The several negative associations of helminths with inflammatory diseases reported in the literature have driven the researchers attention to investigate a role for helminth-derived molecules or even mild infection by worms to treat or prevent allergy and autoimmune diseases.

In this chapter we will be discussing: i) some epidemiological data that point out to the role of helminth infection protecting against immune mediated diseases, especially allergies; ii) the main mechanisms involved in parasite immune modulation and; iii) some pre-clinical and clinical studies using parasite molecules or parasites infection-based immunotherapies for the treatment and prophylaxis of immune-mediated diseases.

2. EPIDEMIOLOGICAL EVIDENCES OF HELMINTH IMMUNE MODULATION

The human immune response to chronic helminth infections is a Th2 type immune response in which $CD4^+$ T cells release interleukin (IL)-4, IL-5, IL-13, increasing significantly the levels of IgE, tissue eosinophils and mastocytosis to control the infection. However, as a resistance mechanism, helminth chronic infections can induce immune regulatory processes in the host, with increased production of regulatory cytokines such as IL-10 and TGF-ß to restrain the local inflammatory response and allow the parasites to survive for long time without causing serious consequences to the host [14].

An epidemiological observation done by our group demonstrated that children living in poorer sanitary conditions are more likely to produce higher levels of IL-10 later in life [15] which in its turn are related to impairment production of Th1 and Th2 cytokines by peripheral blood leukocytes (PBLs) upon mitogen stimulation [6]. It was also demonstrated that children living in hyperendemic exposure to *A. lumbricoides* and/or *T. trichiura* tend to produce spontaneously more immune regulatory cytokines (IL-10 and TGF-β1) [16, 17]. *Schistossoma mansoni* infection also induces down-modulation of immune responses in infected individuals mediated by antigen-driven IL-10 production [18].

Several epidemiological studies have provided evidence that the immune modulation induced by helminth infections may have effects in altering inflammatory responses to antigens unrelated to the parasite, such as potential allergens or self-antigens, possibly leading to control immunologic disorders [14]. According to Cooper *et al.* (2009) [57] these effects may be *time-dependent* (age at infection and duration), *dose-dependent* (*i.e.* the greater the parasitic load, the potent the inhibitory effect is), depending on the helminth parasite and also the host genetics [19-21, 57].

There is a large data from epidemiologic studies supporting a potential protective role of exposures to intestinal parasites against atopic diseases. The *T. trichiura* infection occurring in children with less than three years old may reduce the risk for skin prick test (SPT) positivity to allergens later in childhood even without current infection [22]. Also, individuals living in endemic areas of *Schistosoma* sp. do not respond to SPT to aeroallergens and it has been linked to the reduction of asthma severity [20, 23-25]. However, there is still no consensus so far in the scientific community whether the *A. lumbricoides* reduce the risk of asthma and SPT positivity [19, 23, 26].

There is also an ongoing debate whether infection prevents autoimmune diseases. Various helminth species are shown to limit inflammatory activity in a variety of diseases including diabetes, experimental autoimmune encephalopathy, and Crohn's disease (CrD), mostly in experimental animal models [27-29]. However, there are an increasing number of epidemiologic studies being conducted with this goal. Recently, it has been reported that there is a negative association between antinuclear antibody (ANA) levels and the intensity of *S. mansoni* infections, exerting then a protective role against autoimmune diseases [21].

A direct way to demonstrate the link between helminth infections and immune-mediated disease is through the evaluation of the impact anti-helminthic drugs on the markers and symptoms of disease. The reduction of intestinal parasite infection by helminthic treatment results in a significant increase in both SPT reactivity and serum levels of specific IgE against aeroallergens [18, 30, 31]. Similarly, helminth-infection control using anti-helminthic drugs was associated to increased clinical signs and radiological changes in multiple sclerosis patients as well as a decreased production of $CD4^+CD25^+FoxP3^+$ Treg cells producing TGF-ß and IL-10 in these patients [32]. These findings also must be considered in predicting the long-term consequences of large-scale helminth control programs.

Exposure to helminths may not be able to induce a potent regulatory network, capable of controlling immune disorders, if the host genetic background does not contribute to do so. Individuals carrying genetic variants that elicited Th2 immune response tend to develop allergic responses to helminth and allergens however could also be genetically more resistant to helminth infections [33]. Recently, we have demonstrated that IL-10 genetic polymorphisms can up-regulate the release of such cytokine (IL-10) and consequently contribute to eradicate the helminthic infection. On the other hand, it can also increase the risk of atopy, SPT reactivity, and allergen-specific IgE levels [34].

Taken together epidemiological studies have pointed out by this strong ability to induce immune regulation and thus protect from immunopathologies. The question is how helminth infection can modulate immunopathologies?

3. MECHANISMS INVOLVED IN PARASITE IMMUNE MODULATION

3.1. Induction of Regulatory Cytokines by Helminthes

The revisited hygiene hypothesis has supported the understanding of the modulation of inflammatory disorders may involve not only the bias Th1 *vs* Th2 but, most importantly, the balance between pro-inflammatory immune responses (Th1, Th2 and Th17) through the activation of regulatory mechanisms able control an enhanced immune response [11, 12]. The cytokine IL-10 plays an important role in the regulatory response and its production, as previously mentioned, may be deficient in the absence of exposure to microbial agents during childhood in high-income countries, resulting in an increased prevalence of inflammatory diseases [11, 12]. We have reported the first population-based study in which environmental factors associated with less hygiene (*i.e.* garbage disposal, sewage, and street paving) are able to reduce the production of both Th1 and Th2 cytokines and that these environmental factors are strictly associated to helminth infections, in particular *Ascaris lumbricoides* and *Trichuris trichiura*. Moreover, it has been also shown that such reduction is associated to the increase of IL-10 production. In this way, the exposure to helminth parasites could be one of those environmental effects that could produce such immune modulation [6].

It is well known that helminths parasites suppress the immune response by activating Tregs cells, which are responsible for controlling self-tolerance, prevent the immune response against self-antigens, and avoid enhanced immune responses. Tregs cells are produced mostly in the thymus as a functionally mature subpopulation of T cells but they can also be induced from naive T cells in the periphery. Naturally occurring Tregs cells specifically express the transcription factor Foxp3 (forkhead box P3), a member of the forkhead/winged-helix family of transcription factors. Foxp3 is the major regulator of Treg cells development and function. Foxp3 transduction in naive T lymphocytes also up-regulates CD25 and other Treg markers such as cytotoxic T cell associated antigen-4 (CTLA-4) and glucocorticoid-induced TNF receptor family-related gene/protein (GITR). On the other hand, Foxp3 also suppress the production of IL-2, IFN-γ, and IL-4. Tregs cells mediated suppression can occur: (1) at the time of antigen presentation, antigen-specific Tregs cells compete with antigen-specific naïve T cells for the binding sites presented at dendritic cells; (2) activated Tregs cells reduce the responsiveness of dendritic cells and; (3) in a favorable environment, Tregs cells can secrete immunosuppressive molecules such as perforin and granzymes, in addition to IL-10 and IL-35 [34].

Parasite-driven Tregs activation has been very well explored in literature. One of the main features of helminth-induced immune response, a part from inducing a Th2 profile, is the T-cell hypo-responsiveness induced by these parasites [35]. Lima *et al.* [36] and Ferreira *et al.* [37] demonstrated that immunization of mice with *A. lumbricoides* antigens are able to reduce T-cells activity and also the production of IgM, IgE, IgG1, and IgG2 antibodies. These findings corroborate with others in the literature, which state that during the course of an antihelmintic Th2 immune response, no clinical atopy has been observed, probably, due to the regulatory role of IL-10 and TGF-ß cytokines [36, 38].

TGF-ß is pleiotropic cytokine involved in growth, ECM production and development. TGF-ß1 is a key regulator of inflammation, acting as proinflammatory at low concentrations and anti-inflammatory in high concentrations, depending on the cellular microenvironment [39]. Most models of immune regulation have demonstrated that the role of IL-10 also implicates in TGF-ß function probably by a positive feedback loops in which IL-10 increases TGF-ß expression and *vice versa*. IL-10 may acts in its site of production while TGF-ß are more likely to have a systemic effect on the immune response [40].

Animal models indicate that the immune regulatory role of IL-10 is important to host survival in autoimmune conditions [41]. For example, the treatment of IL-10 neutralizing antibodies in mice with dinitrobenzene sulfonic acid-induced colitis neutralizes the effect of *H. diminuta* infection when this cytokine in blocked [42]. Following the same rational, the presence of IL-10 mRNA correlates positively with the anti-colitis effect of *S. mansoni* eggs [43]. Therefore, the protection for autoimmune, allergic and atopic disorders caused by helminths, such as nematodes and *S. mansoni*, may be dependent on IL-10. Blocking its activity may abolish this effect [25, 44, 45]. Extending the focus on IL-10, Ramaswamy and coworkers [46] have evaluated the anti-inflammatory role of IL-10 produced by Th2 clones and Treg cells after infection with *S. mansoni*. They attributed the immune modulatory effect of this infection as a result of the production of prostaglandin E2 (PGE2), already described as having a suppressor activity, triggered after IL-10 up-regulation [47].

At tissue levels, intestine, for instance, Tregs are pointed out as the main cell type related to limiting inflammation and tissue injury [48]. Moreover, in addition to Treg cells, B cells producing IL-10 are able to suppress fatal anaphylaxis in animals infected with *S. mansoni* [49]. More recently, it has been argued the regulatory role of B cells and whether they influence the function of Treg cells [50].

Regarding to Th17 immune response, it was demonstrated that IL-17 could have a role on immunopathology during *Schistosoma* spp. infection [51] and also IL-10 is implicated in down-regulating the IL-17-driven pathology [51, 52]. Considering the ability of IL-10 producing cells to control inflammation, it is plausible to think that Treg cells assembled in response to helminth infections could, in a bystander manner, limit other inflammatory reactions. It also seems that this immune modulation can be regulated through epigenetics mechanisms since a recent study from our group has demonstrated in a Brazilian population, constantly and historically exposed to helminths, that genetic polymorphisms on *IL10* that determine less production of IL-10 are rare in such population and also, once those SNPs are present, they can predispose to atopic asthma [34]. Further studies are in progress in all over the world trying to better understand both the ability of helminths immune modulate immunopathology and also identifying molecules able to induce this effect.

3.2. Th2 Modified Response and Allergy

The Th2 modified concept was first described by Platts-Mills *et al.* [53]. Accoding to Platts-Mills, it is "alternative hypothesis to how high exposure to inhalant allergens, particularly those derived from domestic animals, can induce a *modified* form of the Th2 response". In that occasion it was considered a form of "immunological tolerance" due to an absence of skin prick test reactivity and also high titers of specific IgG4 antibodies in the body without IgE production [54]. It was proposed that individuals exposed to high doses of cat allergens exhibit important features, which support the 'modified Th2' hypothesis [55]:

- The IgG4 isotype production is stimulated by IL-4;

- Non-allergic individuals do not have SPT reactivity to cat or other common aeroallergens;

- After *in vitro* stimulation with cat antigens, blood cells of these non-allergic individuals produce high levels of IL-10 and IL-5, as well as decreased levels of IFN-γ when compared to controls.

It seems that this 'modified Th2' hypothesis also happens during helminth infection, mostly in chronic phase. We have previously observed that *A. lumbricoides* and *T. trichiura* infections, especially in chronic phases of infection are associated with total IgE and anti-Ascaris IgG4 [16]. We also have shown that children in later childhood with chronic *T. trichiura* infection had less skin reactivity to aeroallergens [22], meanwhile these same children during early childhood, when infected by *T. trichiura* had more atopy and atopic asthma [56]. The suppression of SPT reactivity and allergic responses have been associated with the presence of anti-Ascaris IgG4 antibodies in individuals with chronic infections and/or helminth co-infections. Moreover, the predominance of anti-Ascaris IgG4 on IgE can be attributable to IL-10 [12, 57-61].

3.3. Anti-Helminth Polyclonal IgE and Allergy

Helminths are strong inducers of polyclonal IgE antibodies, which are supposed to protect the parasites against the host-immune response by impairing their capacity to produce specific and effector IgE [62]. This evasion mechanism decreases the antibody dependent cellular citotoxicity (ADCC), which play an important role controlling the parasite burden in the acute phase of helminth infections. Eosinophils and mast cells are the main cells involved in this reaction in tissue and basophils in the blood. It is necessary the specific IgE antibodies cross-linking with antigens in the Fcε receptors of these cells in order for then to degranulate and kill the parasites by expelling toxic molecules for the parasites such as histamine, leucotrienes, prostaglandines, eosinophil basic-protein, inflammatory chemokines and cytokines

[62, 63]. The polyclonal IgE antibody bound to the high-affinity IgE receptor (FcεRI) would saturate the high-affinity FcεRI on basophils, mast cells and eosinophils and block the binding of the parasite specific IgE to the Fcε receptor and consequently the ADCC effector cells degranulation. Since this hypersensitivity reaction type I, which control helminth infection is also the main mechanism of allergic diseases, this would explain why in early phases of parasite infection when the production of polyclonal IgE is low, there is no protection but even exacerbation of allergy in the parasite-infected children [56]. When the parasites overcome this host immune response by producing polyclonal IgE antibodies (together with the Treg cells cytokines) they remain alive, infecting their host for long time.

The hypothesis of polyclonal IgE induced by helminths outcompeting allergen-specific IgE for FcεRI binding on basophils, mast cells and eosinophils decreasing allergy has been postulated since the 1980 decade and Linch and collaborators [64] in the 1990's corroborate this hypothesis in population-based works in highly helminth-infected Venezuelan children. Though, this hypothesis have received many criticism in both epidemiological studies which did not find such association [44, 65] and as well as an experimental study conducted by Mitre and collaborators [66] that showed no association between ratios of mice polyclonal IgE to *Brugia malayi* antigen and from filaria-infected patients (basophil responses to *B. malayi* measured by histamine release). These discrepancies among epidemiological studies may be due to the methodological differences among the studies and differences in genetic background of the studied population. As far as the Mitre and collaborators work is concerned about the use of only one, among several molecules that orchestra the hypersensitivity reaction, it is not enough to discard this hypothesis. Then it is necessary that laboratory works measuring basophils and mast cells degranulation of experimental animals and human cells by polyclonal IgE enriched sera using other markers of these cells degranulation to be carried out in order to clarify the role of polyclonal IgE in parasite infection and in immunomodulation of allergic diseases.

3.4. IgE Cross-Reactivity Between Helminths and Allergen Molecules

Helminth and allergens, mostly those from acarid organism, share IgE reactive molecules. Johansson and colleagues described cross-reactivity between the nematode *Anisakis simplex* and the dust mites *Acarus siro, Lepidoglyphus destructor*, *Tyrophagus putrescentiae* and *Dermatophagoides pteronyssinus* [67]. Acevedo and collaborators [68] study describes cross-reactive between *A. lumbricoides* and *Blomia tropicalis* IgE reacting with tropomyosin and glutathione-S-transferase.

What are the roles of these IgE cross-reactions on protection or exacerbation of atopy and clinical manifestation of allergic diseases? Are they friend or foe? Cross-reactive carbohydrate determinants (CCDs) are sugar moieties of glycoproteins capable of inducing IgE production and also cross-react with different allergens [69]. CCDs are associated to the discrepancy between the presence of specific IgE to pollen and the absence of a positive SPT to it in the same individual, as means of the lack of mast cell degranulation [70].

Our group has reported that cross-reaction between anti-*A. lumbricoides* and *Blomia tropicalis* IgE may be responsible for the discrepancy found in developing countries between the two markers of atopy: *B. tropicalis* allergen specific serum IgE (more positive) and skin hypersensitiviy (less positive) suggesting that these cross-reactive IgE might not participate on the ADCC effector cells degranulation [71]. Although we did not found association between the presence of IgE reactive to carbohydrate and decrease of SPT positivity in 20 studied individuals, using a larger population we have found that IgE from SPT negative children were more reactive to carbohydrate epitopes (data not published). Although the paper mentioned above suggest that the investigated cross-reaction were protective against allergy, one can not discard that if the epitopes involved in the cross-reaction are from molecules able to react with IgE of high avidity, they may participate in the inflammatory immune reaction to both allergens and helminth infection. Further work on identification of cross-reactivity antigens of helminth and mites must be done to disentangle the role of these antibodies on allergic sensitization.

Fig. (**1**) summarizes the main mechanisms (3.1-3.4) whereby helminths could modulate immunopathologies.

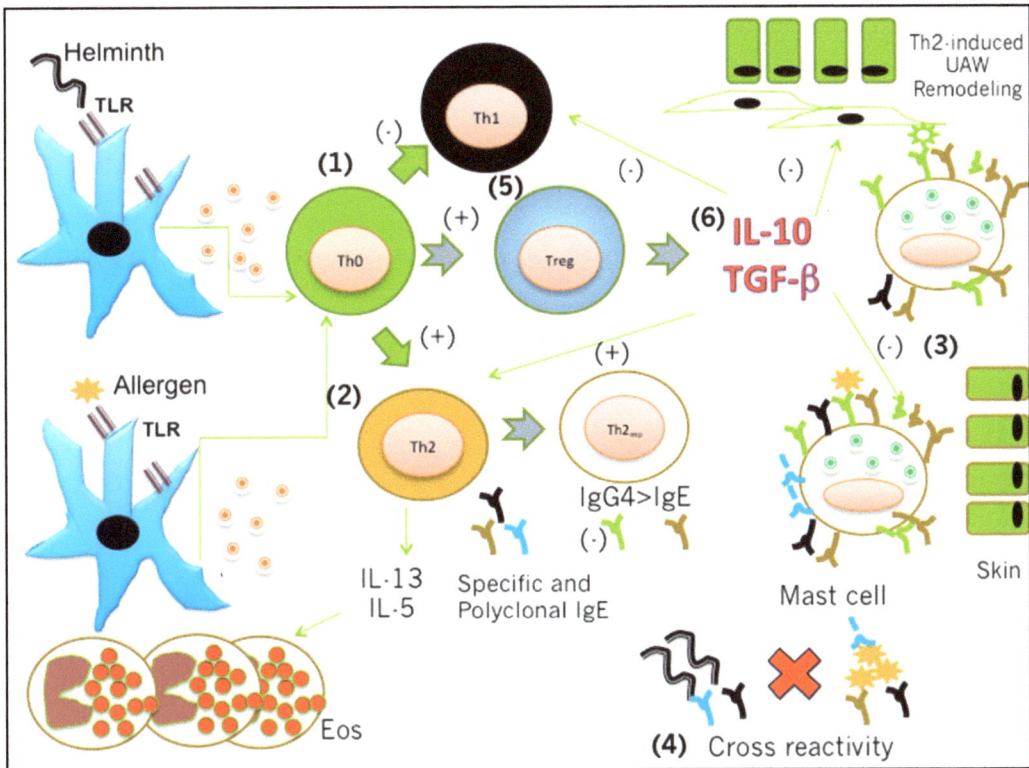

Figure 1: (1) Dendritic cells (DCs) interact with PAMPs from helminths and allergens which modulate DCs and produce cytokines which can differentiate T naïve into (1) Th1 not usually related to helminth infection or Th2 (2) related to both helminth infection and allergic diseases; those clones produce IL-13 and IL-5 which recruits Eosinophils (Eos) and mainly through IL-4 induces IgE production. Helminth infections are also known by its ability to induce polyclonal IgE which in its turns can down-modulate skin reactivity (3). Despite the production of specific IgE against allergens, in infected subjects the polyclonal IgE can cross-react with the allergen which might play a role of specific IgE measurement by commercial techniques (4); however, T naïve lymphocytes can also differentiate into Treg cells (5) whereby through IL-10 and TGF-β production (6) suppress Th1/Th2 immune responses; induce the Th2 modified immune response increasing IgG4 levels which can play a role decreasing skin test reactivity and inducing upper airways remodeling.

3.5. Molecular Mechanisms Involved in Helminth Immune Modulation

Above (3.1 – 3.4) are described the changes in expression of cytokines and antibodies that are actually molecules of the effector immune response. However, they are a result of underlying molecular mechanisms that are early events signaling the immune response to an effector mechanism. TLRs 2 and 4 expression, as well as the molecules suppressor of cytokine signaling-3, expressed by LT CD4$^+$ are related to the maintenance and exacerbation of allergic responses, favoring the production of IgE and production of Th2 cytokines. In both, there is an inverse relationship between helminth infection and its expression, indicating that these, possibly, are early events of the immune response that are inhibited by helminths to achieve its regulatory function [72, 73]. LPS can induce inflammatory cytokine gene expression by macrophages, generally a Th1 pattern, through nuclear factor-κB (NF-κB) and mitogen-activated protein kinase intracellular signaling pathways in macrophages [74]. However, excretory/secretory products from *T. spirallis* prevents the nuclear translocation of NF-κB and induces alternative macrophage activation, which induces expression of Arginase-1 and modulating host immune during helminth infection through IL-10 and TGF-ß [75].

4. PRE-CLINICAL AND CLINICAL STUDIES USING PARASITES-BASED IMMUNOTHERAPY FOR THE TREATMENT AND PROPHYLAXIS OF IMMUNE-MEDIATED DISEASES

The inverse relationship between helminths infection and allergic and autoimmune diseases has led to the completion of preclinical studies and even clinical trials in order to confirm the protection exerted by the helminth extracts, especially excretory and secretory antigens derived from these parasites, or even products already isolated, with *in vitro* activity described on the development of such diseases.

Regarding preclinical trials, very well described murine models of allergic and autoimmune diseases such as asthma/airway hypersensitivity or inflammation, streptozotocin-induced diabetes, type 1 diabetes in NOD mice, experimental autoimmune encephalomyelitis, collagen-induced arthritis and dextran sulphate sodium-induced colitis [76] are available to test the ability of these molecules. The use of such well-defined models enable the study of either prophylactic or therapeutic protocols using products derived from helminths.

To this end we can think about the following strategies: i) the use of natural infections or; ii) parasite-derived isolated molecules.

The protocols involving the use of natural infections, crude extracts or excretory-secretory are not the best alternative to achieve therapeutic success since they consist in complex mixtures which hinders the complete understanding mechanisms by which induce its beneficial effects or not. In addition to that, products would be of difficult standardization and large-scale production. However, as pilot evaluations this strategy can give us the first shot to the discovery of major molecules responsible for such effects. Thus, some experiments in animal models have shown good results. In a murine model of autoimmune encephalomyelitis the adoptive transfer of splenocytes or lymphocytes of mice that were previously infected with *Trichinella spiralis* exhibit a considerable reduction in clinical disease scores in only 3 days which appears to be related to the increased proportion of Treg cells (CD4 + CD25 + Foxp3+) [77]. In another murine model, the NOD (non obese diabetic) mice diabetic at 10 weeks of age, *Heligmossomoides polygyrus* infection was able to completely inhibit the development of disease when the infection occurs in the 5th week of age, but the same protection was not observed when infection occurs from the 7th week, demonstrating the importance of timing in order to achieve protection [78].

Using allergic diseases models, excretory-secretory *Nipostrongylus brasiliensis* products showed significant inhibition on cellularity and histological alterations on ovalbumin-induced airways inflammation, when given prophylactically, probably through reduction of cytokines and chemokines related to the allergic process such as IL-4, IL-5, RANTES, MCP-1 and eotaxin [79].

On the other hand, another work trying to evaluate the effect of helminth-derived complex mixtures on eosinophilic airway inflammation is a typical example of the disadvantages of using such products for immunotherapy. In a fore mentioned work authors have demonstrated the suppressive protein of *Ascaris suum* (PAS-1) which has its immune regulatory activity already described is able to inhibit eosinophilic inflammation induced by APAS-3, a protein also present in *A. suum* extract, however with opposite activity, *i.e.* pro-inflammatory activity. In this way, in this study we could confirm that within a parasite extract we may have molecules with different or even opposite biological effects and also emphasizes that isolated molecules may be better than crude extracts for immunotherapy [80].

Glycoprotein obtained from *Acantocheilonema vitae* (ES-62) is a glycoprotein obtained from *Acantocheilonema vitae*, whose mechanisms of regulatory action has been extensively studied and well understood. It has been used in different models of immune mediated diseases, such as atopic allergy in which the percentage of mast cells degranulation is reduced as well as hyperresponsiveness airway to a cholinergic agent, methacholine [81]. The ES-62 also showed a protective effect against collagen-induced arthritis, where the parameters of disease activity, erosion, hyperplasia and cellular infiltration, were significantly inhibited, recovering articular functionality [82].

Regarding to clinical trials, therapy with *Trichuris suis* ova has been used to treat inflammatory bowel diseases as CrD and ulcerative colitis (UC), in which patients ingest *T. suis* ova resulting in significant clinical improvement in nearly 80% of patients in the CrD however less important effect on UC since clinical manifestations reappear a few weeks after treatment. In this way, this treatment proved to be a safe and effective, but it deserves better understanding and improvement of the therapeutic protocol in order to its use to be expanded [83, 84]. Regarding allergies, the therapy with *T. suis* ova had no therapeutic effect on allergic rhinitis in a randomized, double-blind, placebo-controlled clinical trial [85].

Feary *et al.* conducted the first double-blind placebo-controlled study to measure the effect of hookworm infection in patients with asthma. However, they observed no improvement in clinical symptoms of asthma and suggested changes in the experimental protocol so that the next models better mimic the natural infection [86]. Daveson and colleagues has shown, in a randomized placebo-controlled double-blind clinical trial, the effect of *Necator americanus* in suppressing the gluten induced immunopathology in patients with celiac disease. They concluded that the experimental protocol with *Necator americanus* is safe and can be implemented to evaluate data of autoimmune disorder *in vivo* and *in vitro*, but no benefits for celiac disease has been observed using this model [87]. Recently, in another double-blind clinical trial, Bager *et al.* have shown that after ingestion of *Trichuris suis* eggs, the studied subjects had several undesirable gastrointestinal effects such as moderate to severe bloating, diarrhea and pain in the upper abdomen when compared to the placebo group [88]. Table **1** summarizes some mechanisms whereby helminths would modulate immunopathologies in both pre-clinical and clinical levels.

Table 1: Mechanisms for suppression of immune diseases by helminthes: pre-clinical and clinical data

Disease	Strategies	Helminths	Mechanisms	Refs
Animal Models				
Autoimmune encephalomyelitis	*Adoptive transfer of splenocytes or lymphocytes*	*T. spiralis*	Treg cells (CD4 + CD25 + Foxp3+)	77
Diabetes	Infection	*H. polygyrus*	CD25-and IL-10-independent	78
Allergy	Excretory-secretory products	*N. brasiliensis*	Reduction of cytokines and chemokines	79
Eosinophilic inflammation	Suppressive protein (PAS-1)	*A. suum*	Reduction of cytokines and chemokines	80
Allergy	ES – 62 (glycoprotein)	*A. vitae*	Reduction of mast cells degranulation	81
Clinical trials				
Ulcerative colitis	Ova ingestion	*T. suis*	-	83
Cronh's disease	Ova ingestion	*T. suis*	-	84
Asthma	Cutaneous inoculations	Hookworm	No significant improvement	86
Celiac disease	Cutaneous inoculations	*N. americanus*	No obvious benefit	87

Several reasons explaining why some clinical trials have failed so far, include the following:

- **Biosafety:** For security reasons, the dose used in clinical trials may not be adequate to mimic natural infections;

- **Chronic infection *versus* current infection:** Chronic infection may exerts the modulating effect on immune response, but the randomized, double-blind or placebo-controlled trials implement so far have evaluated recent/current infection only [89];

- **Prophylaxis:** Perhaps clinical trials should use in their models prevention strategies instead of therapeutic strategies, since the parasites could act by preventing immune-mediated diseases rather than curing them.

5. FINAL CONSIDERATIONS

Although scientific evidences indicate that helminth infections protect individuals against allergic and autoimmune diseases, the use of immunotherapies based on such infections still controversial. Helminthiasis, especially in countries of low and middle income, are responsible for causing health many problems in children, such as malnutrition, cognitive and growth deficiencies, which directly affects school performance and immune response to vaccines. Taken all these in consideration, it is clear that the use of helminth infections to prevent or treat immune-mediated disease with curative or preventive purposes is out of perspective [90]. Thus, the identification and isolation of helminth molecules (expressed during the chronic phase especially), with immune regulatory potential and low or absent side effects, are still an important goal to be archived. At the moment, there are already some candidate molecules for immunotherapy. In addition to that, the use of monoclonal antibodies and small molecules, with different actions on Treg cells and effector T cells, has been considered as promising therapeutic agents capable of controlling the balance between Tregs cells and effector T cells.

ACKNOWLEDGEMENTS

We thank the Brazilian agencies CAPES, CNPQ, and FAPESB for funding and providing support for postdoctoral, masters, and doctoral fellowships.

CONFLICT OF INTEREST

The author(s) confirm that this chapter contents have no conflict of interest.

ABBREVIATIONS

ADCC = Antibody-dependent cell-mediated cytotoxicity;

ANA = Antinuclear antibody;

CCDS	=	Cross-reactive carbohydrate determinants;
CrD	=	Cronh's disease;
CTLA-4	=	Cytotoxic T cell associated antigen-4;
ECM	=	Extracellular matrix;
ES-62	=	Glycoprotein obtained from *Acantocheilonema vitae*;
FCεRI	=	High-affinity IgE receptor;
Foxp3	=	Forkhead box P3;
GITR	=	Glucocorticoid-induced TNF receptor family-related gene/protein;
IFN	=	Interferon;
Ig	=	Immunoglobulin;
NF-κB	=	Nuclear factor-κB;
PAS-1	=	Suppressive protein of *Ascaris suum*;
PBLs	=	Peripheral blood leukocytes;
SPT	=	Skin prick test;
TGF-β	=	Transforming growth factor β;
Th	=	T helper;
TNF	=	Tumor necrosis factor;
Treg	=	T regulatory cells;
UC	=	Ulcerative colitis;

REFERENCES

[1] Woolcock AJ, Peat JK. Evidence for the increase in asthma worldwide. Ciba Found Symp 1997; 206: 122-34; discussion 34-9, 57-9.

[2] Upton M, McConnachie A, McSharry C, *et al.* Intergenerational 20 year trends in the prevalence of asthma and hay fever in adults: the Midspan family study surveys of parents and offspring. BMJ 2000; 321: 88-92.

[3] Williams H. Is the prevalence of atopic dermatitis increasing? Clin Exp Dermatol 1992; 17: 385-91.

[4] Braun-Fahrländer C, Riedler J, Herz U, *et al.* Environmental exposure to endotoxin and its relation to asthma in school-age children. N Engl J Med 2002; 347: 869-77.

[5] Barreto ML, Cunha SS, Alcântara-Neves N, *et al.* Risk factors and immunological pathways for asthma and other allergic diseases in children: background and methodology of a longitudinal study in a large urban center in Northeastern Brazil (Salvador-SCAALA study). BMC Pulm Med 2006; 6: 15.

[6] Figueiredo CA, Alcantara-Neves NM, Amorim LD, *et al.* Evidence for a modulatory effect of IL-10 on both Th1 and Th2 cytokine production: the role of the environment. Clin Immunol 2011; 139: 57-64.

[7] Committee IS. Worldwide variation in prevalence of symptoms of asthma, allergic rhinoconjunctivitis, and atopic eczema: ISAAC. The International Study of Asthma and Allergies in Childhood (ISAAC) Steering Committee. Lancet 1998; 351: 1225-32.

[8] Strachan DP. Hay fever, hygiene, and household size. BMJ 1989; 299: 1259-60.

[9] Strachan DP. Family size, infection and atopy: the first decade of the "hygiene hypothesis". Thorax 2000; 55 Suppl 1: S2-10.

[10] Cooke A. Review series on helminths, immune modulation and the hygiene hypothesis: how might infection modulate the onset of type 1 diabetes? Immunology. 2009; 126: 12-7.

[11] Wills-Karp M, Santeliz J, Karp CL. The germless theory of allergic disease: revisiting the hygiene hypothesis. Nat Rev Immunol 2001; 1: 69-75.

[12] Yazdanbakhsh M, Kremsner PG, van Ree R. Allergy, parasites, and the hygiene hypothesis. Science 2002; 296: 490-4.

[13] Bethony J, Brooker S, Albonico M, *et al.* Soil-transmitted helminth infections: ascariasis, trichuriasis, and hookworm. Lancet 2006; 367: 1521-32.

[14] van Riet E, Hartgers FC, Yazdanbakhsh M. Chronic helminth infections induce immunomodulation: consequences and mechanisms. Immunobiology 2007; 212: 475-90.

[15] Figueiredo CA, Alcântara-Neves NM, Veiga R, *et al.* Spontaneous cytokine production in children according to biological characteristics and environmental exposures. Environ Health Perspect 2009; 117: 845-9.

[16] Figueiredo CA, Barreto ML, Rodrigues LC, *et al.* Chronic intestinal helminth infections are associated with immune hyporesponsiveness and induction of a regulatory network. Infect Immun 2010; 78: 3160-7.

[17] Turner JD, Jackson JA, Faulkner H, *et al.* Intensity of intestinal infection with multiple worm species is related to regulatory cytokine output and immune hyporesponsiveness. J Infect Dis 2008; 197: 1204-12.

[18] Cardoso LS, Oliveira SC, Pacífico LG, *et al.* Schistosoma mansoni antigen-driven interleukin-10 production in infected asthmatic individuals. Mem Inst Oswaldo Cruz 2006; 101 Suppl 1: 339-43.

[19] Alcantara-Neves NM, Veiga RV, *et al.* The effect of single and multiple infections on atopy and wheezing in children. J Allergy Clin Immunol 2012; 129: 359-67, 67.e1-3.

[20] Rujeni N, Nausch N, Bourke CD, *et al.* Atopy is inversely related to schistosome infection intensity: a comparative study in Zimbabwean villages with distinct levels of Schistosoma haematobium infection. Int Arch Allergy Immunol 2012; 158: 288-98.

[21] Mutapi F, Imai N, Nausch N, *et al.* Schistosome infection intensity is inversely related to auto-reactive antibody levels. PLoS One 2011; 6: e19149.

[22] Rodrigues LC, Newcombe PJ, Cunha SS, *et al.* Early infection with Trichuris trichiura and allergen skin test reactivity in later childhood. Clin Exp Allergy 2008; 38: 1769-77.

[23] Cardoso LS, Costa DM, Almeida MC, *et al.* Risk factors for asthma in a helminth endemic area in bahia, Brazil. J Parasitol Res 2012; 2012: 796820.

[24] Araujo MI, Hoppe B, Medeiros M, *et al.* Impaired T helper 2 response to aeroallergen in helminth-infected patients with asthma. J Infect Dis 2004; 190: 1797-803.

[25] Araújo MI, Hoppe BS, Medeiros M, *et al.* Schistosoma mansoni infection modulates the immune response against allergic and auto-immune diseases. Mem Inst Oswaldo Cruz 2004; 99: 27-32.

[26] Ponte EV, Lima F, Araújo MI, *et al.* Skin test reactivity and Der p-induced interleukin 10 production in patients with asthma or rhinitis infected with Ascaris. Ann Allergy Asthma Immunol 2006; 96: 713-8.

[27] Kuijk LM, Klaver EJ, Kooij G, *et al.* Soluble helminth products suppress clinical signs in murine experimental autoimmune encephalomyelitis and differentially modulate human dendritic cell activation. Mol Immunol 2012; 51: 210-8.

[28] Zaccone P, Fehérvári Z, Jones FM, *et al.* Schistosoma mansoni antigens modulate the activity of the innate immune response and prevent onset of type 1 diabetes. Eur J Immunol 2003; 33: 1439-49.

[29] La Flamme AC, Canagasabey K, Harvie M, *et al.* Schistosomiasis protects against multiple sclerosis. Mem Inst Oswaldo Cruz 2004; 99: 33-6.

[30] Lynch NR, Hagel I, Perez M, *et al.* Effect of anthelmintic treatment on the allergic reactivity of children in a tropical slum. J Allergy Clin Immunol 1993; 92: 404-11.

[31] van den Biggelaar AH, Rodrigues LC, van Ree R, *et al.* Long-term treatment of intestinal helminths increases mite skin-test reactivity in Gabonese schoolchildren. J Infect Dis 2004; 189: 892-900.

[32] Correale J, Farez MF. The impact of parasite infections on the course of multiple sclerosis. J Neuroimmunol 2011; 233: 6-11.

[33] Smits HH, Everts B, Hartgers FC, *et al.* Chronic helminth infections protect against allergic diseases by active regulatory processes. Curr Allergy Asthma Rep 2010; 10: 3-12.

[34] Figueiredo CA, Barreto ML, Alcantara-Neves NM, *et al.* Coassociations between IL10 polymorphisms, IL-10 production, helminth infection, and asthma/wheeze in an urban tropical population in Brazil. 2013; 131: 1683-90.

[35] Smits HH, Hartgers FC, Yazdanbakhsh M. Helminth infections: protection from atopic disorders. Curr Allergy Asthma Rep 2005; 5: 42-50.

[36] Lima C, Perini A, Garcia ML, *et al.* Eosinophilic inflammation and airway hyper-responsiveness are profoundly inhibited by a helminth (Ascaris suum) extract in a murine model of asthma. Clin Exp Allergy 2002; 32: 1659-66.

[37] Ferreira AP, Faquim ES, Abrahamsohn IA, *et al.* Immunization with Ascaris suum extract impairs T cell functions in mice. Cell Immunol 1995; 162: 202-10.

[38] Yazdanbakhsh M, van den Biggelaar A, Maizels RM. Th2 responses without atopy: immunoregulation in chronic helminth infections and reduced allergic disease. Trends Immunol 2001; 22: 372-7.

[39] Letterio JJ, Roberts AB. Regulation of immune responses by TGF-beta. Annu Rev Immunol 1998; 16: 137-61.

[40] Mottet C, Golshayan D. CD4+CD25+Foxp3+ regulatory T cells: from basic research to potential therapeutic use. Swiss Med Wkly 2007; 137: 625-34.

[41] Schopf LR, Hoffmann KF, Cheever AW, et al. IL-10 is critical for host resistance and survival during gastrointestinal helminth infection. J Immunol 2002; 168: 2383-92.

[42] Hunter MM, Wang A, Hirota CL, et al. Neutralizing anti-IL-10 antibody blocks the protective effect of tapeworm infection in a murine model of chemically induced colitis. J Immunol 2005; 174: 7368-75.

[43] Elliott DE, Li J, Blum A, et al. Exposure to schistosome eggs protects mice from TNBS-induced colitis. Am J Physiol Gastrointest Liver Physiol 2003; 284: G385-91.

[44] van den Biggelaar AH, van Ree R, Rodrigues LC, et al. Decreased atopy in children infected with Schistosoma haematobium: a role for parasite-induced interleukin-10. Lancet 2000; 356: 1723-7.

[45] Wohlleben G, Trujillo C, Müller J, et al. Helminth infection modulates the development of allergen-induced airway inflammation. Int Immunol 2004; 16: 585-96.

[46] Ramaswamy K, Kumar P, He YX. A role for parasite-induced PGE2 in IL-10-mediated host immunoregulation by skin stage schistosomula of Schistosoma mansoni. J Immunol 2000; 165: 4567-74.

[47] O'Garra A, Vieira P. Regulatory T cells and mechanisms of immune system control. Nat Med 2004; 10: 801-5.

[48] Groux H, O'Garra A, Bigler M, et al. A CD4+ T-cell subset inhibits antigen-specific T-cell responses and prevents colitis. Nature 1997; 389: 737-42.

[49] Mangan NE, Fallon RE, Smith P, et al. Helminth infection protects mice from anaphylaxis via IL-10-producing B cells. J Immunol 2004; 173: 6346-56.

[50] Wei B, Velazquez P, Turovskaya O, et al. Mesenteric B cells centrally inhibit CD4+ T cell colitis through interaction with regulatory T cell subsets. Proc Natl Acad Sci U S A 2005; 102: 2010-5.

[51] Mbow M, Larkin BM, Meurs L, et al. T-helper 17 cells are associated with pathology in human schistosomiasis. J Infect Dis 2013; 207: 186-95.

[52] Larkin BM, Smith PM, Ponichtera HE, et al. Induction and regulation of pathogenic Th17 cell responses in schistosomiasis. Semin Immunopathol 2012; 34: 873-88.

[53] Platts-Mills T, Vaughan J, Squillace S, Woodfolk J, Sporik R. Sensitisation, asthma, and a modified Th2 response in children exposed to cat allergen: a population-based cross-sectional study. Lancet 2001; 357: 752-6.

[54] Perzanowski MS, Rönmark E, Platts-Mills TA, et al. Effect of cat and dog ownership on sensitization and development of asthma among preteenage children. Am J Respir Crit Care Med 2002; 166: 696-702.

[55] Platts-Mills TA, Woodfolk JA, Erwin EA, et al. Mechanisms of tolerance to inhalant allergens: the relevance of a modified Th2 response to allergens from domestic animals. Springer Semin Immunopathol 2004; 25: 271-9.

[56] Alcântara-Neves NM, Badaró SJ, dos Santos MC, et al. The presence of serum anti-Ascaris lumbricoides IgE antibodies and of Trichuris trichiura infection are risk factors for wheezing and/or atopy in preschool-aged Brazilian children. Respir Res 2010; 11: 114.

[57] Cooper PJ. Interactions between helminth parasites and allergy. Curr Opin Allergy Clin Immunol 2009; 9: 29-37.

[58] Maizels RM, Yazdanbakhsh M. Immune regulation by helminth parasites: cellular and molecular mechanisms. Nat Rev Immunol 2003; 3: 733-44.

[59] Ponte EV, Lima F, Araújo MI, et al. Skin test reactivity and Der p-induced interleukin 10 production in patients with asthma or rhinitis infected with Ascaris. Ann Allergy Asthma Immunol 2006; 96: 713-8.

[60] Rodrigues LC, Newcombe PJ, Cunha SS, et al. Early infection with Trichuris trichiura and allergen skin test reactivity in later childhood. Clin Exp Allergy 2008; 38: 1769-77.

[61] Moore KW, de Waal Malefyt R, et al. Interleukin-10 and the interleukin-10 receptor. Annu Rev Immunol 2001; 19: 683-765.

[62] McSorley HJ, Maizels RM. Helminth infections and host immune regulation. Clin Microbiol Rev 2012; 25: 585-608.

[63] McSorley HJ, Hewitson JP, Maizels RM. Immunomodulation by helminth parasites: Defining mechanisms and mediators. Int J Parasitol 2013; 43: 301-10.

[64] Lynch NR, Hagel IA, Palenque ME, et al. Relationship between helminthic infection and IgE response in atopic and nonatopic children in a tropical environment. J Allergy Clin Immunol 1998; 101: 217-21.

[65] Scrivener S, Yemaneberhan H, Zebenigus M, et al. Independent effects of intestinal parasite infection and domestic allergen exposure on risk of wheeze in Ethiopia: a nested case-control study. Lancet 2001; 358: 1493-9.

[66] Mitre E, Norwood S, Nutman TB. Saturation of immunoglobulin E (IgE) binding sites by polyclonal IgE does not explain the protective effect of helminth infections against atopy. Infect Immun 2005; 73: 4106-11.

[67] Johansson E, Aponno M, Lundberg M, et al. Allergenic cross-reactivity between the nematode Anisakis simplex and the dust mites Acarus siro, Lepidoglyphus destructor, Tyrophagus putrescentiae, and Dermatophagoides pteronyssinus. Allergy 2001; 56: 660-6.

[68] Acevedo N, Sánchez J, Erler A, et al. IgE cross-reactivity between Ascaris and domestic mite allergens: the role of tropomyosin and the nematode polyprotein ABA-1. Allergy 2009; 64: 1635-43.

[69] van Ree R. Carbohydrate epitopes and their relevance for the diagnosis and treatment of allergic diseases. Int Arch Allergy Immunol 2002; 129: 189-97.

[70] Mari A, Iacovacci P, Afferni C, et al. Specific IgE to cross-reactive carbohydrate determinants strongly affect the *in vitro* diagnosis of allergic diseases. J Allergy Clin Immunol 1999; 103: 1005-11.

[71] Ponte JC, Junqueira SB, Veiga RV, et al. A study on the immunological basis of the dissociation between type I-hypersensitivity skin reactions to Blomia tropicalis antigens and serum anti-B. tropicalis IgE antibodies. BMC Immunol 2011; 12: 34.

[72] Hartgers FC, Obeng BB, Kruize YC, et al. Lower expression of TLR2 and SOCS-3 is associated with Schistosoma haematobium infection and with lower risk for allergic reactivity in children living in a rural area in Ghana. PLoS Negl Trop Dis 2008; 2: e227.

[73] Ozaki A, Seki Y, Fukushima A, et al. The control of allergic conjunctivitis by suppressor of cytokine signaling (SOCS)3 and SOCS5 in a murine model. J Immunol 2005; 175: 5489-97.

[74] Tominaga K, Saito S, Matsuura M, et al. Lipopolysaccharide tolerance in murine peritoneal macrophages induces downregulation of the lipopolysaccharide signal transduction

pathway through mitogen-activated protein kinase and nuclear factor-kappaB cascades, but not lipopolysaccharide-incorporation steps. Biochim Biophys Acta 1999; 1450: 130-44.

[75] Bai X, Wu X, Wang X, et al. Regulation of cytokine expression in murine macrophages stimulated by excretory/secretory products from Trichinella spiralis in vitro. Mol Cell Biochem 2012; 360: 79-88.

[76] Osada Y, Kanazawa T. Parasitic helminths: new weapons against immunological disorders. J Biomed Biotechnol 2010; 2010: 743758.

[77] Gruden-Movsesijan A, Ilic N, Mostarica-Stojkovic M, et al. Mechanisms of modulation of experimental autoimmune encephalomyelitis by chronic Trichinella spiralis infection in Dark Agouti rats. Parasite Immunol 2010; 32: 450-9.

[78] Liu Q, Sundar K, Mishra PK, et al. Helminth infection can reduce insulitis and type 1 diabetes through CD25-and IL-10-independent mechanisms. Infect Immun 2009; 77: 5347-58.

[79] Trujillo-Vargas CM, Werner-Klein M, Wohlleben G, i Helminth-derived products inhibit the development of allergic responses in mice. Am J Respir Crit Care Med 2007; 175: 336-44.

[80] Itami D, Oshiro T, Araujo C, et al. Modulation of murine experimental asthma by Ascaris suum components. Clin Exp Allergy 2005; 35: 873-9.

[81] Melendez AJ, Harnett MM, Pushparaj PN, et al. Inhibition of Fc epsilon RI-mediated mast cell responses by ES-62, a product of parasitic filarial nematodes. Nat Med 2007; 13: 1375-81.

[82] McInnes IB, Leung BP, Harnett M, et al. A novel therapeutic approach targeting articular inflammation using the filarial nematode-derived phosphorylcholine-containing glycoprotein ES-62. J Immunol 2003; 171: 2127-33.

[83] Summers R, Elliott D, Urban JJ, et al. Trichuris suis therapy for active ulcerative colitis: a randomized controlled trial. Gastroenterology 2005; 128: 825-32.

[84] Summers R, Elliott D, Urban JJ, et al. Trichuris suis therapy in Crohn's disease. Gut 2005; 54: 87-90.

[85] Bager P, Arnved J, Ronborg S, et al. Trichuris suis ova therapy for allergic rhinitis: a randomized, double-blind, placebo-controlled clinical trial. J Allergy Clin Immunol 2010; 125: 123-30.e1-3.

[86] Feary JR, Venn AJ, Mortimer K, et al. Experimental hookworm infection: a randomized placebo-controlled trial in asthma. Clin Exp Allergy 2010; 40: 299-306.

[87] Daveson AJ, Jones DM, Gaze S, et al. Effect of hookworm infection on wheat challenge in celiac disease--a randomised double-blinded placebo controlled trial. PLoS One 2011; 6: e17366.

[88] Bager P, Kapel C, Roepstorff A, et al. Symptoms after ingestion of pig whipworm Trichuris suis eggs in a randomized placebo-controlled double-blind clinical trial. PLoS One 2011; 6: e22346.

[89] Smits HH, Everts B, Hartgers FC, et al. Chronic helminth infections protect against allergic diseases by active regulatory processes. Curr Allergy Asthma Rep 2010; 10: 3-12.

[90] Cooper PJ, Chico ME, Guadalupe I, et al. Impact of early life exposures to geohelminth infections on the development of vaccine immunity, allergic sensitization, and allergic inflammatory diseases in children living in tropical Ecuador: the ECUAVIDA birth cohort study. BMC Infect Dis 2011; 11: 184.

CHAPTER 10

The Impact of Helminths on the Human Microbiota: Therapeutic Correction of Disturbed Gut Microbial Immunity

Thea Magrone[1], Emilio Jirillo[1,*] and Giuseppe Miragliotta[2]

[1]*Department of Basic Medical Sciences, Neuroscience and Sensory Organs and* [2]*Department of Interdisciplinary Medicine, University of Bari, Bari, Italy*

Abstract: Intestinal microbiota is in strict relationship with gut immune cells and a good balance between both components is able to guarantee a condition of healthy status in the host. Helminths tend to alter the host immune system *via* release of anti-inflammatory cytokines and, in particular, interleukin (IL)-10. IL-10 release by FoxP3+ T regulatory (Treg) cells, in turn, down-regulates T helper (h)2 cells, which instead protects the host against helminths. At the same time, helminths are able to interact with intestinal microbiota, thus leading to either harmful or protective effects. Therapeutically, polyphenols have been shown to modulate gut microbiota, also interfering with helminth development. In this context, our studies using polyphenols from red wine and fermented grape marc have shown anti-inflammatory activities exerted by these compounds, even including expansion and activation of Treg cells. Since evidence has been provided that Treg cell activation with production of IL-10 can attenuate immunopathology in the later phase of helminth infections, dietary polyphenols may be beneficial in the chronic stage of parasitoses.

Keywords: Antigen presenting cells, bacteria, basophils, cytokines, dendritic cells, eosinophils, helminths, interferon, interleukins, immunopathology, lipopolysaccharides, macrophages, microbiota, monocytes, neutrophils, polymorphonuclear cells, polyphenols, T helper cells, T regulatory cells, Toll like receptors.

INTRODUCTION

Microbes are widespread in our body and, particularly, in those areas heavily exposed to the environment. Skin, mouth and vagina are colonized by microbes but the gut harbors the most elevated number of microbial communities [1].

In our body, all the complexes of microbial cells have been named microbiota and

*Corresponding author **Emilio Jirillo:** Department of Basic Medical Sciences, Neuroscience and Sensory Organs, Policlinico, Piazza Giulio Cesare, 11-70124 Bari, Italy; Tel: +39 080 5478492; Fax: +39 080 5478488; E-mail: emilio.jirillo@uniba.it

the genes they encode are known as microbiome. *Bacteroidetes* and *Firmacutes* are the major *phyla* in the adult human gut [2] but type of diet and use of antibiotics can perturb the composition of microbiota [3,4]. For instance, abuse of antibiotics in humans causes an increase of antibiotic resistant genes [5], and, moreover, perturbation of intestinal microbiota has been reported in inflammatory pathologies such as diabetes, obesity and Crohn's disease (CD) [6] (see Fig. **1**).

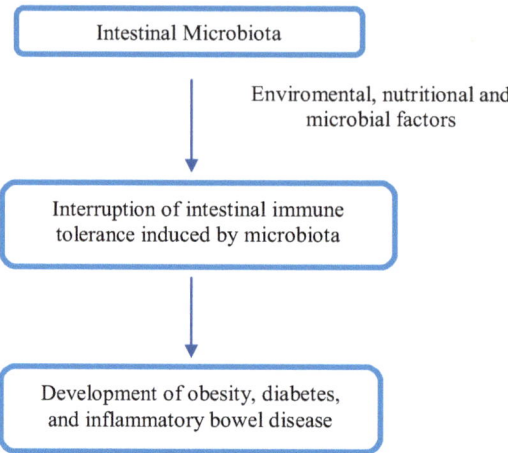

Figure 1: Interruption of gut immune tolerance and development of diseases.

In this context, evidence has been provided that *Akkermansia (A.) muciniphila*, a mucin-degrading bacterium (representing 3-5% of the microbial community), is reduced in obese and type 2 diabetic mice [7]. Quite interestingly, *A. muciniphila* administration in these mice could normalize some parameters related to high-fat diet such as fat-mass gain, endotoxemia, adipocytes, inflammation and insulin resistance. With regard to CD, some reports have demonstrated the presence of adherent/invasive *Escherichia (E.) coli* in ileal specimens in CD patients [8,9]. Other studies have provided evidence for either an increase in *Enterobacteriaceae* in CD patients [10] or reduced numbers of *Faecalibacterium prausnitzii* in ileal CD [11]. However, it is hard to state whether altered gut microbiota in CD represents the cause or the consequence of this pathology. Experimentally, *Citrobacter rodentium* [12], and *Helicobacter trognotum* [13] are able to cause severe colitis in mice with a subversion of anaerobic bacteria in the context of the gut microbiota and overgrowth of *Enterobacteriaceae*. This evidence indicates the existence of a strict relationship between intestinal microbiota and gut immune cells whose equilibrium is of paramount importance in the maintenance of a healthy status [14]. In particular, bacterial components [lipopolysaccharides (LPS) and peptidoglycans] interact with the so-called microbe-associated molecular patterns such as Toll-like receptors (TLRs) and Nod-like receptors (NLRs) [15,16]. TLRs are able to suppress inflammation, thus inducing a condition of immune tolerance. NLRs, in turn, recognizing microbial components, generate inflammasomes which represent sensors of damage-associated patterns. For instance, deficiency of NLRP6 gives rise to a reduced release of interleukin (IL)-18, alteration of the microbiota and intestinal hyperplasia [17]. With regard to adaptive immune system, *Bacteroides (B.) fragilis*, another component of the gut microbiota, induces production of IL-10 by FoxP3+ T regulatory (Treg) cells, thus inhibiting the inflammatory subset T helper (h)-17 [18]. In this direction, *Clostridium* species also promotes switch of Treg cells [19]. In addition, Lactobacilli and Bifidobacteria can induce less mature undifferentiated phenotypes of dendritic cells (DCs) [20]. Other gut bacteria binding to TLRs suppress the NF-κB pathway, while enhancing the production of defensins [21]. In the course of intestinal parasitoses, and, in particular, of infections with eukaryotes, many evidences of their interaction with intestinal bacterial community have been reported. *Giardia (G.) lamblia* grows very slowly in the presence of Lactobacillus, and *G. lamblia* cells harboring endosymbionts undergo destruction by Paneth cells [22]. *Entamoeba histolytica* has been shown to become more invasive in the presence of pathogenic strains of *E. coli* and *Shigella (S.) dysenteriae* [23]. *Trichomonas (T.) vaginalis* is associated with *Mycoplasma hominis*, which acts as an endosymbiont, thus leading to co-infection by transferring *Mycoplasma* to epithelial cells [24]. Quite interestingly, infection with *T. vaginalis* can expose individuals to other infections, such as bacterial vaginosis and HIV [25].

Interactions Between Helminths and Gut Microbiota

A number of helminths harbor the human gut, such as flatworms (*e.g., Taenia, Fasciolopsis* and *Schistosoma*) and nematodes (*e.g., Ascaris, Trichuris* and *Strongyloides*) [26]. Therefore, helminths living in close contact with mucosa and intestinal lumen automatically interact with components of the microbiota. In mice, infection with *Heligmosomoides (H.) polygyrus* causes a change of the microbiota in the ileum but not in the colon with a prevalence of Lactobacilli with attenuation of inflammation and modulation of the epithelial barrier function [27]. In pigs, *Trichuris (T.) suis* leads to a modification of the gut microbiota with a decrease of *Fibrobacter* and *Ruminococcus* [28]. Important metabolic changes have been detected in the course of *Schistosoma (S.) mansoni* infection. In particular, elevated urinary excretions of trimethylamine, phenylacetylglucine and p-cresol-glucoronide suggest an alteration of the gut microbiota [29]. Also in the case of *S. japonicum* infection, ^{1}H NMR spectroscopy revealed metabolic alterations in terms of lipid metabolism, elevated glycolysis, and down-regulation of trycarboxylic acid cycle [30]. In addition, elevated urinary levels of 4-cresol-glucoronide and phenylacetylglycine (PAG) and depression of hyppurate, as microbial metabolites, strongly indicate an alteration of the gut microbiota. These results were also confirmed by Balog *et al.* [31] in rodent and human *S. mansoni* infection and by Li *et al.* [32], who detected 12 urinary and 5 faecal metabolites as biomarkers of infection and evidence of gut microbiota disturbance. In this framework, metabolic profiling of *Echinostoma (E.) caproni* murine infection has provided further evidence for an altered gut microbiota in the course of this parasitosis [33]. In *E. caproni* infected mice, the decrease of the short chain fat acids (SFA) in stool is an index of an altered microbiota since food derived carbohydrates are fermented by colonic bacteria to acetate, propionate and butyrate. In particular, *Clostridium (C.) aminovalericum* produces and degrades 5-aminovalerates to propionate and acetate in the bowel [34]. Therefore, it is likely that *E. caproni* in the gut may be able to depress the growth of *C. aminovalericum*. Furthermore, in *E. caproni* infected mice, the urinary increase of trimethylamine-N-oxide (TMAO) by choline degrading bacteria with a decrease of the choline/glycerophosphocholine in the plasma has been reported. This may represent a further evidence of the microbiota disturbance in *E. caproni* infection. Similar results have been obtained in hamsters co-infected with *S. japonicum* and *Necator (N.) americanus* in terms of diminished concentration of hyppurate, TMAO, 3-hydroxyphenylpropionic acid (HPPA) and high levels of 4-cresol-glucoronide and PAG [35]. With regard to helminth infections and related metabolic modifications, in a recent report Yang and associates [36] have demonstrated that in mouse models of obesity and concomitant infection with nematodes a dramatic drop of fasting blood glucose, fatty liver disease, leptin and insulin occurred. In general terms, co-infection between helminths has been shown to lead to either enhancement or suppression of clinical manifestations. For instance, *S. mansoni* infection limits *T. muris* infection and *Strongyloides venezuelensis* viability [37,38]. In mice co-infected with *Litomosoides (L.) sigmodontis* and *Leishmania major*, the latter parasitosis clinical course was attenuated [39]. In conclusion, co-infection may modulate host immune responses either in terms of protection or further damage. Therefore, a link between helminth infections, change of the gut microbiota and host immune response needs to be stressed out. In this respect, a recent report [40] has emphasized the ability of hookworm to inhibit protective Th1 and Th17 responses in latent tuberculosis, thus promoting the development of active tuberculosis in humans.

Cross Talk between Intestinal Microbiota and Helminths in the Modulation of Gut Immunity

Both microbial components of the microbiota and helminths share the ability to profoundly regulate the gut immune cells. Therefore, in this section we will describe the immune activities of microbiota, on the one hand, and, the influence of helminths on the gut immune system, on the other hand. Finally, we will highlight how the cross talk between bacteria and helminths with intestinal immune cells can polarize gut immunity.

Studies in germ free (GF) animals lacking microbiota have demonstrated abnormal numbers of immune cells, with spleens and lymph nodes poorly formed, even including, Peyer's patches (PP) [41] and intestinal lymphoid follicles (ILF) [42]. In GF animals, IgA-producing plasma cells as well as levels of IgA and IgG [41] were dramatically reduced and abnormal levels of cytokines have been detected, thus leading to an impaired oral tolerance [43]. GF animals lack expansion of CD4+ T-cell populations and this deficiency can be completely reversed by treatment with polysaccharide A (PSA) of *B. fragilis* [44].

B. fragilis, as a component of the microbiota, hampers Th17 induction, promoting release of IL-10 by Treg cells which recognize PSA *via* TLR-2. At the same time, in GF animals with a systemic polarization towards a Th2 type cytokine, PSA treatment reverses such an abnormality [45]. Also, various *Lactobacilli spp*. are able to modulate DC function with consequent influence on the mucosal Th1/Th2/Treg cell cytokine profile [46], as well as to activate natural killer (NK) cells [47]. Furthermore, peptidoglycan, as a component of the cell wall of Lactobacilli, leads to the formation of isolated LF *via* NOD1 (an NLR) signaling with further maturation of ILF into B cell clusters [42]. In the gut, DCs preferentially induce differentiation of resident T cells into Treg cell subsets [48], thus leading to a more tolerogenic state. This tolerogenic phenotype expressed by DCs is dependent on the stimulation of intestinal epithelial cells (IECs) with different *Lactobacillus spp.* and different *E. coli* strains [49]. Moreover, this stimulation induces secretion of thymic stromal lymphopoietin and transforming growth factor (TGF)-β by IECs [49], with Lactobacilli more effective than *E. coli* in the modulation of DCs. Another effective mechanism of tolerance is exerted by *B. thetaiotaomicron*, which prevents activation of the NF-κB [50].

Segmented filamentous bacteria (SFB) can induce murine Th17 cells *via* production of IL-23 from DCs [51]. By contrast, colonization with SFB did not lead to increased expression of FoxP3+ cells. Furthermore, SFB strongly stimulated IgA induction in the gut [52]. Of note, also Bacteroides and Lactobacilli were able to induce intestinal secretory IgA production but not to the same extent of SFB [53].

Helminths interact with the intestinal immune system, suppressing the Th2 response mounted by the host against their invasion. Anti-helminth protective innate immunity promoted by Th2 cytokines and innate lymphoid cells (nuocytes) include release of the Muc5ac mucin and the resistin-like molecule-β, which inhibit motility and feeding [54,55]. Furthermore, granulocytes, mastcells, eosinophils, and macrophages armed by specific antibodies can attack and kill parasites. In particular, larvae into the skin can be destroyed by IL-5-activated eosinophils, whereas bloodstream microfilariae are eliminated by IgM-mediated mechanisms [54,56,57]. However, microfilariae can escape immune response down regulating Langherans cell and keratinocyte function at skin levels [58]. A recent report has shown that regulatory granulocytic cells accumulation correlates with protection in murine neurocystercosis [59]. These Th2-dependent mechanisms are down-regulated by the rapid rise of FoxP3+ Treg cell responses in murine helminth infections [54]. Helminths *per se* can also increase the expression of activation markers on FoxP3+ Treg cells, such as CD103 [60]. These evidences are further supported by depletion of Treg cells prior to infection which increases Th2 responses and clearance of *Filariae* and *Strongyloides rattii* parasites [61,62]. In murine *S. mansoni* and *T. spiralis* infections, anti-CD25 depletion of Treg cells leads to reduction of egg numbers, even if this treatment resulted to be ineffective in the chronic phase [63,64]. In *L. sigmodontis* infection later depletion of Treg cells was beneficial only if associated with CTLA-4 or through co-stimulation with glucocorticoid-induced TNFR family related gene (GITR) [65]. In humans, the role of FoxP3+ Treg cells in helminth infections is more difficult to be interpreted. In fact, in individuals co-infected with T-cell lymphotropic virus 1 and *S. stercoralis* an increase in FoxP3+ Treg cells positively correlated with severity of infection [66]. By contrast, in *Onchocerca volvulus* infection increase in FoxP3+Treg cells was rather associated to dead parasites, thus attributing a protective role to Treg cells [67]. Quite interestingly, FoxP3+ Treg cells also control Th2-dependent immune pathology in helminth infections. For instance, the severity of egg-induced liver pathology in *S. mansoni* infection negatively correlates with number of FoxP3+ Treg cells [68]. In mice with impaired FoxP3+ Treg cell functions, there is evidence for an increased granuloma formation and liver damage which can be recovered by transfer of CD4+CD25+ Treg cells [68]. In *T. muris* and *H. polygyrus* infections, depletion of FoxP3+ Treg cells aggravated intestinal inflammation [69,70]. Also in human filarial infection, lymphoedema is associated with reduction in FoxP3, CTLA-4 and TGF-β and increase in Th1 and Th17-type responses [71].

Both natural and adaptive FoxP3+ Treg cells seem to participate to immunity to helminths. Natural Treg cells intervene in the early phase of infection, while adaptive Treg cells appear later in infection and limit immunopathology in *S. mansoni* infection [54]. Quite interestingly, in the case of *H. polygyrus* infection, this parasite is able to secrete a TGF-β mimic which induces adaptive Treg cells that may suppress protective immunity in later infection [53].

Over the past few years, the role of IL-22 [72,73] has been emphasized as a link between helminths, intestinal microbiota and related immune responses [74]. IL-22 has been reported to be over-expressed in the bowel in certain intestinal infections with nematodes, *e.g.*, *T. trichuria*. In one case of treatment of ulcerative colitis with *T. trichuria,* improvement of clinical symptoms correlated with an increased release of IL-22 and Th2-related cytokines [75]. This immune mechanism has been found to confer protection to the infected host, thus leading to the expulsion of the parasite. Also in patients infected with *N. americanus,* in intestinal biopsies an increased of IL-22 expression has been shown, thus suggesting a putative role of this cytokine in human infections with these parasites. However, further studies are required for confirming this hypothesis [76]. In murine models, the role of IL-22 in helminth infections has been investigated by experiments using IL-22 deficient animals or neutralizing antibodies against IL-22 [77]. However, in *S. mansoni* infection, wild type mice and IL-22 deficient mice developed similar hepatic and intestinal granulomas and survival, thus indicating that IL-22 has played a negligible role in the pathogenesis of schistomiasis. These murine models need to be used in the case of other intestinal helminth infections to confirm the role of IL-22.

H. polygyrus causes a chronic intestinal infection with an increase of Lactobacillaceae family which, in turn, was able to decrease colitis as well a type 1 diabetes [78]. However, it is also possible that *H. polygyrus* needs commensal bacteria for its development [79].

T. muris represents a mouse model of *T. trichuria* infection in humans in terms of mucosal immunity involvement. In this respect, studies have allowed to clarify the mechanisms of resistance or susceptibility to this infection. In the expulsion of *T. muris,* a prevalent Th2 type response has been detected and characterized by an increased release of IL-4, IL-9 and IL-13 [80]. However, basophils and innate lymphoid cells seem to act as an early source of Th2-derived cytokines, thus facilitating Th2 response in the later phase. In addition, IL-13 seems to be involved in the secretion of mucin which inhibits the attachment of the parasites to the epithelium. In resistant animals, the mucin Muc5ac is increased, thus acting on worm viability. Finally, IL-9 is able to increase contractility of the muscle in the gut, thus leading to parasite expulsion. On the other hand, susceptibility to infection depends on a Th1 response with production of interferon (IFN)-γ, thus leading to a decreased epithelial cell turnover and muscle contractility. In this context, a decrease of Muc5ac production has been reported. The exaggerated Th1 response provokes colitis and Treg cells seem to play a role in *T. muris* infection.

Therapeutic Approaches

Th2 response failure seems to be the major dysfunction of the intestinal immunity in the course of helminth infections. In addition, both helminths and intestinal microbiota collaborate to maintain a condition of Th2 suppression. In fact, in human studies drug eradication of helminths or neutralization of TGF-β and IL-10 *in vitro* partially restores Th2 subset function [81,82]. However, despite curative drug therapy, protective immunity does not fully recover and patients may undergo re-infections since Th2 cells continuously exposed to antigenic pressure and immune suppression become hyporesponsive or anergic [83]. In experimental and human filariasis as well in murine schistosomiasis, evidence has been provided for a condition of intrinsic unresponsiveness of Th2 cells towards parasitic antigens, since neutralization of IL-10 or depletion of FoxP3+ cells does not restore Th2 function [54]. However, in filarial patients and filarial murine models, blockade of CTLA-4 has been shown to render Th2 cells less hyporesponsive [54].

Mechanisms of Treg cell related immune-responsiveness are depicted in Fig. (2).

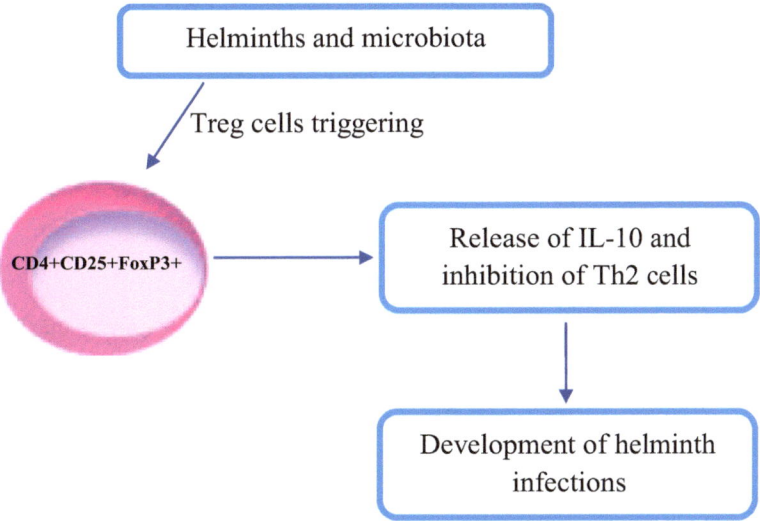

Figure 2: Mechanisms of Th2 dysfunction in helminth infections.

In this framework, another issue is represented by a condition of exhaustion of Th2 cells following their early priming as in the case of *S. mansoni* infection.

Murine studies have demonstrated that exhaustion can be mediated by inhibitory receptors, such as PD-1 and TIM-1, and PD-L1 and PD-L2 expressed on macrophages in the course of *S. mansoni* and *Nippostrongylus brasiliensis* infections [84-86]. This is also confirmed by the evidence that in murine schistosomiasis, Th2 cell hyporesponsiveness is linked to gene related to anergy in lymphocytes (GRAIL) expression [61]. Of note, GRAIL is an E3 ubiquitin ligase associated with T cell tolerance [87].

It has been hypothesized that recovery of hyporesponsive Th2 cells in the course of helminth infections may occur through different modalities. One possibility is to replace anergic/exhausted cells by expanding the remaining Th2 cells or priming new T cells. In alternative, neutralization of inhibitory molecules (PD-1, CTLA-4) or induction of cytokine like IL-5 or GITR co-stimulation have been envisaged [54].

Quite interestingly, in *S. mansoni* ugandan patients treated with praziquantel (PZQ), boosting of fresh protective Th2 cells with new parasitic epitopes has apparently been achieved [88]. PZQ by disrupting schistosome tegument (Teg) allows exposure of Teg antigens to the host immune system. Newly exposed Teg antigens are able to trigger a greater release of Th2 cytokines, such as IL-4, IL-5, IL-10 and IL-13 in comparison to that evoked by soluble egg antigen (SEA). In conclusion, new epitopes from Teg seem to mount a protective immunity in endemic areas for schistosomiasis, while limiting severe reactions to SEA, *e.g.*, liver granulomatosis.

It is well known that several natural products exert anti-helmintic activities and, in many plant extracts mostly the presence of flavonoids has been revealed, such as genistein, kaemperol, rutin, quercetin *et cetera* [89]. In particular, curcumin is able to exert a strong adulticidal effect on *S. mansoni* at 50 and 100 μM concentrations [90], acting on the ubiquitin-proteasome pathway. In addition, in animals treated with curcumin a reduction of hepatic granuloma and collagenesis was observed [91]. The *in vitro* effects of curcumin against eggs, cercariae, pre-adults, and adults of *S. japonicum* have been investigated [92]. Curcumin showed time- and dose-dependent schistosomicidal effects on every life stages of *S. japonicum*. In addition, curcumin exhibited an optimal activity against the adult stage with no differential sensitivity between male and female worms. Schistosome eggs antigens are able to elicit pro-inflammatory responses in trophoblast thus, compromising pregnancy. In endemic areas for schistosomiasis curcumin treatment may represent a prevention treatment in pregnant women [93].

Genistein has been proven to exert anti-helminthic activities in cestodes and trematodes infections with a major effect on tegumental enzymes [94]. In *Fasciolopsis ruski,* genistein *in vitro* induces elevated production of nitric oxide (NO) [95], which may be responsible for neurotoxicity, with myo-inhibition and paralysis of flukes [96]. At higher doses, genistein as well as kaemperol and quercetin can induce generation of NO from activated macrophages, thus implying an intervention of the immune system [97].

Another important aspect of polyphenol activity is represented by their ability to modulate gut microbiota. In this respect, evidence has been provided that in human volunteers, six-week intake of *Vaccinium angustifolium* (a wild blueberry) increased *Bifidobacterium spp.* [98]. Using the NMR-based metabolite profile, the activity of the intestinal microbiota in fecal samples of human healthy volunteers, who consumed either a grape juice extract or both grape juice and wine extract *vs* placebo was determined. Grape juice and wine extract mix reduced isobutyrate levels, thus indicating a modification of the intestinal microbiota [99]. In ten healthy male volunteers, assuming red wine or gin for 20 days each, alterations in fecal microbiota were assessed on total fecal DNA by means of PCR [100]. Increase in *Bacteroides*, *Bifidobacterium*, *Enterococcus*, *Prevotella* organisms and decrease in cholesterol and CRP correlated with bifidobacteria number increase.

Finally, many evidences have supported a number of anti-inflammatory activities exerted by polyphenols, and therefore, it is important discussing their potential application in patients with helminth infections. In our studies, we have demonstrated an increased *in vitro* release of NO from human circulating monocytes stimulated by red wine polyphenols [101-103]. Therefore, at mucosal level NO released by lamina propria macrophages in the presence of ingested polyphenols may account for cytoxicity of helminths, as described in the case of genistein. Also, in animal models, polyphenols from fermented grape marc (FGM) were are able to attenuate experimental murine colitis, also decreasing intestinal release of TNF-α and IL-1β [104].

In very recent studies, we have described the ability of FGM polyphenols to induce expression and activation of FoxP3+ Treg cells in human peripheral T lymphocytes [105,106]. This finding apparently is not in favour of the host infected with helminths since production of IL-10 by Treg cells may promote the escape of parasites from protective Th2 immune responses. However, as discussed in the previous sections of this chapter, Treg function may be important in the reduction of immunopathology due to schistosoma infection *e.g.,* evolution of liver granuloma (see Fig. **3**).

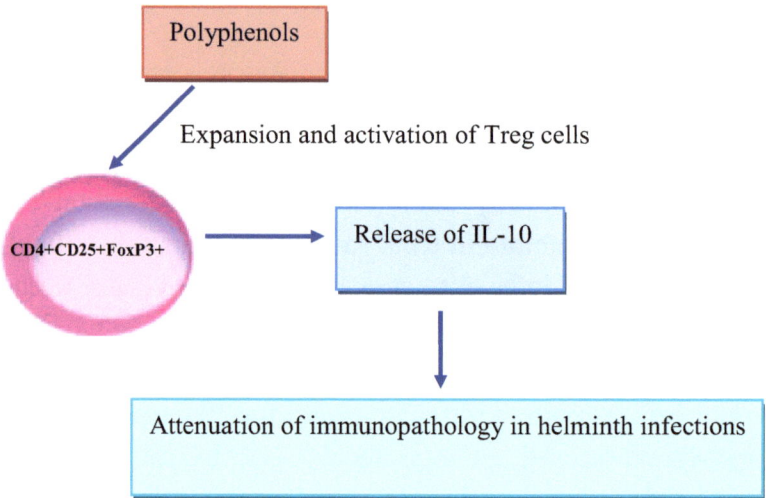

Figure 3: Putative role of dietary polyphenols in the course helminth infections.

Therefore, studies determining the amounts of polyphenols and their metabolites able to maintain immune homeostasis in the host are needed. In this respect, in our *in vitro* experiments with red wine polyphenols we have found increased production of IgG and IgA, thus indicating a preserved function of Th2 cells [107].

In conclusion, it appears that a treatment with polyphenols may be beneficial in the course of a consolidated chronic helminth infection, rather than in the earlier phase of disease.

In terms of prevention, daily intake of polyphenols may directly act on helminths, causing their death and also shaping the gut microbiota, thus promoting a protective immune response.

This means that lack of dietary polyphenols may favor helminth infections.

ACKNOWLEDGEMENTS

Thea Magrone is a recipient of a contract in the context of the project "Bioscience and Health (B&H) (PONa3_00395).

CONFLICT OF INTEREST

The author(s) confirm that this chapter contents have no conflict of interest.

ABBREVIATIONS

CD	=	Cronh's disease;
DCs	=	Dendritic cells;
GF	=	Germ free;
GITR	=	Glucocorticoid-induced TNFR family related gene;
HPPA	=	3-hidroxyphenylpropionic acid;
IFN	=	Interferon;
IL	=	Interleukin;
ILF	=	Intestinal lymphoid follicles;
LPS	=	Lipopolysaccharides;
NK	=	Natural killer;
NLRs	=	Nod-like receptors;

NO = Nitric oxide;

PAG = Phenylacetylglycine;

PP = Peyer's patches;

PSA = Polysaccharide A;

PZQ = Praziquantel;

SFA = Short fatty acid;

SFB = Segmented filamentous bacteria;

TGF = Transforming growth factor;

Th = T helper;

TLRs = Toll-like receptors;

TMAO = Trimetylamine-N-oxide;

Treg = T regulatory.

REFERENCES

[1] Costello EK, Lauber CL, Hamady M, *et al*. Bacterial community variation in human body habitats across space and time. Science 2009; 326: 1694-7.
[2] Turnbaugh PJ, Ley RE, Mahowald MA, *et al*. An obesity-associated gut microbiome with increased capacity for energy harvest. Nature 2006; 444: 1027-31.
[3] Turnbaugh PJ, Ridaura VK, Faith JJ, *et al*. The effect of diet on the human gut microbiome: a metagenomic analysis in humanized gnotobiotic mice. Sci Transl Med 2009; 1: 6ra14.
[4] Dethlefsen L, Huse S, Sogin ML, *et al*. The pervasive effects of an antibiotic on the human gut microbiota, as revealed by deep 16S rRNA sequencing. PLoS Biol 2008; 6: e280.
[5] Sommer MO, Dantas G, Church GM. Functional characterization of the antibiotic resistance reservoir in the human microflora. Science 2009; 325: 1128-31.
[6] Clemente JC, Ursell LK, Parfrey LW, *et al*. The impact of the gut microbiota on human health: an integrative view. Cell 2012; 148: 1258-70.
[7] Everard A, Belzer C, Geurts L, *et al*. Cross-talk between Akkermansia muciniphila and intestinal epithelium controls diet-induced obesity. Proc Natl Acad Sci U S A 2013; 110: 9066-71.

[8]   Darfeuille-Michaud A, Boudeau J, Bulois P, et al. High prevalence of adherent-invasive Escherichia coli associated with ileal mucosa in Crohn's disease. Gastroenterology 2004;127: 412-21.

[9]   Martinez-Medina M, Aldeguer X, Lopez-Siles M, et al. Molecular diversity of Escherichia coli in the human gut: new ecological evidence supporting the role of adherent-invasive E. coli (AIEC) in Crohn's disease. Inflamm Bowel Dis 2009;15: 872-82.

[10] Sartor RB. Microbial influences in inflammatory bowel diseases. Gastroenterology 2008; 134: 577-94.

[11] Sokol H, Pigneur B, Watterlot L, et al. Faecalibacterium prausnitzii is an anti-inflammatory commensal bacterium identified by gut microbiota analysis of Crohn disease patients. Proc Natl Acad Sci U S A 2008; 105: 16731-6.

[12] Lupp C, Robertson ML, Wickham ME, et al. Host-mediated inflammation disrupts the intestinal microbiota and promotes the overgrowth of Enterobacteriaceae. Cell Host Microbe 2007; 2: 119-29.

[13] Whary MT, Danon SJ, Feng Y, et al. Rapid onset of ulcerative typhlocolitis in B6.129P2-IL10tm1Cgn (IL-10-/-) mice infected with Helicobacter trogontum is associated with decreased colonization by altered Schaedler's flora. Infect Immun 2006; 74: 6615-23.

[14] Magrone T, Jirillo E. The interplay between the gut immune system and microbiota in health and disease: nutraceutical intervention for restoring intestinal homeostasis. Curr Pharm Des 2013; 19: 1329-42.

[15] Kawai T, Akira S. TLR signaling. Cell Death Differ 2006; 13: 816-25.

[16] Strober W, Murray PJ, Kitani A, et al. Signalling pathways and molecular interactions of NOD1 and NOD2. Nat Rev Immunol 2006; 6: 9-20.

[17] Elinav E, Strowig T, Kau AL, et al. NLRP6 inflammasome regulates colonic microbial ecology and risk for colitis. Cell 2011; 145: 745-57.

[18] Round JL, Mazmanian SK. Inducible Foxp3+ regulatory T-cell development by a commensal bacterium of the intestinal microbiota. Proc Natl Acad Sci U S A 2010; 107: 12204-9.

[19] Sansonetti PJ. To be or not to be a pathogen: that is the mucosally relevant question. Mucosal Immunol 2011; 4: 8-14.

[20] Davies JM, Sheil B, Shanahan F. Bacterial signalling overrides cytokine signalling and modifies dendritic cell differentiation. Immunology 2009; 128(1Suppl): e805-15.

[21] Zeng H, Wu H, Sloane V, et al. Flagellin/TLR5 responses in epithelia reveal intertwined activation of inflammatory and apoptotic pathways. Am J Physiol Gastrointest Liver Physiol 2006; 290: G96-G108.

[22] Müller N, von Allmen N. Recent insights into the mucosal reactions associated with Giardia lamblia infections. Int J Parasitol 2005; 35: 1339-47.

[23] Galván-Moroyoqui JM, Del Carmen Domínguez-Robles M, Franco E, et al. The interplay between Entamoeba and enteropathogenic bacteria modulates epithelial cell damage. PLoS Negl Trop Dis 2008; 2: e266.

[24] Rappelli P, Carta F, Delogu G, et al. Mycoplasma hominis and Trichomonas vaginalis symbiosis: multiplicity of infection and transmissibility of M. hominis to human cells. Arch Microbiol 2001; 175: 70-4.

[25] Soper D. Trichomoniasis: under control or undercontrolled? Am J Obstet Gynecol 2004; 190: 281-90.

[26] Berrilli F, Di Cave D, Cavallero S, et al. Interactions between parasites and microbial communities in the human gut. Front Cell Infect Microbiol 2012; 2: 141.

[27] Walk ST, Blum AM, Ewing SA, et al. Alteration of the murine gut microbiota during infection with the parasitic helminth Heligmosomoides polygyrus. Inflamm Bowel Dis 2010; 16: 1841-9.

[28] Wu S, Li RW, Li W, et al. Worm burden-dependent disruption of the porcine colon microbiota by Trichuris suis infection. PLoS One 2012; 7: e35470.

[29] Wang Y, Holmes E, Nicholson JK, et al. Metabonomic investigations in mice infected with Schistosoma mansoni: an approach for biomarker identification. Proc Natl Acad Sci U S A 2004; 101: 12676-81.

[30] Wu JF, Xu WX, Ming ZP, et al. Metabolic changes reveal the development of schistosomiasis in mice. Plos Negl Trop Dis 2010; 4: e807.

[31] Balog CI, Meissner A, Göraler S, et al. Metabonomic investigation of human Schistosoma mansoni infection. Mol Biosyst 2011; 7: 1473-80.

[32] Li JV, Holmes E, Saric J, et al. Metabolic profiling of a Schistosoma mansoni infection in mouse tissues using magic angle spinning-nuclear magnetic resonance spectroscopy. Int J Parasitol 2009; 39: 547-58.

[33] Saric J, Li JV, Wang Y, et al. Metabolic profiling of an Echinostoma caproni infection in the mouse for biomarker discovery. PLoS Negl Trop Dis 2008; 2: e254.

[34] Ramsay IR, Pullammanappallil PC. Protein degradation during anaerobic wastewater treatment: derivation of stoichiometry. Biodegradation 2001; 12: 247-57.

[35] Wu JF, Holmes E, Xue J, et al. Metabolic alterations in the hamster co-infected with Schistosoma japonicum and Necator americanus. Int J Parasitol 2010; 40: 695-703.

[36] Yang Z, Grinchuk V, Smith A, et al. Parasitic nematode-induced modulation of body weight and associated metabolic dysfunction in mouse models of obesity. Infect Immun 2013; 81: 1905-14.

[37] Curry AJ, Else KJ, Jones F, et al. Evidence that cytokine-mediated immune interactions induced by Schistosoma mansoni alter disease outcome in mice concurrently infected with Trichuris muris. J Exp Med 1995; 181: 769-74.

[38] Yoshida A, Maruyama H, Yabu Y, et al. Immune response against protozoal and nematodal infection in mice with underlying Schistosoma mansoni infection. Parasitol Int 1999; 48: 73-9.

[39] Lamb TJ, Graham AL, Le Goff L, et al. Co-infected C57BL/6 mice mount appropriately polarized and compartmentalized cytokine responses to Litomosoides sigmodontis and Leishmania major but disease progression is altered. Parasite Immunol 2005; 27: 317-24.

[40] Parakkal JV, Anuradha R, Kumaran PP, et al. Modulation of mycobacterial-specific Th1 and Th17 cells in latent tuberculosis by coincident hookworm infection. *J Immunol* 2013; 190: 5161-8.

[41] Macpherson AJ, Harris NL. Interactions between commensal intestinal bacteria and the immune system. *Nat Rev Immunol* 2004; 4: 478-85.

[42] Bouskra D, Brézillon C, Bérard M, et al. Lymphoid tissue genesis induced by commensals through NOD1 regulates intestinal homeostasis. Nature 2008; 456: 507-10.

[43] O'Hara AM, Shanahan F. The gut flora as a forgotten organ. Embo report 2006; 7: 688-93.

[44] Ishikawa H, Tanaka K, Maeda Y, et al. Effect of intestinal microbiota on the induction of regulatory CD25+ CD4+ T cells. Clin Exp Immunol 2008; 153: 127-35.

[45] Mazmanian SK, Liu CH, Tzianabos AO, et al. An immunomodulatory molecule of symbiotic bacteria directs maturation of the host immune system. Cell 2005; 122: 107-18.

[46] Christensen HR, Frøkiaer H, Pestka JJ. Lactobacilli differentially modulate expression of cytokines and maturation surface markers in murine dendritic cells. J Immunol 2002; 168: 171-8.

[47] Fink LN, Zeuthen LH, Christensen HR, et al. Distinct gut-derived lactic acid bacteria elicit divergent dendritic cell-mediated NK cell responses. Int Immunol 2007; 19: 1319-27.

[48] Kelsall BL, Leon F. Involvement of intestinal dendritic cells in oral tolerance, immunity to pathogens, and inflammatory bowel disease. Immunol Rev 2005; 206: 132-48.

[49] Zeuthen LH, Fink LN, Frokiaer H. Epithelial cells prime the immune response to an array of gut-derived commensals towards a tolerogenic phenotype through distinct actions of thymic stromal lymphopoietin and transforming growth factor-beta. Immunology 2008; 123: 197-208.

[50] Kelly D, Campbell JI, King TP, et al. Commensal anaerobic gut bacteria attenuate inflammation by regulating nuclear-cytoplasmic shuttling of PPAR-gamma and RelA. Nat Immunol 2004; 5: 104-12.

[51] Ivanov II, Atarashi K, Manel N, et al. Induction of intestinal Th17 cells by segmented filamentous bacteria. Cell 2009; 139: 485-98.

[52] Ivanov II, Littman DR. Segmented filamentous bacteria take the stage. Mucosal Immunol 2010; 3: 209-12.

[53] Macpherson AJ, Geuking MB, McCoy KD. Homeland security: IgA immunity at the frontiers of the body. Trends Immunol 2012; 33: 160-7.

[54] Taylor MD, van der Werf N, Maizels RM. T cells in helminth infection: the regulators and the regulated. Trends Immunol 2012; 33: 181-9.

[55] Scalfone LK, Nel HJ, Gagliardo LF, et al. Participation of MyD88 and interleukin-33 as innate drivers of Th2 immunity to Trichinella spiralis. Infect Immun 2013; 81: 1354-63.

[56] Liu AY, Dwyer DF, Jones TG, et al. Mast cells recruited to mesenteric lymph nodes during helminth infection remain hypogranular and produce IL-4 and IL-6. J Immunol 2013; 190: 1758-66.

[57] Vukman KV, Adams PN, Metz M, et al. Fasciola hepatica tegumental coat impairs mast cells' ability to drive Th1 immune responses. J Immunol 2013; 190: 2873-9.

[58] Boyd A, Bennuru S, Wang Y, et al. Quiescent innate response to infective filariae by human Langerhans cells suggests a strategy of immune evasion. Infect Immun 2013; 81: 1420-9.

[59] Mishra PK, Morris EG, Garcia JA, et al. Increased accumulation of regulatory granulocytic myeloid cells in mannose receptor C type 1-deficient mice correlates with protection in a mouse model of neurocysticercosis. Infect Immun 2013; 81: 1052-63.

[60] Layland LE, Mages J, Loddenkemper C, et al. Pronounced phenotype in activated regulatory T cells during a chronic helminth infection. J Immunol 2010; 184: 713-24.

[61] Taylor MD, van der Werf N, Harris A, et al. Early recruitment of natural CD4+ Foxp3+ Treg cells by infective larvae determines the outcome of filarial infection. Eur J Immunol 2009; 39: 192-206.

[62] Blankenhaus B, Klemm U, Eschbach ML, et al. Strongyloides ratti infection induces expansion of Foxp3+ regulatory T cells that interfere with immune response and parasite clearance in BALB/c mice. J Immunol 2011; 186: 4295-305.

[63] Layland LE, Rad R, Wagner H, et al. Immunopathology in schistosomiasis is controlled by antigen-specific regulatory T cells primed in the presence of TLR2. Eur J Immunol 2007; 37: 2174-84.

[64] Beiting DP, Gagliardo LF, Hesse M, et al. Coordinated control of immunity to muscle stage Trichinella spiralis by IL-10, regulatory T cells, and TGF-beta. J Immunol 2007; 178: 1039-47.

[65] Taylor MD, Harris A, Babayan SA, et al. CTLA-4 and CD4+ CD25+ regulatory T cells inhibit protective immunity to filarial parasites in vivo. J Immunol 2007; 179: 4626-34.

[66] Montes M, Sanchez C, Verdonck K, et al. Regulatory T cell expansion in HTLV-1 and strongyloidiasis co-infection is associated with reduced IL-5 responses to Strongyloides stercoralis antigen. PLoS Negl Trop Dis 2009; 3: e456.

[67] Korten S, Badusche M, Büttner DW, et al. Natural death of adult Onchocerca volvulus and filaricidal effects of doxycycline induce local FOXP3+/CD4+ regulatory T cells and granzyme expression. Microbes Infect 2008; 10: 313-24.

[68] Baumgart M, Tompkins F, Leng J, et al. Naturally occurring CD4+Foxp3+ regulatory T cells are an essential, IL-10-independent part of the immunoregulatory network in Schistosoma mansoni egg-induced inflammation. J Immunol 2006; 176: 5374-87.

[69] Rausch S, Huehn J, Loddenkemper C, et al. Establishment of nematode infection despite increased Th2 responses and immunopathology after selective depletion of Foxp3+ cells. Eur J Immunol 2009; 39: 3066-77.

[70] D'Elia R, Behnke JM, Bradley JE, et al. Regulatory T cells: a role in the control of helminth-driven intestinal pathology and worm survival. J Immunol 2009; 182: 2340-8.

[71] Babu S, Bhat SQ, Pavan Kumar N, et al. Filarial lymphedema is characterized by antigen-specific Th1 and th17 proinflammatory responses and a lack of regulatory T cells. PLoS Negl Trop Dis 2009; 3: e420.

[72] Zenewicz LA, Yin X, Wang G, et al. IL-22 deficiency alters colonic microbiota to be transmissible and colitogenic. J Immunol 2013; 190: 5306-12.

[73] Lee Y, Kumagai Y, Jang MS, et al. Intestinal Lin-c-Kit+NKp46-CD4- population strongly produces IL-22 upon IL-1β stimulation. J Immunol 2013; 190: 5296-305.

[74] Leung JM, Loke P. A role for IL-22 in the relationship between intestinal helminths, gut microbiota and mucosal immunity. Int J Parasitol 2013; 43: 253-7.

[75] Broadhurst MJ, Ardeshir A, Kanwar B, et al. Therapeutic helminth infection of macaques with idiopathic chronic diarrhea alters the inflammatory signature and mucosal microbiota of the colon. PLoS Pathog 2012; 8: e1003000.

[76] McSorley HJ, Gaze S, Daveson J, et al. Suppression of inflammatory immune responses in celiac disease by experimental hookworm infection. PLoS One 2011; 6: e24092.

[77] Wilson MS, Feng CG, Barber DL, et al. Redundant and pathogenic roles for IL-22 in mycobacterial, protozoan, and helminth infections. J Immunol 2010; 184: 4378-90.

[78] Mishra PK, Patel N, Wu W, et al. Prevention of type 1 diabetes through infection with an intestinal nematode parasite requires IL-10 in the absence of a Th2-type response. Mucosal Immunol 2013; 6: 297-308.

[79] Reynolds LA, Filbey KJ, Maizels RM. Immunity to the model intestinal helminth parasite Heligmosomoides polygyrus. Semin Immunopathol 2012; 34: 829-46.

[80] Klementowicz JE, Travis MA, Grencis RK. Trichuris muris: a model of gastrointestinal parasite infection. Semin Immunopathol 2012; 34: 815-28.

[81] Sartono E, Kruize YC, Kurniawan A, *et al.* Elevated cellular immune responses and interferon-gamma release after long-term diethylcarbamazine treatment of patients with human lymphatic filariasis. J Infect Dis 1995; 171: 1683-7.

[82] King CL, Mahanty S, Kumaraswami V, *et al.* Cytokine control of parasite-specific anergy in human lymphatic filariasis. Preferential induction of a regulatory T helper type 2 lymphocyte subset. J Clin Invest 1993; 92: 1667-73.

[83] Black CL, Mwinzi PN, Muok EM, *et al.* Influence of exposure history on the immunology and development of resistance to human Schistosomiasis mansoni. PLoS Negl Trop Dis 2010; 4: e637.

[84] Wherry EJ. T cell exhaustion. Nat Immunol 2011; 12: 492-9.

[85] Huber S, Hoffmann R, Muskens F, *et al.* Alternatively activated macrophages inhibit T-cell proliferation by Stat6-dependent expression of PD-L2. Blood 2010; 116: 3311-20.

[86] Smith P, Walsh CM, Mangan NE, *et al.* Schistosoma mansoni worms induce anergy of T cells *via* selective up-regulation of programmed death ligand 1 on macrophages. J Immunol 2004; 173: 1240-8.

[87] Ichikawa D, Mizuno M, Yamamura T, *et al.* GRAIL (gene related to anergy in lymphocytes) regulates cytoskeletal reorganization through ubiquitination and degradation of Arp2/3 subunit 5 and coronin 1A. J Biol Chem 2011; 286: 43465-74.

[88] Joseph S, Jones FM, Walter K, *et al.* Increases in human T helper 2 cytokine responses to Schistosoma mansoni worm and worm-tegument antigens are induced by treatment with praziquantel. J Infect Dis 2004; 190: 835-42.

[89] Middleton E, Kandaswami CH, Theoharides TC. The effects of plant flavonoids on mammalian cells: Implications for inflammation, heart disease, and cancer. Pharmacol Rev 2000; 52: 673-751.

[90] Magalhães LG, Machado CB, Morais ER, *et al. In vitro* schistosomicidal activity of curcumin against Schistosoma mansoni adult worms. Parasitol Res 2009; 104: 1197-201.

[91] Allam G. Immunomodulatory effects of curcumin treatment on murine schistosomiasis mansoni. Immunobiology 2009; 214: 712-27.

[92] Chen YQ, Xu QM, Li XR, *et al. In vitro* evaluation of schistosomicidal potential of curcumin against Schistosoma japonicum. J Asian Nat Prod Res 2012; 14: 1064-72.

[93] McDonald EA, Kurtis JD, Acosta L, *et al.* Schistosome egg antigens elicit a proinflammatory response by trophoblast cells of the human placenta. Infect Immun 2013; 81: 704-12.

[94] Pal P, Tandon V. Anthelmintic efficacy of Flemingia vestita (Leguminoceae): genisteininduced alterations in the activity of tegumental enzymes in the cestode, Raillietina echinobothrida. Parasitol Int 1998; 47: 233-43.

[95] Pfarr KM, Qazi S, Fuhrman JA. Nitric oxide synthase in filariae: demonstration of nitric oxide production by embryos in Brugia malayi and Acanthocheilonema viteae. Exp Parasitol 2001; 97: 205-14.

[96] Kar PK, Tandon V, Saha N. Anthelmintic efficacy of Flemingia vestita: genistein-induced effect on the activity of nitric oxide synthase and nitric oxide in the trematode parasite, Fasciolopsis buski. Parasitol Int 2002; 51: 249-57.

[97] Hämäläinen M, Nieminen R, Vuorela P, *et al.* Anti-inflammatory effects of flavonoids: Genistein, kaempferol, quercetin, and daidzein inhibit STAT-1 and NF-κB activations, wherwas flavone isorhamnetin, naringenin, and Pelargonidin inhibit only NF-κB activation

along with their inhibitory effect on iNOS expression and NO production in activated macrophages. Mediat Inflamm 2007; 2007: 45673.

[98] Vendrame S, Guglielmetti S, Riso P, et al. Six-week consumption of a wild blueberry powder drink increases bifidobacteria in the human gut. J Agric Food Chem 2011; 59: 12815-20.

[99] Jacobs DM, Deltimple N, van Velzen E, et al. (1)H NMR metabolite profiling of feces as a tool to assess the impact of nutrition on the human microbiome. NMR Biomed 2008; 21: 615-26.

[100] Queipo-Ortuño MI, Boto-Ordóñez M, Murri M, et al. Influence of red wine polyphenols and ethanol on the gut microbiota ecology and biochemical biomarkers. Am J Clin Nutr 2012; 95: 1323-34.

[101] Magrone T, Kumazawa Y, Jirillo E. Polyphenol-mediated beneficial effects in healthy status and disease with special references to immune-based mechanisms. In: Watson RR, Preedy VR, Zibaldi S. Polyphenols in Human Health and Disease. Eds. Elsevier. 2014; Vol. 1, 467-79.

[102] Magrone T, Tafaro A, Jirillo F, et al. Red wine consumption and prevention of atherosclerosis: an in vitro model using human peripheral blood mononuclear cells. Curr Pharm Des 2007; 13: 3718-25.

[103] Magrone T, Candore G, Caruso C, et al. Polyphenols from red wine modulate immune responsiveness: biological and clinical significance. Curr Pharm Des 2008; 14: 2733-48.

[104] Kawaguchi K, Matsumoto T, Kumazawa Y. Effects of antioxidant polyphenols on TNF-alpha-related diseases. Curr Top Med Chem 2011; 11: 1767-79.

[105] Marzulli G, Magrone T, Kawaguchi K, et al. Fermented grape marc (FGM): immunomodulating properties and its potential exploitation in the treatment of neurodegenerative diseases. Curr Pharm Des 2012; 18: 43-50.

[106] Marzulli G, Magrone T, Vonghia L, et al. Immunomodulating and anti-allergic effects of Negroamaro and Koshu Vitis vinifera fermented grape marc (FGM). Curr Pharm Des 2014; 20: 864-8.

[107] Magrone T, Tafaro A, Jirillo F, et al. Elicitation of immune responsiveness against antigenic challenge in age-related diseases: effects of red wine polyphenols. Curr Pharm Des 2008; 14: 2749-57.

Subject Index

A

Anisakis 163, 164, 169, 170, 172, 222
Antigen presenting cells 55, 194, 235

B

Basophils 55, 63, 64, 95, 123, 133, 163, 167, 168, 180, 220, 221, 235, 242
B cells 33, 76, 81, 95, 97, 105, 112, 133, 179, 180, 183, 184, 185, 219

C

Complement 6, 33, 39, 77, 78, 83, 99
Cytokines 3,4, 7, 8, 10, 11, 13, 19, 20, 27, 32, 62, 63, 69,74,76,81,99, 101, 103, 104, 112, 125, 132, 133, 145, 166, 167, 168, 180, 181, 182, 184, 185, 188, 193, 194, 215, 217, 218, 221, 223, 225, 227, 235, 240, 242, 244

D

Dendritic cells 51, 54, 56, 57, 58, 59, 62, 77, 78, 96, 100, 125, 167, 168, 179, 186, 193, 218, 223, 235, 237

E

Echinococcosis 69, 82
Echinococcus 8, 69, 73, 75, 77, 78, 79, 84, 191, 192, 195

F

Fasciola 51, 53, 54, 56, 62, 63, 109, 200

G

Granulocytes 31, 146, 180, 240

M

Macrophages 11, 12, 33, 36, 41, 51, 55, 56, 57, 59, 60, 61, 63, 74, 79, 95, 96, 103, 112, 125, 135, 136, 197, 198, 179, 180, 183, 185, 186, 188, 189, 192, 224, 235, 240, 244, 245

Mast cells 12, 33, 36, 51, 55, 56, 57, 61, 62, 63, 64, 96, 125, 129, 131, 144, 163, 167, 168, 180, 220, 221, 226, 227
Microbiota 97, 235, 236, 237, 238, 239, 241, 243, 245

N

Neutrophils 32, 40, 41, 55, 74, 77, 78, 82, 84, 95, 112, 125, 136, 145, 168, 191, 200, 235
NK cells 33, 240

S

Schistosoma 6, 7, 10, 42, 52, 58, 93, 94, 95, 96, 97, 99, 103, 106, 108, 109, 111, 112, 113, 185, 189, 192, 199, 216, 219, 237, 238, 246
Schistomiasis 242

T

T lymphocytes 8, 79, 81, 82, 106, 163, 167, 168, 217, 246
Toxocara 27, 28, 30, 33, 35, 36, 38, 42, 43, 182, 214
Trichinellosis 125, 138, 142, 144, 146, 147-149